Medical Group Practice and Health Maintenance Organizations

Robert G. Shouldice *and*
Katherine Henneberger Shouldice

INFORMATION RESOURCES PRESS

WASHINGTON, D.C.   1978

Information Resources Press
2100 M Street, N.W.
Washington, D.C. 20037

Library of Congress Catalog Card Number 78-53824

ISBN 0-87815-020-X

ii

Foreword

I have been acquainted with Robert Shouldice and his studies of medical group practice and HMOs since 1972. He and his wife and coauthor, Katherine, have managed to compile—in one volume—information that should be of interest and value as a resource text to managers and health care professionals engaged in developing and operating HMOs, as well as to government officials and serious students in the field of health care administration.

In reading the text, one should be aware that the material therein was accumulated during a very dynamic six-year period for prepaid group practice plans—a period marked by the first specific recognition of this method of health care delivery in law: P.L. 92-603, the Social Security Amendments of 1972; and P.L. 93-222, the Health Maintenance Organization Act of 1973. These two acts, although meant to be helpful, still pose serious problems for operating HMOs, and were painfully slow in being implemented by government. Amendments to and regulations based on P.L. 93-222 are, at this time, still in the process of development. The attempt to put together and constantly update a comprehensive textbook encompassing the history, law, organizational structure, and operating principles regarding prepaid group practice during such a highly fluid period represents real dedication on the part of the authors.

It should be recognized that the book documents the methods and operating styles of many organizations, from newly developed, insurance-sponsored prototypes subscribing to insurance principles to the classic community-rated prepaid group practice prototype based on Saward's Genetic Code. The new insurance models are relatively untested, and HMO managers and administrators using the text should explore the limited operating experience of such models carefully before attempting to emulate them.

I believe health care administrators and other health care professionals, as well as students, will find this text a valuable addition to their resource library and will return to it, again and again, in their search for useful operating information. Thank you, Bob and Katherine for your contribution to our field.

Harold F. Newman, M.D., M.P.H.
Vice President, Kaiser Foundation
Health Plan, Inc.

Preface

In the 1960s, health industry leaders began to recognize the potential of prepaid group practice plans as mechanisms to contain the dramatic rise in health services costs. Studies of existing plans completed in the 1950s and 1960s provided clear evidence that medical group practice and prepaid group practice were effective in controlling costs and the quality of care. The Federal Government, in attempting to restrain the runaway costs of the Medicare and Medicaid programs, provided impetus for expanding the number of prepaid health plans. President Nixon's administration coined the phrase Health Maintenance Organization to describe the prepaid health plan models, and introduced and supported legislation to develop and expand HMOs. Each succeeding president has supported the concept of the HMO program as a major element of the nation's health programs.

Recently, the emphasis has been shifting away from traditional institutional inpatient care toward ambulatory and preventive services, which creates a need to study the management of group practice and prepaid group practice of medicine. This book is the product of a course in the development and managment of HMOs, conducted by the graduate program in health care administration at The George Washington University. The course, first offered in 1972, was structured around the numerous studies and articles written about prepaid group practice, but it lacked a comprehensive text on the subject. Over the next six years, the present book was shaped to fit the needs of students in the program, managers in the field, and government officials. As the text was developed and revised, the several hundred students who used the rough copies provided extremely valuable criticisms and suggestions to improve its effectiveness.

v

While this book is designed primarily for students of medical group practice and HMOs, it also should be helpful to managers of developing HMOs and those interested in establishing new prepaid health plans. A glance at the table of contents reveals that the major issues of HMOs are introduced, not for exhaustive treatment, but for the purpose of pointing out the most important and useful elements on the subject. We suggest that the reader also make use of the footnotes and bibliographies at the end of each chapter for further information.

We acknowledge the comments and criticisms of the numerous students at George Washington University while the text was being developed, and the constant encouragement of Departmental Chairman, Leon Gintzig, Ph.D., for us to commit the extra effort. We are grateful to the following students for the original research they provided: William R. Niehoff and Salvatore J. Profita for Chapter 2, Donald Moulton for Chapter 6, Michael Broom and Todd Peterson for Chapter 8, Ronald R. Peterson for Chapter 9, and Todd Peterson for Chapter 10. Mrs. Gladys Shimasagi, as always, did a superb job of typing the manuscript. Finally, we are indebted to the editors at Information Resources Press, Gene Allen and Nancy Moran, who made the text readable.

Contents

1

The Health Maintenance
Organization Concept

Free enterprise in the health care industry has fostered the development of several delivery structures. Traditionally, physicians and hospitals provided services for fees paid directly by those who received the care or through the philanthropy of private citizens. As the structure of American society became more complex, the traditional one-to-one delivery system developed into today's integrated system of complicated, highly technological delivery components with several sophisticated payment structures. A basic discussion of the health maintenance organization (HMO) as a health-delivery concept first requires an understanding of the five common delivery and financing systems available.

Health-Delivery Structures

PRIVATE PAY

In 1973, approximately 10 percent of the civilian population was without some form of private health insurance.[1] Although these self-responsible persons may have had some public financing of health care, many of them continued to be directly responsible for payment of their medical care, as indicated in Figure 1. Health care administrators frequently state that many private-pay patients not only are unable to

---

[1]Health Insurance Institute. *Source Book of Health Insurance Data 1974–75.* New York, 1975, p. 19.

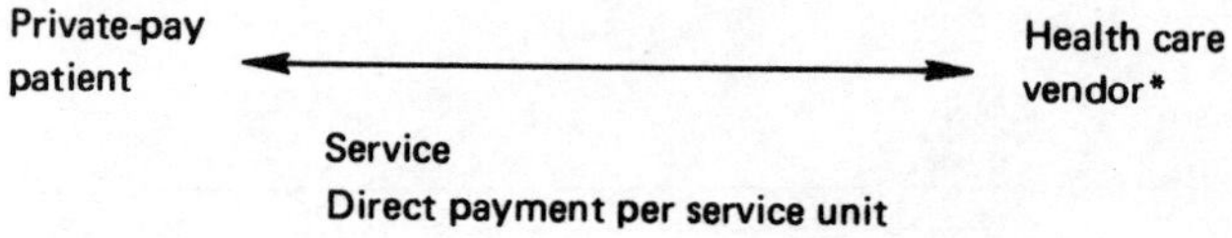

Private-pay   Health care
patient   ◄───────────────────────►   vendor*

Service
Direct payment per service unit

*The term "health care vendor" encompasses all providers of health
care—physicians and other health care personal providers, hospitals,
and other institutions, clinics, and delivery programs.

Figure 1   Private-pay health care structure.

pay out-of-pocket expenses for required health care, they cannot afford
to purchase adequate health insurance. Only a small minority of
private-pay patients are sufficiently affluent to pay upon receipt of
care. Generally, the self-responsible, private-pay patient, because no
third party such as government or an insurer is involved in payment to
providers, has become the "balancing factor" for most provider institutions; payments from such patients are the only ones that hospitals, for example, can vary as the financial situation demands without
third-party approval or interference. In the states with rate-review
commissions, even charges to the private-pay patients are being monitored and controlled.

SERVICE PLANS

Blue Cross and Blue Shield (BC/BS) plans are known as "service
plans." The Great Depression of 1929 forced the nation's hospitals to
depend less on philanthropic revenues and more on patient-payment
revenues for their services. Hospitals were faced with declining occupancy rates and losses of revenue. Concurrently, patients were faced
with substantial losses in income and mounting debts, including those
for medical care. A device was needed by the middle class to protect
themselves from the economic consequences of hospitalization. Consequently, several innovative approaches, including the "service
plan," were developed to protect families from high hospitalization
costs and to stabilize the financial situation of hospitals.

The Baylor Hospital experiment in Dallas, Texas is credited with the
origin of the Blue Cross movement. Led by Justin Ford Kimball, a
group of 1,250 school teachers banded together to form an arrangement
with Baylor Hospital to provide themselves with hospital care on a
prepayment basis. The considerations of social responsibility and
humanitarianism inherent in the Baylor Hospital experiment also were
incorporated into the Blue Cross plans that were based on the experi-

ment. It is from the social-insurance function of income redistribution and risk assumption by the local Blue Cross plans that the present Blue Cross programs have evolved. This service-plan concept had a profound effect on the traditional writers of insurance—commercial insurance carriers—by introducing insurance for hospital and surgical care. By 1933, the Blue Cross service plan and the group hospitalization prepayment principle had been adopted by the American Hospital Association.

Autonomous local Blue Cross plans were loosely joined through the national Blue Cross Association. Boards of directors represented hospitals, physicians, and the general public. This local control by boards of trustees permitted quicker, more accurate, and more acceptable responses to local situations than a national body could provide. All Blue Cross employees were placed on salaries, with no commissions offered to sales personnel. Most important, the Blue Cross plans placed emphasis on hospital benefits in the form of service rather than a cash indemnity (a benefit, usually cash, paid by an insurer for an insured loss).[2] In addition, Blue Cross plans provided for a "full service" benefit in recognition of a perceived responsibility to provide *total* hospital expense coverage to subscribers. These characteristics have changed very little over the 40 years that Blue Cross plans have been in existence.

As nonprofit, hospital-service organizations, Blue Cross plans affiliate on a contractual basis with local hospitals; in essence, hospitals entering into such an association with Blue Cross agree to accept the Blue Cross reimbursement schedule for hospital services provided to Blue Cross member patients, and are usually paid directly by Blue Cross. Three basic reimbursement formulas are used by Blue Cross:[3]

1. Reimbursement based on the retail charges of the hospital for services provided.
2. Reimbursement based on the cost of the services provided.
3. Reimbursement based on a uniform daily rate to all hospitals.

Blue Shield plans, like hospital-service plans, are nonprofit medical-service organizations which have developed along the lines of the Blue Cross model. Prior to the Great Depression, the lack of

[2]Sylvia A. Law. *Blue Cross: What Went Wrong?* 2nd Edition. New Haven, Conn., Yale University Press, 1976, pp. 6–25.

[3]Fredric R. Hedinger. *The Social Role of Blue Cross as a Device for Financing the Cost of Hospital Care: An Evaluation.* Health Care Research Series No. 2. Ames, Iowa, Graduate Program in Hospital and Health Administration, University of Iowa, 1966, p. 74.

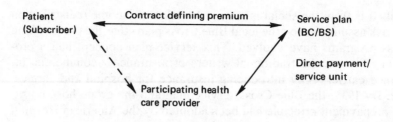

Figure 2   Blue Cross/Blue Shield plans—financing.

adequate medical resources in the northwest United States encouraged the growth of various industrial contract practices. In Washington State, the lumber industry had been contracting with physicians for care of its workers since the early 1900s. In response to the growing number of private physician/employer contracts, county Medical Service Bureaus were established "through which all medical contracts were to be channeled so that free choice would be preserved and the profession might have at least some nominal control over the practices."[4] The ultimate objectives of the Medical Service Bureaus were to meet and, if possible, control the competition of employer-sponsored medical-service programs. Thus, the Medical Service Bureaus became the forerunners of the present local medical societies as well as of the Blue Shield plans.

In 1934, following the example of the American Hospital Association in adopting the group hospitalization prepayment principle, the American Medical Association's (AMA) House of Delegates adopted a set of principles to provide guidance in the development of medical-service (Blue Shield) plans. By 1938, AMA recommended that its local medical societies develop medical-service plans—the first of which were the California Physicians' Service and the County Medical Society in Oregon and Washington. It is now recognized that these activities were principally undertaken by AMA to prevent the Blue Cross plans from underwriting physician services.

Blue Shield complements Blue Cross hospital coverage. Individual enrollment in a Blue Shield plan provides coverage for physician services as identified in a contract between the individual and Blue Shield. All physicians in the local medical society are usually eligible to participate in the local Blue Shield plan; physicians who do participate agree to accept direct payment for the services they provide to their patients.

[4]William A. MacColl. *Group Practice and Prepayment of Medical Care.* Washington, D.C., Public Affairs Press, 1966, p. 37.

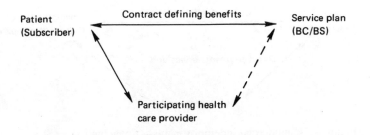

Figure 3   Blue Cross/Blue Shield plans—health-services delivery.

Reimbursement by Blue Shield follows a prenegotiated reimbursement schedule based on service units provided or a "profile" of previous levels of physician services.

The relationships described in the preceding paragraphs are illustrated in Figures 2 and 3.

INDEMNITY PLANS

Prior to the Great Depression, insurance companies were interested in insuring individuals against loss of income due to inability to work as a result of sickness, accident, or the loss of life. With the development of the "Blues" family in the 1930s, commercial carriers recognized the great market for health insurance and realized that their expertise in risk pooling and actuarial techniques would be of great advantage in entering this new market. Beginning in 1940, both life and casualty carriers entered the health insurance field.

Unlike BC/BS arrangements, commercial carriers do not establish working agreements with, or profiles of, hospitals or physicians. The individual subscriber enters into a contractual agreement with the private insurance company or indemnity carrier. The carrier identifies the illness risk of its subscribers by statistically determining the probability that they will become ill or disabled. The company is then able to accurately predict its costs and to calculate the premiums it must charge. Monthly or other periodic premium payments based on these costs are then "prepaid by the subscriber"; that is, they are paid prior to receiving health care services.

Indemnity plans reimburse the insured patient (or beneficiary) with stipulated sums of money to be applied against expenditures for the insured risks. Note that the insurance company has a contractual arrangement with the patient only; therefore, it pays the patient directly. These payments, as stipulated in the policy, can be either reimbursement for the patient's expenditures for health services and/or cash

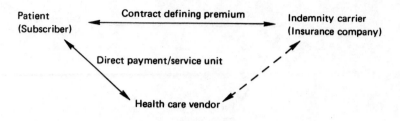

Figure 4   Commercial indemnity plans—financing.

benefits for loss of income during illness. The provision of health services is an indirect part of this financing system: Subscribers are solely
responsible for identifying their need for care, locating the providers of
such care, and, in most instances, paying for this care. It is only after
care has been received and paid for that the indemnity carrier reimburses the patient. The vendor of care has an indirect relationship with
the insurance company with regard to provision and payment for that
care, as indicated by the broken lines in Figures 4 and 5.

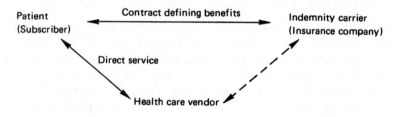

Figure 5   Commercial indemnity plans—health-services delivery.

As these figures show, the major difference between Blue Cross
plans and commercial insurers is that the former have contractual arrangements with hospitals and, through Blue Shield, with physicians,
while commercial carriers have no such relationships. Both delivery
systems do provide the patient/enrollee with free choice of vendor,
although the Blue Cross patient is limited to those hospitals that participate, and Blue Shield subscribers are limited to participating physicians. These limitations are minimal, however; 91 percent of the short-
term nonfederal hospitals are affiliated with a local Blue Cross plan.[5]
Although cash benefits for services usually are paid to the insured
patient by commercial carriers, they also can be made directly to the
provider of care through an arrangement called an *assignment of,* or

---

[5]American Hospital Association. *Hospital Statistics.* Chicago, 1973, p. 200.

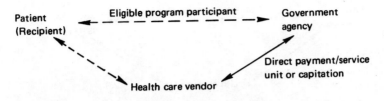

Figure 6   Government-sponsored programs—financing.

authorization to pay, benefits.

Three concepts are basic to Blue Cross plans: service benefits, full-coverage benefit packages, and community-rating methods.[6] Although these terms will be explained more fully later in this book, it is important to realize that Blue Cross plans, to compete with commercial carriers, will provide, under certain conditions, service and/or cash benefits and partial coverage, and they may use experience-rating methods. Thus, the practices of Blue Cross and commercial insurers may be slowly converging.

GOVERNMENT-SPONSORED PROGRAMS

Federal, state, and local governments have assumed a large role in health care financing. In fiscal 1971, of the total national health expenditures of $75 billion, 37.9 percent consisted of public funds.[7] Included in this figure are funds for Medicare and Medicaid programs, Public Health Service programs, the CHAMPUS program, the Federal Employees Health Benefits program, and county and state welfare-assistance programs, among others. Under these programs, service benefits are provided to recipients who have met eligibility requirements, with fees generally paid directly to the provider of care by the government agency. In some instances, the recipient is required to pay a nominal charge for the services rendered. Figures 6 and 7 illustrate the patient, health care vendor, and paying agency relationships under government-sponsored programs.

[6]Hedinger. *The Social Role of Blue Cross,* p. 47.

[7]B. S. Cooper and N. L. Worthington. "National Health Expenditures, Fiscal Year 1971." *Research and Statistics Notes.* Note No. 13. Washington, D.C., Office of Research and Statistics, Social Security Administration, U.S. Department of Health, Education, and Welfare, 1971. (Spending for health and medical care is increasing dramatically each year; it has increased from $75.6 billion in 1971 to $94.1 billion in 1973 and an estimated $118 billion in 1975. In 1975, the government portions were 42 percent, with much of this coming from the Federal Government (28 percent). Marjorie Smith Mueller. "National Health Expenditures, Fiscal Year 1975." *Social Security Bulletin.* Washington, D.C., U.S. Department of Health, Education, and Welfare, 1976.)

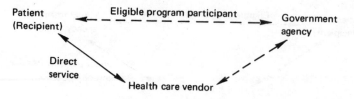

Figure 7 Government-sponsored programs—health-services delivery.

DIRECT-SERVICE PLANS

The final method of health delivery available in the United States is through direct-service plans, frequently called health maintenance organizations (HMOs). These organizations have been referred to by various other titles: prepaid group practice plans, prepaid individual practice plans, prepaid health plans, independent health insurance plans, or health insurance plans other than Blue Cross or Blue Shield plans or insurance companies.[8] To simplify terminology, health maintenance organization or HMO will be used to identify direct-service plans.

Compared to the "Blues" and commercial carriers, HMOs are a relatively small group of health insurers/providers. In 1973, approximately 5 percent of all persons who had private insurance coverage for hospital care and 10 percent of those having physician office and home visit coverage were HMO subscribers.[9] HMO health plans combine the functions of the insurance carrier and the providers of service in a single organization, including hospital care and physicians' services. Consequently, HMOs compete directly with BC/BS plans and commercial insurers, as well as with major providers (solo and group practices and hospitals). Competitive activity before the 1970s had been limited to rather localized geographic areas, primarily the Far West and Northwest, Detroit, Cleveland, District of Columbia, and New York City.

As illustrated in Figure 8, subscribers pay their health insurance premiums to the HMO (health plan). The HMO establishes close relationships with both inpatient and outpatient providers of care—usually via contractual agreements. Thus, when care is required, the HMO can directly furnish services through its professional staff and affiliate organizations, as shown in Figure 9. Since all fees have been prepaid in

[8]Louis Reed and Maureen Dwyer. *Directory of Health Insurance Plans Other than Blue Cross or Blue Shield Plans or Insurance Companies, 1970 Survey.* Washington, D.C., Office of Research and Statistics, Social Security Administration, U.S. Department of Health, Education, and Welfare, 1971.

[9]Marjorie Smith Mueller. *Independent Health Insurance Plans in 1973.* Note No. 15. Washington, D.C., Office of Research and Statistics, Social Security Administration, U.S. Department of Health, Education, and Welfare, 1975.

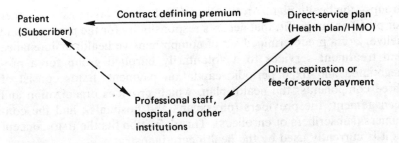

Figure 8 Health Maintenance Organization—financing.

the form of a premium, the HMO does not charge for specific services rendered to its subscribers; therefore, the patient does not directly pay the providers for care rendered. Hospitals and physicians may have contractual relationships with the health plan and are usually paid by the HMO, either on a per-unit-of-service basis or a capitation basis. *Capitation* is the price charged by the actual health care vendor for providing service *per person* for a specified time period, for example, $30 per person per month.

This close association between the providers and the health plan exemplifies one of the fundamental characteristics of HMOs—for the subscriber/patient, the HMO is not merely an insurer but *is the provider* of care. The HMO must guarantee the availability of care described in the subscriber contract; unlike the BC/BS or private insurance carrier arrangements, it is the responsibility of the HMO to furnish the providers of health care as well as to pay them for providing such care.

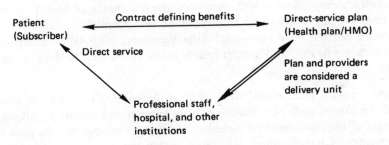

Figure 9 Health Maintenance Organization—health-services delivery.

The HMO Concept

The HMO concept combines a financing mechanism and a delivery system under the control and direction of a single management group—the health plan. An HMO is defined as any organization, either for profit or nonprofit, that accepts responsibility for the provision and delivery of a predetermined set of comprehensive health maintenance and treatment services to a voluntarily enrolled group for a pre-negotiated and fixed periodic capitation payment. HMOs consist of three components: the health plan, which provides organization and management; the providers (physicians and hospitals); and the consumers (subscribers or enrollees). This definition fits the HMO concept as it is currently used by the health care industry.

Two other, more specific definitions are provided in

1. The HMO Act of 1973, Public Law 93-222, which details the specific requirements that must be met before certification of an organization as a qualified HMO by the Federal Government. Chapter 3 discusses these regulations in detail.

2. The Genetic Code, originated by Ernest Saward, M.D., which outlines the tried and proven method of organizing an HMO under a medical group practice arrangement.[10]

Based on experience of the Kaiser-Permanente Medical Care Program, the code includes the following elements:

Prepayment—usually by community-rated monthly dues, which are paid by a variety of organizations.
Medical group practice—a group of full-time, autonomous, and self-governing physicians, who are paid through a capitation arrangement.
Medical center—with integrated inpatient and ambulatory health care facilities.
Voluntary enrollment—with members given a choice of health plans.
Capitation payment—both to physicians and hospitals.
Comprehensive coverage—including inpatient, outpatient, extended care, home health, and mental health services, as well as drug coverage.

As a purist, Dr. Saward states that, if the code is violated, the plan will be unsuccessful or defective in its growth and maturity. All elements of the code must be included; if one part is omitted, the plan is permanently handicapped. He states further that

---

[10]Ernest W. Saward. *The Relevance of Prepaid Group Practice to the Effective Delivery of Health Services.* Washington, D.C., Health Services and Mental Health Administration, U.S. Department of Health, Education, and Welfare, 1969, pp. 8–10.

It is fundamental that the program be non-profit and that it be self-sustaining without philanthropy or tax support, although the poor and the elderly need tax support to participate in the system. The program must be conducted in the paramount interest of the membership. The principal characteristic of the program is the assumption of the responsibility, by the providers of medical services, for the organization and delivery of such services on a prepaid basis. It is not an insurance program that trades dollars of premiums for benefits. Dollars are only available for use as services.[11]

The HMO Umbrella

The Genetic Code, describing the purest form of an HMO, allows for no variations in form or style. It is the intent of the federal program, however, to allow experimentation with the HMO form within the guidelines of the law. The strength of the HMO concept appears to be its great flexibility in sponsorship, method of payment, delivery, coverage, and profit status.[12] Although the Kaiser-Permanente plan, model for Saward's Genetic Code, has been eminently successful since the early 1940s, there are other successful HMO plans that differ in various aspects from his code, including such plans as

1. The community/consumer-sponsored Group Health Cooperative of Puget Sound in Washington State and the Group Health Association in the District of Columbia
2. The union-sponsored Community Health Association of Detroit (now the Metro Health Plan) and the "miners' clinics" of Pennsylvania, Ohio, and West Virginia
3. Private group clinics, such as the Ross-Loos Medical Clinic of Los Angeles and the Palo Alto Medical Clinic, Palo Alto, California
4. Individual practice plans, such as the Foundation for Medical Care of San Joaquin County, California

The term HMO, therefore, is an umbrella term that includes all prepaid health plans. Two general types of HMOs can be included under the HMO umbrella, according to a classification by type of physician participation: prepaid group practice plans and prepaid individual practice plans.

[11]*Ibid.*, p. 9.
[12]President Richard M. Nixon. *Health Message from the President of the United States: Relative to Building a National Health Strategy* (February 18, 1971). 92nd Congress, 1st Session. Washington, D.C., U.S. Government Printing Office, 1971, p. 4.

A *prepaid group practice plan* (PGP) is developed around a medical group practice of physicians and dentists, usually in a multispecialty arrangement. As defined by the American Medical Association, medical group practice describes the provision of medical service by a number of physicians working in systematic association, with the joint use of equipment and technical personnel and centralized administration and financial organization. The PGP may be sponsored by the group practice; the physicians develop the insuring mechanism and make it available to their patients and others either on an individual or a group basis. Premium payments are pooled, and physician salaries are drawn from this income. The PGP also may be sponsored by nonphysician groups; the Health Insurance Plan (HIP) of Greater New York is an example of a prepaid group practice plan developed by a city. HIP, as the responsible organization, contracts with physician groups throughout metropolitan New York City to provide care to HIP subscribers. Payment to physicians is on a capitation basis.

Prepaid individual practice plans (PIPs), in contrast, use the services of individual, solo practitioners in their private office settings. Currently, two types of sponsorship are being used to develop individual practice HMOs. In the first type, local and state medical societies have developed PIPs, called Foundations for Medical Care (FMCs), or Individual Practice Associations (IPAs). These foundations are associations of physicians (usually a local medical society) that organize and develop a management and fiscal structure and determine a fee schedule for individual physicians who join the foundation. (Foundations will be reviewed in more detail in Chapter 4.) The foundation, usually a separate corporation controlled by the medical society, is the managing organization (health plan) that establishes benefit and premium structures, markets benefits, and completes peer review and payment of claims. All medical society members are eligible for participation in the HMO; the physician is paid by the foundation, not by the patient, on a *fee-for-service basis*, unlike other HMO types, which usually compensate their providers via a capitation arrangement.

The second type of PIP, which might be called a "community individual practice plan," is a program established by community residents as a health-ensuring mechanism for such residents. Subscribers are given a free choice of any available private practitioner in the area. The plan either pays the provider directly on a fee-for-service basis or may reimburse the subscriber for charges incurred, who then pays the provider. This type of PIP does not qualify as a direct-service plan as defined here, because it does not guarantee health care service.

TABLE 1   HMO Organizations and Enrollments for Selected Years*

Month and Year	Estimated Number of Plans	Estimated Enrollments
1960	20	—
January 1970†	33	—
December 1972	72	4,500,000
October 1974	142	5,300,000
May 1975	173	5,734,000
December 1975	166	5,851,000
July 1976	176	6,016,443

*Estimates are provided in the several Health Maintenance Organization Service's *Program Status Reports, 1972–1976,* and the *Annual Reports to the Congress, 1971–* (Washington, D.C., Health Services Administration, U.S. Department of Health, Education, and Welfare). Additional estimates are reported by Rhona L. Wetherille and Jean M. Nordby in *A Census of HMOs: October 1974 (Including Further HMO Act Survey Results and HMO Enrollment Estimates).* Minneapolis, Minn., InterStudy, 1974. The latter estimates are somewhat higher than those reported by DHEW and in Group Health Association of America. *National HMO Census Survey 1977.* Washington, D.C. 1977.

†Reed and Dwyer, in the *Directory of Health Plans Other than Blue Cross or Blue Shield Plans or Insurance Companies* (p. 81), also provide estimates of plans for 1970 and earlier. Their January 1970 estimates suggest that there were a total of 59 HMO organizations in existence, of which 39 were prepaid group practice plans and 20 were prepaid individual practice plans (3 foundation and 17 community). Reed and Dwyer report four additional subcategories of plans—two types are sponsored, developed, and operated by jointly managed union/employer welfare funds, employers' employee-benefit associations, or unions for the exclusive benefit of the employee groups and their dependents (pp. 5–6) and include 427 programs. Membership in these plans is limited to employees of the unions, associations, or companies and, perhaps, their dependents. According to P.L. 93-222, these organizations do not meet the open-enrollment requirement (i.e., they do not enroll persons who are broadly representative of the various age, social, and income groups within the service area, nor do they provide an open enrollment period during which the plan accepts individuals, up to its capacity, in the order in which they apply for enrollment). Two additional subcategories are limited to the practice of prepaid dentistry (Reed and Dwyer, p. 6) and do not meet the "basic health services" section of the law. These latter groups include 20 private dental clinics or corporations.

Table 1 shows the estimated number of HMO organizations and the estimated total enrollment levels for selected years.

Beverlee Myers, former Assistant Administrator for Resources Development, Health Services and Mental Health Administration, U.S. Department of Health, Education, and Welfare, stated in an April 1971 speech that an HMO is a four-way arrangement between the enrolled population; a medical group—solo practitioners, hospital(s), and other health facilities; a management organization; and a financing mechanism.[13] These HMO components might be arranged as shown in Figure

[13]Beverlee A. Myers. *Health Maintenance Organizations: Objectives and Issues.* Washington, D.C., U.S. Government Printing Office, 1972.

10. An interested group of physicians and laymen joins together with a common intent—HMO development. The group develops the prepaid plan, first identifying and obtaining financing. Gradually, over a period of from one to five years, the management group formulates a benefit package and corresponding premium structures, and identifies target populations to whom the plan will be marketed. The benefit package is then marketed to that audience. Premiums collected from enrollees are deposited into the system to defray the cost of care provided. This cyclical process continues as the plan is marketed, as new members are enrolled, and as enrollee care is financed. Health care is guaranteed by the plan through its contractual relationships with the plan's physicians and other health vendors. As the plan grows with the addition of new enrollees, it generates new resources to provide more services and/or to reduce the cost of the existing benefit package; that is, it improves the "product"—comprehensive health services.

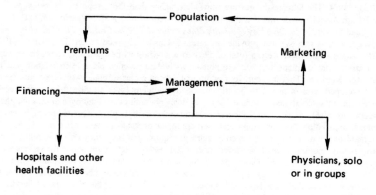

Figure 10   HMO schema.

Prepayment: Fee-for-Service Versus Capitation

The traditional method of providing ambulatory health services is a one-to-one relationship between private solo physicians and their patients. Charges for care are paid by the patients or their insurance programs on a fee-for-service (unit-of-service) basis. The more units of service provided, the greater the total fee collected by the physician. When BC/BS and commercial insurers enter into a relationship, the patient prepays for his health services, which may or may not be required at a later date. Responsibility for obtaining care remains with the subscriber, but payment flows from the insurer on a *per-unit-of-service* basis.

If Blue Cross and Blue Shield plans and private insurance carriers are prepaid by periodic premiums, how do these delivery structures differ from HMOs, whose subscribers also prepay on a periodic basis? As Figure 11 shows, there is little difference between the systems. Enrollees pay premiums to their insurance plans: individuals pay their own premiums, and persons included in group contracts have their premiums totally or partly paid on a capitation basis. The difference between the systems is in the interaction of the specific plan and the providers of care. Again, an HMO stresses the total-system, direct-service approach; that is, the HMO comprises both the health plan and the health provider. Within this structure, the providers can be paid on a salary or retainer, per capita, or fee-for-service basis. Applying the Genetic Code definition of an HMO, providers should be paid by contract, capitation, or salary. The HMO law, however, allows for a fee-for-service payment, which is considered by many early prepayment advocates as an illegitimate HMO model associated with the medical foundation and individual practice association approach.

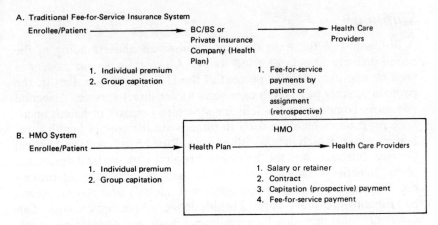

Figure 11   Premium movement.

Setting aside the foundation model for the time being,[14] the major difference between the traditional fee-for-service system and the HMO system centers on the providers' incentives in the fee-for-service system: the more units of service rendered, the greater the provider's revenue. Conversely, under the HMO system, the fewer units of service provided, the greater the savings to the plan. These savings may be

[14]The foundation or IPA approach is a compromise between the traditional fee-for-service, solo practitioner system and the prepaid, group or solo practitioner system. The foundation system is described in Chapter 4.

shared with the providers as incentive payments, may be used to provide additional benefits to the subscribers, or may be used to reduce the premium. Under the HMO system, the incentive payment to physicians is used as an inducement for providers to function more efficiently, to reduce overuse where possible, and to help control costs. Cost containment within the concepts of good patient care is one of the major goals of the HMO movement. Thus, the change to the capitation mechanism is one of the methods used by HMOs to control their operating costs. The purpose of Figure 11, however, is to identify the major differences between the two systems, and, more importantly, to emphasize the parallelism between them. This similarity is further emphasized when one considers the fee-for-service foundation approach and the fact that both systems use common components of the industry. Thus, the HMO is not a *new delivery system* but a *new delivery concept*—a different way of thinking about and arranging the current health-delivery components.

Summary

A discussion of the HMO concept requires an understanding of the health-delivery structures used today. A *private-payment system* is used by approximately 10 percent of the U.S. population; that is, the patients directly pay health care vendors for direct service. A second and more common health-delivery structure consists of health insurance programs which are used to underwrite the cost of health care. *Service plans,* which include Blue Cross, Blue Shield, and the Medical Service Bureaus, are the available hospital and medical insurance plans. Benefits usually are provided in the form of fees to the providers. Subscribers to these plans are free to identify and choose among participating providers. A third health-delivery structure consists of an *indemnity plan* provided by commercial insurance companies or private carriers who, following the lead of BC/BS, insure the costs of both physician and hospital care. Subscribers are free to select their providers of care and are reimbursed for the cost of the care; under certain conditions, patients may assign this cash payment to the provider. A fourth health-delivery structure consists of *government-sponsored programs.* Within this group are federal, state, and local government-financed programs, including Medicare, Medicaid, the Federal Employees Health Benefit program, CHAMPUS, and county and state welfare programs. Eligible program participants receive service benefits, and their fees generally are paid directly to the provider of care by the government. A fifth method of health delivery is the *direct-service plan* or health maintenance organization. HMOs comprise a relatively small group of health insurers/providers—approximately 5 percent of all private hospital insurance coverage in 1973. These plans are characterized by the unique development of one organization to provide both the insurance coverage and the provider service, including inpatient, outpatient, and other health services. Thus, the HMO concept is both a financing mechanism and a delivery system under the control of a single management group. The HMO may be defined as either a for-profit or nonprofit organization that accepts the responsibility for the provision and delivery of a prenegotiated set of comprehensive health care services to a voluntarily enrolled group for a periodic premium.

HMO is an umbrella term that identifies several models. Most narrowly defined, an HMO may take the form of a prepaid group practice plan (PGP) as described by the Genetic Code of prepayment. In this configuration, an HMO has the following elements: a medical group practice of physicians, a medical center with integrated inpatient and ambulatory-care facilities, voluntary enrollment, capitation, prepayment to all providers, and comprehensive coverage. The broader HMO definition includes the prepaid individual practice plans (PIP), individual practice associations (IPA), and medical foundations. The major differences between the group practice and individual practice plans are in the areas of sponsorship, physician practice patterns, and provider reimbursement. PGPs are sponsored by private physician or non-medical groups, whereas PIPs usually are sponsored by local medical societies. Physicians practice as a group in PGPs versus as individuals in PIPs and foundations. Finally, capitation is used as the payment mechanism for PGP physicians, while the traditional fee-for-service approach is used in PIPs. Thus, identifying an HMO is somewhat complicated, because of the variety of models available. This flexibility in sponsorship, delivery, and payment, however, is one of the characteristics that makes the HMO concept attractive and strong.

All HMO organizations are a four-way arrangement between the enrolled population, a group of providers, a management organization, and a financing mechanism. The objective of these plans is to organize the health-delivery components so the plan can market its product—the benefit package—and provide direct, comprehensive health services to its enrollees. Moreover, in the process of providing services, the goal of HMOs is to reduce and/or to contain the costs of furnishing health care by providing incentives to the providers to use appropriate levels and types of health care services, including health maintenance. One mechanism used by the prepaid group practice HMO model to help control costs and to provide efficiency incentives is capitation—the price charged by the health care vendor for providing service per person for a specified time period.

Both the fee-for-service and the HMO systems use prepayment in the form of health insurance. The HMO system is the only one that uses capitation payments for both physicians and hospitals; however, fee-for-service reimbursement to providers, similar to the traditional system, also is used by one HMO model—the foundation approach. The use of identical components, such as medical group practice and prepaid health insurance, emphasizes the parallelism between the two systems. Thus, the HMO does not create new delivery components, but provides an alternative method of arranging the current ones.

References

Dearing, Walter P. *Developments and Accomplishments of Comprehensive Group Practice Prepayment Programs.* Washington, D.C., Group Health Association of America, Inc., 1963, pp. 1–10.

Hedinger, Fredric R. *The Social Role of Blue Cross as a Device for Financing the Cost of Hospital Care: An Evaluation.* Health Care Research Series No. 2. Ames, Iowa, Graduate Program in Hospital and Health Administration, University of Iowa, 1966, pp. 1–13, 17–18, 34–49, 73–76, 82–84.

Law, Sylvia A. *Blue Cross: What Went Wrong?* 2nd Edition. New Haven, Conn., Yale University Press, 1976.

Myers, Beverlee A. *Health Maintenance Organizations: Objectives and Issues.* Washington, D.C., U.S. Government Printing Office, 1972. DHEW Publ. No. (SHM) 73-13002.

Nixon, President Richard M. *Health Message from the President of the United States: Relative to Building a National Health Strategy* (February 18, 1971). 92nd Congress, 1st Session. Washington, D.C., U.S. Government Printing Office, 1971, p. 4.

Reed, Louis, and Dwyer, Maureen. *Directory of Health Insurance Plans Other than Blue Cross or Blue Shield Plans or Insurance Companies, 1970 Survey.* Washington, D.C., Office of Research and Statistics, Social Security Administration, U.S. Department of Health, Education, and Welfare, 1971.

Saward, Ernest W. *The Relevance of Prepaid Group Practice to the Effective Delivery of Health Services.* Washington, D.C., Health Services and Mental Health Administration, U.S. Department of Health, Education, and Welfare, 1969.

University of Chicago, Graduate Program in Hospital Administration, Center for Health Administration Studies, Graduate School of Business. *Health Maintenance Organization: A Reconfiguration of the Health Services System. Proceedings of the Thirteenth Annual Symposium on Hospital Affairs.* Chicago, 1971, pp. 2–10.

U.S. Department of Health, Education, and Welfare. *Health Maintenance Organizations: The Statements of President Richard M. Nixon and Secretary Elliot L. Richardson of the U.S. Department of Health, Education, and Welfare.* Rockville, Md., 1971.

_____ . *Towards a Comprehensive Health Policy for the 1970's: A White Paper.* Washington, D.C., U.S. Government Printing Office, 1971, pp. 31–37.

_____ . Health Services and Mental Health Administration. *Health Maintenance Organization. The Concept and Structure.* Rockville, Md., 1971.

2

History, Philosophy, and Objectives

The concepts upon which today's HMOs are structured have been a part of the medical care delivery system for many years. In this country, early efforts to provide prepaid group practice medical care were undertaken by the Federal Government on behalf of military personnel and merchant seamen. The Merchant Marine Hospital system, which is now a part of the Public Health Service, provides medical care on a group basis for merchant marines, who are continually traveling. The HMO-like organizations for the civilian population began to evolve during the beginning of the twentieth century, with the industrialization of the western United States. Railroads and the associated railroad workers' unions realized that it was necessary to provide medical care for the crews as they moved farther away from established medical service. Medical arrangements also were developed in the "company towns" by the mining, lumber, and manufacturing industries. Historical evidence suggests that prepaid group practice plans were established for workers to fill the void when adequate, solo fee-for-service medical care was not available.

Medical Group Practice Development

Together with provisions for medical care for specific groups of people, sponsored by employers, the government, and unions, another major HMO element appeared—medical group practices sponsored by physicians. The first medical group practice, a partnership between Dr.

W. W. Mayo and his two sons, W. J. and C. H. Mayo, was formed in Rochester, Minnesota in 1887. The physical properties of the clinic ultimately became the Mayo Properties Association in 1920. As a charitable corporation without capital stock, the association leased the plant and equipment to the Mayo Clinic and appointed a board of governors. By 1929, the clinic employed 386 physicians and dentists and 895 lay persons and provided care on a fee-for-service basis.[1]

During this same year, 1929, Drs. Donald E. Ross and H. Clifford Loos established the Ross-Loos group practice clinic in Los Angeles. Described by some writers as the first HMO prototype, the Ross-Loos Medical Clinic contracted with the Los Angeles Water and Power Department to provide care for its 400 employees. Within a year, several other groups had applied to participate in the program, and, by 1932, membership had increased twentyfold. Between 1929 and 1936, the clinic functioned strictly as the partnership of Ross and Loos. In 1936, 16 physicians on the staff were admitted into the partnership. By 1973, prepaid membership had grown to more than 120,000 members served by 150 physicians, 48 of whom are partners in the plan. It now is the largest private, physician-owned, prepaid group practice health plan in the United States.[2]

Also in 1929, another notable group practice was formally organized—the Palo Alto Medical Clinic in Palo Alto, California. Originally a partnership between Drs. Thomas William and George DeForest Barnett, formed in 1924, it was gradually expanded to handle an increasing patient load. In 1929, the clinic was composed of eight physicians, with Dr. Russell V. Lee as its medical director. According to Dr. Lee, the most important development at the clinic during the years 1930 to 1941 was the emergence among the physician partners of "a true feeling for the essential principles of group practice as contrasted with solo practice."[3] Palo Alto Medical Clinic entered into prepaid medical care in 1947, when it agreed to provide complete medical care to the Stanford University student body and to various nursing and long-term care facilities in the Palo Alto area. In 1970, with 112 full-time physicians, the clinic served approximately 16 percent of its patients on a prepaid basis.[4]

[1]C. Rufus Rorem. *Private Group Clinics.* New York, Milbank Memorial Fund, 1971, pp. 115–118. (Reprint)
[2]Leon Gintzig and Robert G. Shouldice. "Prepaid Group Practice—A Comparative Study." Part I, Vol. 2. Washington, D.C., The George Washington University, 1971, chap. 11, pp. 1–2. Mimeographed.
[3]Russell V. Lee. "Palo Alto Medical Clinic." *Group Practice, XI:*510, August 1962.
[4]Gintzig and Shouldice. "Prepaid Group Practice." Part I, Vol. 2, chap. 10, pp. 1–3.

Probably the oldest prepaid group practice plan was the Western Clinic in Tacoma, Washington. It was organized in 1906 as a partnership by Drs. James R. Yocum and Thomas B. Curran and originally was based on the fee-for-service system. Within a few years, however, the clinic became the pioneer in the field of prepaid medicine. Although the exact date when the first prepaid contract was signed is unknown, such an arrangement was developed between the Western Clinic and the lumber industry around 1910.

Tacoma was the lumber capital of the world in the early 1900s. The owners of the mills, their employees, or both, entered into contracts with Drs. Yocum and Curran, under which the physicians offered to provide medical care for a premium of 50 cents per member per month. Almost simultaneously, another physician, Dr. Bridge, founded a clinic and established prepaid contracts with other groups of employees in Tacoma. Most employees in the area were soon covered by a prepaid contract at one of the clinics. To compete for patients in the Tacoma area, other physicians banded together and, in 1917, formed the Pierce County Medical Bureau, the first locally organized medical group in the country. The Western Clinic, in 1975, had 44 contracts with groups of employees and unions, serving more than 12,000 prepaid members. Medical care was provided by 18 physicians who also served 40 percent of their patients on a fee-for-service basis.[5] Because of its inability to compete financially with other providers, the Western Clinic decided, in 1976, not to renew their contracts for prepaid service and gradually reverted to a totally fee-for-service operation.

After the opening of his small clinic in Tacoma in about 1911, Dr. Bridge organized a chain of approximately 20 group practice industrial clinics in the Washington and Oregon areas, staffed by local physicians and offering medical care to male employees of the lumber industry on a prepaid basis. These clinics, owned by the Bridge Company, became the predecessors of several of today's prepaid group practice plans. Before his death in 1946, Dr. Bridge arranged for the physicians staffing the clinics to be eligible to purchase the clinics from his estate. Two Bridge clinics in Seattle were purchased by staff physicians and continued with prepaid programs—the Community Medical Services (CMS) of Seattle and the Medical Securities Clinic (MSC). CMS was purchased by Doctors Hospital of Seattle in 1972, and MSC combined its resources with a consumer organization to become the Group Health Cooperative of Puget Sound in 1947.[6]

[5]*Ibid.*, Part I, Vol. 3, chap. 13, pp. 1–2.
[6]*Ibid.*, Part I, Vol. 1, chap. 4, pp. 1–3.

Although many other group practices evolved during the early 1900s, these clinics—Ross-Loos, Western, Palo Alto, and the Bridge clinics—were the first to offer their services on a prepaid basis to groups of employees and others.

Prepayment as a Social Movement

During the mid-1920s, the prosperity of the nation was reflected by a change in the national emphasis from wartime programs to social programs and domestic health issues. This emphasis was sharpened by the financial plight of the general hospital and the lack of available medical care and its rising cost to the individual. By 1927, it was clear that some kind of action was necessary to control health costs and to review the system. During that year, several foundations provided funds for a study of the American health system. The Committee on the Costs of Medical Care was formed, and the services of several outstanding individuals in the health industry were obtained. The committee's report, *Medical Care for the American People,* published in 1933, predicted the major economic health problems of today; but the report also suggested some possible solutions for these problems. Five general conclusions were presented:

1. Medical service, both preventive and therapeutic, should be furnished largely by organized groups of physicians and other associated personnel in order to maintain high standards and to develop or preserve a personal relationship between patient and physician.
2. All basic public health services should be extended so they will be available to the entire population according to its needs.
3. The cost of medical care should be placed on a group prepayment basis—by insurance and/or taxation. An individual fee basis should be continued for those who prefer the present method.
4. The study, evaluation, and coordination of medical service should be considered important functions for every state and local community.
5. Increased emphasis should be given to the training of physicians, dentists, pharmacists, nurses' aids, nurse-midwives, and hospital and clinic administrators.[7]

[7]Committee on the Costs of Medical Care. *Medical Care for the American People.* Chicago, University of Chicago Press, 1933. (Reprint ed., Washington, D.C., Community Health Service, Health Services and Mental Health Administration, U.S. Department of Health, Education, and Welfare, 1970, pp. 109–138.)

In the discussion concerning the first conclusion, the committee further stated that

. . . organized groups of consumers [should] unite in paying into a common fund agreed annual sums, in weekly or monthly installments, and in arranging with organized groups of medical practitioners working as private group clinics, hospital medical staffs, or community medical centers, to furnish them and their families with virtually complete medical services. By "organized groups of consumers" the Committee means industrial, fraternal, educational or other reasonably cohesive groups.[8]

These conclusions were presented at a time when the effects of the Great Depression were being strongly felt. As William MacColl states, the American public had been seriously challenged to look at the whole social structure under which it lived and to reexamine many of the traditional values and habits threatened with change.[9] The depression created both an insecurity that prompted Americans to look for new solutions to their problems and an atmosphere in which change could take place. People were looking for solutions that would bring stability to their daily lives, and the first recommendation of the Committee on the Costs of Medical Care was most appropriate.

The Cooperative Society

Joint action through the use of "organized groups of consumers" had been used for many years in Europe as a means of handling problems of instability. In an attempt to relieve some of the hardships and abuses of an industrialized society, factory workers joined together in consumers' (or producers') cooperatives. Their objective was the "substitution of common ownership and operation of trade and industry for individual or capitalistic ownership."[10] The cooperative is a voluntary association whose members organize to supply their needs through mutual action. The motive of production and distribution is service. As cooperative societies grew, they took many forms: consumer cooperatives in England, rural farm cooperatives in Denmark, credit cooperatives in Germany, producer cooperatives in Norway.

---

[8]*Ibid.*, p. 121.

[9]William A. MacColl. *Group Practice and Prepayment of Medical Care.* Washington, D.C., Public Affairs Press, 1966, p. 14.

[10]James Ford. *Co-operation in New England.* New York, Survey Associates, Inc., 1913, p. 8. The co-op member seeks common ownership *not* through government, as does the socialist, but through voluntary association of producers or consumers.

One of the most important cooperatives was the Rochdale Cooperative of England. Its objective was to lower the cost of living for its members, since wages could not be increased. In 1844, the cooperative was founded with 28 members. Their guiding philosophy included voluntary membership, one vote per member, service not profit, continuing education for members, regular reporting from elected executives, and full financial disclosure.[11] As surpluses were accumulated, they were used to support educational activities and, to a lesser extent, to underwrite various charitable activities for ill or unemployed members. The nature of this closed philanthropy was primarily goods and services "in kind," such as free groceries and the gratuitous services of medical or nursing practitioners in the employ of the cooperative society. It was not until the Great Depression that European cooperatives followed the Rochdale model and provided health care services as customary benefits for its members. Most of the concepts of HMO-like organizations were included; the traditional physician-patient relationship was maintained, but the cost of the practitioner's services to the member was lessened by "regularizing" doctors' incomes—ostensibly by providing them with a fixed capitation fee and permitting a token copayment for each use of their services.[12]

In the United States, group action during the depression manifested itself in the form of credit unions—buying clubs similar to the English and European cooperatives—and the expansion of labor unions hastened by passage of the Wagner Act. Health care became a negotiable item at the bargaining table. Employers were forced to pay for at least part of their employees' health care and were, therefore, interested in the development and control of new health care programs. Moreover, as noted in Chapter 1, the financial crises for providers of medical care brought about the development and expansion of hospital and medical insurance. The Blue Cross plans were initiated by the American Hospital Association in 1929 to help stabilize and ensure the sources of funds for member hospitals. A few years later, the American Medical Association was instrumental in establishing Blue Shield plans, following the organizational patterns developed by Blue Cross.

The movement to organize medicine, first at the local levels and then by the formation of the national American Medical Association, had its origin in the pressures of competition from the early prepaid group practice plans. Although the early prepaid plans were conceptualized in terms of *assurance* of service and financing—rather than as insur-

[11]P. H. Casselman. *The Cooperative Movement and Some of Its Problems*. New York, The Philosophical Library, 1952, p. 2.

[12]J. Baker. *Cooperative Enterprise*. New York, Vanguard Press, 1937, pp. 100–101.

ance programs—the effect of the plans was to capture a moderate share of the local health care market. Other physicians, outside the plans, viewed plan activities as attempts to control all local health care delivery. To meet this threat, whether imagined or real, nonplan physicians joined together to form medical societies—such as the Pierce County Medical Bureau. Blue Shield-like plans were then established by these local societies as *insurance* programs. The effect was to control the payment for service and thus the delivery of that service. The confrontations between the prepaid group practice plans and organized medicine culminated in long court battles over restraint of trade under the terms of the Sherman Antitrust Act. Courts ruled in favor of the prepaid plans in all of the cases.

The objectives of the American health care cooperative movement parallel those of the Rochdale Society models. Both the society and the prepaid health plans were organized by group action for the betterment of their members. Their joint action was directed toward stabilizing society, increasing the value obtained from limited incomes, and obtaining products and services as good as or better than those they could obtain as individuals. As with the Rochdale Society, the originators of the new health plans desired a voice in the development of the plans—on an equal basis with the providers of care. They wanted assurances of quality, fiscal responsibility, availability, and most important, security from financial loss. This system, however, could only be effective if the providers also were assured of financial stability through salary arrangements. Elimination of fee-for-service payments allowed the physicians to concentrate on professional activities that would, hopefully, enhance the quality of medical care. Finally, the goal of the prepaid health plan was the development of parallel interests of patients and physicians—a program designed to promote good care, preventive and treatment services, and stability in financing.

The year 1929 was important in the development of cooperative prepaid group practice plans. During that year, Dr. Michael A. Shadid helped organize a group of families in Elk City, Oklahoma to form a health cooperative, the Community Hospital Association. After some initial setbacks, the association began to grow. In 1934, the Farmers' Union agreed to take over sponsorship of the organization. Under the new name, Farmers' Union Cooperative Hospital Association, the program continued to expand, but not without harassment from the county and state medical associations. After 20 years of confrontations with the medical societies, an antitrust suit for $100,000 in damages was filed by the association. The case was settled out of court, in an almost complete victory for the association.

During the early years of the Elk City operation, Dr. Shadid played an advocacy role in the development and establishment of several pre-paid plans, spanning locations from the Midwest to the Pacific Coast and from Texas to Canada. The Elk City operation and these plans influenced the development of the health cooperative movement in the United States. They also were a tribute to the ideals and efforts of Michael Shadid, who died in 1966 at age 85.

The Pre-HMO Period

The period between the development of group practices and health plans (prior to 1930) and the evolution of federally influenced and spon-sored plans (1970) was one of moderate expansion in prepaid group practice plans. Their development is well documented in the litera-ture.[13] Table 2 provides a list of many of these plans. The early plans had a great influence on the development of the philosophy of prepaid medical care and the development of the HMO concepts included in P.L. 93-222.

Prior to 1929, most plans were started by physicians as a sole propri-etorship or two- to three-person medical partnership and were later developed into multispecialty medical group practices. All provided prepaid medical services to employees of local industry through con-tracts with employers or employee groups. By 1929, however, the insecurity of daily living had brought people together, and the first cooperatives were developed. The Elk City program and the several cooperatives that were patterned on Dr. Shadid's early model have been mentioned earlier. The forerunner of the Group Health Coopera-tive of Puget Sound (GHC) began during 1935 as the Medical Securities Clinic. As a medical partnership, this clinic originally had been organ-ized to provide services to the lumber industry and logging unions. During World War II, membership dropped substantially. A group composed of the Washington State Grange and several unions ap-proached the physicians associated with the Medical Securities Clinic, and a merger between the two groups was effected. Approximately 300 families were involved in the formation of GHC. They combined their resources into a cooperative and purchased the assets and hospital of

---

[13]The history of many of the plans is given in MacColl. *Group Practice and Prepay-ment of Medical Care,* pp. 24–54; Jerome L. Schwartz. "Early History of Prepaid Medical Care Plans." *Bulletin of the History of Medicine, 39:*450–475, September–October 1965; and Gintzig and Shouldice. "Prepaid Group Practice." Part I, Vols. 1–3.

TABLE 2   Selected HMO Organizations from 1900 to 1975

Plan	Date of Establishment	Sponsor
Western Clinic, Tacoma, Washington	1906, 1910*	Medical partnership
Bridge Clinics in Oregon and Washington†	1911	Individual practitioner
Palo Alto Medical Clinic, Palo Alto, California	1929, 1947*	Medical partnership
Ross-Loos Clinic, Los Angeles	1929	Medical partnership
Community Hospital Association, Elk City, Oklahoma	1929	Cooperative
Group Health Cooperative of Puget Sound (1947), Seattle (formerly Medical Securities Clinic)	1935	Cooperative (originally a medical partnership)
Group Health Association, Washington, D.C.	1937	Cooperative
Physicians Association of Clackamus County, Gladstone, Oregon	1938	Medical partnership
Kaiser Foundation Health Plan, Oakland, California and Portland, Oregon	1942	Industry
Community Health Center, Two Harbors, Minnesota	1944	Union cooperative
Labor Health Institute, St. Louis	1945	Teamsters Union
"Miners' clinics"—nine group practice plans in Pennsylvania, Ohio, and West Virginia	1946	United Mine Workers Union
Health Insurance Plan of Greater New York, New York City	1947	City, physicians, and community
Foundation for Medical Care of San Joaquin County, Stockton, California	1954	Medical society
Community Health Association of Detroit	1956	United Auto Workers Union
Group Health Plan of St. Paul, Minnesota	1957	Indemnity insurance company
Community Medical Services, Seattle†	1960	Sole proprietorship/ medical partnership
Columbia Plan, Columbia, Maryland	1969	Connecticut General Life Insurance Company, The Johns Hopkins University and Hospital, and the Rouse Company
Harvard Community Health Plan, Boston	1969	University
Kaiser Foundation Health Plan, Denver	1969	Industry, community
Greater Marshfield Community Health Plan, Marshfield, Wisconsin	1971	Physician
Geisinger Health Plan, Danville, Pennsylvania	1972	Hospital

TABLE 2 (continued)

Plan	Date of Establishment	Sponsor
New Mexico Health Care Corporation, Albuquerque	1973	Hospital
Group Health of Arizona, Tucson	1974	Carrier
U.S. Community Health Services, Canoga Park, California	1974	Physician
North Communities Health Plan, Inc., Evanston, Illinois	1975	Consumer

*The second figure is the date the prepayment plan was first offered. The Western Clinic decided to end its capitated contracts in 1976.

†Bridge Clinic, established in 1911, was purchased by Dr. John Pieroth in 1946 and then sold in 1952 to Dr. Irwin S. Neiman. In 1960, Dr. Neiman incorporated the clinic as the Community Medical Services of Seattle (CMS). In 1972, CMS was purchased by Doctors Hospital of Seattle.

the Medical Securities Clinic; in turn the 18 physicians on the staff of the clinic agreed to work with the cooperative toward development of a prepaid program. The Group Health Cooperative of Puget Sound was formed in 1947 as a truly cooperative venture. Today it is the most successful of all the prepaid group practice plans.

The Group Health Association (GHA) in Washington, D.C. also was established during the 1930s. One of the outstanding consumer cooperatives, GHA was formed by a group of federal employees of the Home Owners' Loan Corporation as a voluntary, mutual association that would provide for their members' health needs. Membership was opened to employees of the Federal Reserve Board, Farm Credit Administration, and Social Security Administration. Within the next year (1938), 10 additional federal agencies were declared eligible for health coverage in GHA.

The Kaiser Foundation Health Plan evolved during the late 1930s to meet a need for providing health services to isolated construction projects in the Southern California desert and the Grand Coulee Dam site in the state of Washington. Dr. Sidney Garfield is credited with engineering the Kaiser health idea. He felt that if he were provided with a regular source of income, he would be able to budget his expenses and, thus, to provide care to the Kaiser construction workers. But, he also knew that the workers saved none of their earnings to pay for their medical care. With the help of Mr. A. B. Ordway and an indemnity firm sponsored by Henry Kaiser, Dr. Garfield successfully negotiated a capitation rate to cover the construction workers' medical needs.

World War II

World War II created unusual pressures on the domestic fee-for-service health system. The war brought a rapid influx of shipyard workers into the San Francisco Bay and Portland, Oregon areas and into the employ of Kaiser. Again, Dr. Garfield's ideas were used to meet the health care needs of Kaiser employees. In August 1942, two separate but similar Permanente Foundations were inaugurated for the Kaiser Industry employees and their families—one in Oakland, California and the second in Portland, Oregon. With the end of the war, membership in the plans declined drastically. A decision was made to open the plans to the community, and the Kaiser-Permanente Medical Care Program was well on its way to becoming the largest private prepaid hospital and medical care program in the United States. It provides care for more than 3.5 million subscribers through six regional Kaiser Foundation Health Plans.

Two problems resurfaced with World War II, one of access to health care and the other of rising costs of medical services and hospitalization. The conclusions of the Committee on the Costs of Medical Care were as relevant in 1942 as they were in 1932; attention was directed to methods of financing and organizing medical care. Higher personal disposable income, greater health awareness, financial insecurity, and fear of catastrophic illness provided the stimulus for the growth of both private health insurance programs and prepaid group practice plans. The wage-price freeze instituted during the war also proved to be a boon for health insurance programs, including prepaid health care plans. Health insurance continued to be one of the major negotiable fringe benefits available to employers in their efforts to attract reliable high-quality employees in a tight labor market. It also was considered an important element at the bargaining table by union groups. In fact, unions were to play a large role in the development of many HMO-like organizations during the 1940s, including the Community Health Center of Two Harbors, Minnesota; the Labor Health Institute of St. Louis; the nine "Miners' Clinics" in Pennsylvania, Ohio, and West Virginia; and the Community Health Association in Detroit, Michigan (in 1956).

The Two Decades from 1950 to 1970

The 20 years between 1950 and 1970 provide evidence of continued innovative approaches to prepaid health care delivery. The role of

TABLE 3   Number of Persons with Health Insurance Protection by
Type of Coverage in the United States (in millions)

Year Ended	Hospital Expenses	Surgical Expenses	Regular Medical Expenses
1950	76,639	54,156	21,589
1955	101,400	85,681	53,038
1960	122,500	111,525	83,172
1965	138,671	130,530	109,560
1970	158,847	151,440	138,658
1973	167,147	158,624	146,342
1974	171,760	162,571	151,780

Source: Health Insurance Institute. *Source Book of Health Insurance Data 1975–76*. New York,
1976, p. 22.

labor in these efforts was great, as collectively bargained health and
welfare funds began to spread. During this period, disposable personal
income grew to all-time high levels, with a resultant growth in the
ability to pay for and use private health insurance. Tables 3 and 4
illustrate the dramatic increases in both disposable real income and

TABLE 4   Disposable Personal Income (in billions of dollars)

Year	Disposable Personal Income	
	Current	Constant (1958 dollars)
1950	206.9	249.6
1955	275.3	296.7
1960	350.0	340.2
1965	473.2	435.0
1968	591.0	499.0
1969	634.4	513.6
1970	689.5	533.2
1971	744.4	554.7
1972	802.5	578.5
1973	903.7	602.9
1974	979.7	619.4

Source: U.S. Department of Commerce. *Statistical Abstracts of the U.S.* Washington, D.C., U.S.
Government Printing Office, 1976, p. 324.

numbers of persons covered by health insurance. Health insurance was extended not only to a greater number of Americans but also to a larger cross-section of the population. New types of health plans emerged, some sponsored by the traditional cooperatives and physician partnerships, and several new organizational arrangements appeared. Indemnity insurance companies and Blue Cross/Blue Shield plans sponsored the development of HMO-like organizations. Examples include the Group Health Plan of St. Paul and the Columbia Plan, Columbia, Maryland. The latter, at its inception, was considered to be a *consortium plan,* in that a triumverate sponsorship—the Connecticut General Life Insurance Company, The Johns Hopkins University and The Johns Hopkins University Hospital, and the Rouse Company (builders and developers of Columbia)—were joint sponsors. Universities, Blue Cross associations, private companies, and cities all have been involved in developing innovative HMO approaches.

During 1954, the medical society in San Joaquin County, California established the first medical foundation. Now recognized by the HMO law as a valid HMO model, the Foundation for Medical Care of San Joaquin County has been used as a model for many other foundation HMOs and individual practice associations (IPAs).

The HMO movement grew at an accelerated rate during this 20-year period. The number of operational HMOs with open-community enrollment increased from approximately 20 in 1950 to approximately 33 in 1970 and to 166 in 1975. Some HMO organizations, however, either were dissolved or discontinued during this period. The Community Hospital Association of Elk City and at least four other physician-sponsored group practice plans were some of the casualties.[14]

Federal Government Interest

Costs of health care increased dramatically between 1950 and 1970. In 1950, the average hospital cost per patient day was $15.62, and the total cost of an average hospital stay was $126.52. By 1960, these costs had increased to $32.33 and $244.95, respectively. In 1970, these figures had escalated to $81.01 and $668.67, respectively. For 1974, total expenses per patient day were $127.81, and expenses per admission were a staggering $992.42. Similarly, in 1950, individuals spent 4.6 percent of their disposable personal incomes for health care, including health insurance. By 1975, this percentage had increased to 8.3 percent. The

[14]Jerome L. Schwartz. *Medical Plans and Health Care.* Springfield, Ill., Charles C Thomas, Publisher, 1968, p. 23.

Consumer Price Index also shows that, over the years, medical costs increased more rapidly than any major category of personal expenses. Since 1962, medical costs have risen 59 percent.

Both private groups and public agencies began to look for mechanisms that would reduce and contain costs. Some of the new federal programs initiated include the Regional Medical Programs, Community Health Centers, and Comprehensive Health Planning programs. Several national studies suggested possible solutions to the cost-of-care crisis. In particular, the 1967 *Report to the President*[15] recommended, among other things, that "group practice, especially prepaid group practice, should be encouraged." The gestation period for the federal program was relatively short: by March 9, 1970, a position paper was completed by Paul M. Ellwood, Jr. and his associates at the American Rehabilitation Foundation, wherein he coined the phrase "Health Maintenance Organization."[16] As described in the paper, the HMO concept was to become a major portion of the Nixon Administration's health program.

The first announcement by the administration of its HMO program was by John C. Veneman, Under Secretary of the Department of Health, Education, and Welfare (DHEW), before an executive session of the House Ways and Means Committee on March 23, 1970. At that time, the administration's proposal was a method of containing the escalating cost of Medicare and Medicaid programs only. In a March 25, 1970 press release, DHEW Secretary Robert H. Finch introduced Alternative C, as the proposal was called. Legislation would be introduced that would authorize the Social Security Administration to enter into contracts with HMOs guaranteeing comprehensive health service for the elderly at a fixed annual rate. The HMO idea was again emphasized when President Nixon, during his February 1971 health message, stated that the HMOs would play a key role in his national health strategy. This strategy was fully outlined in a White Paper issued by the Department of Health, Education, and Welfare in May 1971.[17] The administration's bill, designed to help establish HMOs, was introduced in March 1971.

[15]U.S. Department of Health, Education, and Welfare. *A Report to the President on Medical Care Prices*. Washington, D.C., U.S. Government Printing Office, 1967, pp. 4–5.

[16]Paul M. Ellwood, Jr. "The Health Maintenance Strategy." Minneapolis, Minn., InterStudy, 1970. Mimeographed.

[17]U.S. Department of Health, Education, and Welfare. *Towards a Comprehensive Health Policy for the 1970's: A White Paper*. Washington, D.C., U.S. Government Printing Office, 1971, pp. 31–37.

Summary

The HMO philosophy has evolved over the past 70 years. It grew out of a need to obtain adequate health care, usually where the traditional fee-for-service system could not cope with the demand. Although several plans began prior to 1929, the major growth of HMO organizations came after that date. Pre-1929 plans usually were developed around a group practice of physicians for particular groups of employees and were initiated by the employees themselves or by their employers. These group practices generally were formed as partnerships; early medical group practices include the Mayo Clinic, the Palo Alto and Ross-Loos Medical clinics, the Bridge clinics, and the Western Clinic.

The Great Depression of 1929 was instrumental in changing the social structure of American life, including the financing and delivery of health care. Health insurance was introduced by the American Hospital Association in the form of Blue Cross plans to finance hospital care and thus to stabilize the critical financial plight of hospitals. Individual Americans were faced with serious financial problems and lack of access to acceptable medical care. Using the English and European cooperative society concept as their model, Americans joined together in a common effort; with strength and stability in numbers, health cooperatives began to appear. The first American cooperatives were the rural health cooperatives, such as the Elk City, Oklahoma Community Hospital Association established by Dr. Michael Shadid.

The early cooperative philosophy stressed stability and security in group action—*assurance* of health care services rather than *insurance* against loss due to illness or accident. It was not until competitive pressures were felt from Blue Cross and Blue Shield and the private insurance companies that the prepaid health plans began to identify one of their objectives as an insurance function. The early cooperative experiments regarded the function of pooling individual resources for the good of the group as a method for controlling the cost of medical care and a way of including economics in health delivery. Over time, individual members would save money—their limited financial resources would go farther. The cooperatives were described as a socialized approach—not in the political sense of a federal social program but in terms of a group action approach of "self-help."

The passage of the Wagner Act hastened the expansion of labor unions and the resultant bargaining for health benefits by union employees. For the first time, many employers were forced to participate in financing health care for their employees and in developing new health care plans. Union- and employer-sponsored prepaid health plans appeared throughout the country. This interest in negotiable health benefits was heightened during World War II, when such benefits were used as a method of attracting employees from a limited civilian labor force. Employer and union awareness of prepaid health plans has influenced sound management principles in the provision of quality care to employees and the delivery of health care by prepaid plans.

Quality care has been a major objective of the prepaid plans. The early plans also sought stability—a comprehensive rather than a piecework, fee-for-service approach to health care. The prepaid plans' objectives of quality and comprehensive care required that both consumers and providers hold joint and parallel objectives. This compromise approach between a totally federal socialized system and a totally fee-for-service solo practice system further required that the health system have controls to safeguard the interests of both vendor and patient. The cooperative members needed total financial disclosure and quality care in exchange for prospective monthly payments. The physicians needed an environment where they could practice their profession without the financial constraints of a fee-for-service system and could demand a salary or retainer comparable to yearly fee-for-service income. The physicians also were interested in using joint action with the objective of providing quality care—the thesis being that medical care is not only a long-term joint venture among providers but also between the providers and the health plan members. Ultimately, the interests of the medical group became the interests of their community.

Comprehensive care was described as total care early in prepaid health plan development. It was to include prevention, care, education, supervision of health delivery, rehabilitation, and guidance in health maintenance. The physician's role was that of manager of the plan members' health needs. Increasingly, the early plans found it difficult to provide all the services and still continue to compete with Blue Cross/Blue Shield and private insurance carriers. By the 1960s, most plans had standard benefit packages similar to those offered by Blue Cross/Blue Shield plans.

The history of HMOs is filled with the names and activities of notable men and plans. Drs. Shadid, Bridge, Ross, Loos, Lee, Yocum, Curran, and Garfield all contributed their efforts to the prepaid experiments. Plans such as Group Health Cooperative of Puget Sound, Western Clinic, Kaiser Foundation Health Plan, Group Health Association, Ross-Loos, and the Community Hospital Association of Elk City all colored the HMO philosophy. By 1967, HMO activities were recognized by health care experts as a possible method for controlling the rapid increase in the cost and utilization of medical care. The Federal Government acknowledged the potential usefulness of prepaid health plans in their fight against rising health costs in *A Report to the President on Medical Care Prices* in 1967. By 1970, the Nixon Administration had adopted the prepaid health care concept—the Health Maintenance Organization—as a key part of its health strategy. In March 1971, the administration's first HMO bill was introduced in Congress.

References

Casselman, P. H. *The Cooperative Movement and Some of Its Problems.* New York, The Philosophical Library, 1952.

Chase, Stuart. *The Story of Toad Lane.* Chicago, The Cooperative League of the U.S.A., 1969.

Committee on the Costs of Medical Care. *Medical Care for the American People.* Chicago, University of Chicago Press, 1933. Reprint. Washington, D.C., Community Health Service, Health Services and Mental Health Administration, U.S. Department of Health, Education, and Welfare, 1970, pp. v–xii, 103–144.

Ford, James. *Co-operation in New England.* New York, Survey Associates, Inc., 1913.

Gintzig, Leon, and Shouldice, Robert G. "Prepaid Group Practice—A Comparative Study." Part I. 3 Vols. Washington, D.C., The George Washington University, 1971. Mimeographed.

MacColl, William A. *Group Practice and Prepayment of Medical Care.* Washington, D.C., Public Affairs Press, 1966, pp. 10–56.

McCaffree, Kenneth M. "How Organized Medical Programs Have Been Established: The Urban Cooperative Plan." *Proceedings of the 9th Group Health Institute.* Chicago, Group Health Association of America, 1969, pp. 31–34.

Rorem, C. Rufus. *Private Group Clinics.* New York, Milbank Memorial Fund, 1971, pp. 115–118. (Reprint)

Schwartz, Jerome L. *Medical Plans and Health Care.* Springfield, Ill., Charles C Thomas, Publisher, 1968.

University of Chicago, Graduate Program in Hospital Administration, Center for Health Administration Studies, Graduate School of Business. *Health Maintenance Organization: A Reconfiguration of the Health Services System. Proceedings of the Thirteenth Annual Symposium on Hospital Affairs.* Chicago, 1971, pp. 2–10.

U.S. Department of Health, Education, and Welfare. *A Report to the President on Medical Care Prices.* Washington, D.C., U.S. Government Printing Office, 1967.

3

Legislative Activity

The history of the HMO movement from the early 1900s to 1970 is continued in this chapter with a review of legislative activity and the efforts of Congress and the Nixon Administration to pass and implement a federal law designed to foster HMO development. The legislative proposals introduced from 1970 through 1974 are reviewed first, then the present law (P.L. 93-222), its amendments (P.L. 94-460), and its regulations are discussed.

Three Major Problems

In Chapter 2, the major objectives of HMOs were described—to provide access to care, to stabilize the financing and cost of care for both the consumer and the provider, and to assure a high level of health care. The Federal Government has taken an active legislative role in HMOs because of the problems involved in meeting these three objectives. First, government has recognized that there is widespread *maldistribution of health resources* in specific geographic areas throughout the country and among selected socioeconomic groups of citizens. Included in this resource category are the providers of care—physicians, paramedical personnel, hospitals, and other health care institutions. The Federal Government initiated steps to facilitate distribution of health resources as early as 1946, when the Hill-Burton program (P.L. 79-725, Hospital Survey and Construction Act) was used to expand rural hospitals. Although the program generated many small rural hospitals, it did little to influence coordination among hospitals and other health facilities or to increase the economic stability of such facilities. More recently, the federal role in coordinating health facilities development was expanded by the passage of P.L. 89-749 (the Comprehensive Health Planning and Public Health Service Amendments Act of 1966) and P.L. 93-641 (the National Health Planning and Resources Development Act of 1974). The latter establishes Health Systems Agencies that are responsible for national planning and development in health service areas designated by state governors. In addition to developing the planning structures at the regional, state, and local levels, the Federal Government is the major voice in the process of allocating monies to be invested in medical education, including medical schools and training of paramedical personnel; it has played a major role in strengthening the health planning and resource allocation process and in making health care more accessible.

The second problem addressed by the Federal Government is the *escalation in the cost of health care,* which has increased from 4.6 percent of the gross national product in 1950 to approximately 7 percent in 1970. This represents an average increase of 7.3 percent per year as compared to an average increase in salaries and wages of only 4.3 percent per year. The cost to the Federal Government of Medicare and Medicaid also has increased sharply; payments to or on behalf of Part A and B enrollees totaled $3.2 billion during the first full year of operation (1967). In comparison, during fiscal year 1972, total benefits rose to $8.4 billion. By 1974, total payments were $12.4 billion.[1] These higher payments have resulted from increasing demands for services because of population growth, rising incomes, technological advances, prevailing insurance coverage, and pressure by the public that quality medical care be available to all Americans. In addition, the costs to the providers of care also have accelerated—wages are rising in a tight labor market and prices are higher for goods and services.

Economists advise that two methods are available for moderating or controlling increases in medical care costs: reduce the demand for, or increase the supply of, care (i.e., medical facilities and manpower); and increase productivity of the present resources. The Federal Government has suggested both methods and has been active in their implementation. Recently, the Department of Health, Education, and Welfare suggested that the benefit packages of both Medicare and

[1]U.S. Department of Health, Education, and Welfare. *Medicare Fiscal Years 1968–1972, Selected State Data.* Rockville, Md., Office of Research and Statistics, Social Security Administration, 1974, p. v; and Health Insurance Institute. *Source Book of Health Insurance Data 1975–76.* New York, 1976, p. 15.

Medicaid be limited and that the supplementary payments required of recipients be extended—a method of reducing demand for services. On the supply side, the Federal Government has actively supported the training of medical personnel through project grants, traineeships, and support of medical schools, in addition to other programs. Increasing productivity has been a more difficult task; federal funds have been made available for research directed toward improving internal operations of hospitals, for identifying cost-reducing methods of reorganizing the delivery system, for reviewing Medicare and Medicaid reimbursement formulas, for identifying incentives to contain costs, and for increasing the use of prepaid group and individual practice plans.

The third problem—*controlling the quality of care*—has been by far the most difficult to solve. There are no national standards for measuring quality; but even when broadly defined, quality of care varies among geographic areas of the country and among socioeconomic groups. Federal efforts to assure high quality of care are evidenced through the passage of P.L. 92-603, which mandates the development of Professional Standards Review Organizations, and P.L. 93-222, the Health Maintenance Organization Act. Both laws attempt to control the quality of care through the use of peer review, both formally and informally.

The Potential HMO Solution

The HMO strategy was developed as part of the Nixon Administration's program to provide federal solutions to the aforementioned three problems. Paul M. Ellwood, Jr., M.D. and his associates at the Health Services Research Center, Institute for Interdisciplinary Studies, American Rehabilitation Foundation are credited with the development of the HMO strategy.[2] In his Spring 1970 position paper, "The Health Maintenance Strategy," Dr. Ellwood states that

. . . the health maintenance strategy envisions a series of government and private actions designed to promote a highly diversified, pluralistic and competitive health industry in which:

—Many different types of Health Maintenance Organizations would provide comprehensive services needed to keep people healthy, offering consumers—both public and private—a choice between such service and traditional forms of care.

[2]Paul M. Ellwood, Jr. is the executive director of the Institute for Interdisciplinary Studies, now known as InterStudy (123 East Grant Street, Minneapolis, Minnesota 55403).

—Services would be purchased annually from such organizations through Health Maintenance Contracts (capitation), at rates agreed upon before illness has occurred, with the provider sharing the economic risk of ill health.[3]

Dr. Ellwood and his associates set forth the following steps that should be taken by the Federal Government over a 5- to 10-year period to implement the strategy:

1. Adopt the health maintenance strategy and require both private enterprise and public agencies to join the health industry in implementing the national objective of health maintenance.

2. Provide incentives for creation of health maintenance organizations.

3. Foster the elimination of any legal barriers that may block creation of such organizations.

4. Begin purchasing services under Medicare, Medicaid, and other federal reimbursement programs by health maintenance contracts rather than by present methods of paying for individual medical services.

5. Build into these contracts a sufficient return to support necessary investments in manpower, facilities, and health services research by the contracting health maintenance organizations.

6. Review the Federal Government's activities in the health field to determine how they currently contribute to, or frustrate, the health maintenance strategy and initiate necessary modifications to support it.[4]

Since 1970, at least the first four of these steps have been instituted. More importantly, it appears likely that all of Dr. Ellwood's proposed steps will be accomplished in the next few years.

The Administration's HMO Disclosures

Drawing upon the HMO strategy proposed by Dr. Ellwood, the Department of Health, Education, and Welfare developed its own health strategy, which included the HMO concept. In February 1970, Robert H. Finch, Secretary of DHEW, announced that it was the Nixon Admin-

---

[3]Paul M. Ellwood, Jr. "The Health Maintenance Strategy." Minneapolis, Minn., InterStudy, 1970, pp. 1–2. Mimeographed.
[4]*Ibid.*, p. 2.

istration's intention to reshape the health-delivery system. Initially, the administration was concerned with whether the beneficiaries of Medicare and Medicaid would receive care through HMO arrangements— ostensibly, it was believed that federal funds would be saved by using HMOs as the providers of care for these two groups. Toward this end, John G. Veneman, Under Secretary of DHEW, testified before an executive session of the House Ways and Means Committee on March 23, 1970, during which the administration's Health Cost Effectiveness bill was presented. The bill became known as Alternative C, and was designed to permit the HMO option to be inserted in the Medicare legislation. Alternative C was to "bring together all the resources of the Medicare patient needs."[5]

In a March 25, 1970 press release, Secretary Finch publicly introduced Alternative C. He noted that the legislation to be introduced in Congress ". . . would authorize the Social Security Administration to enter into contracts with HMOs guaranteeing comprehensive health service for the elderly [and poor] at a fixed annual rate."[6] Parts A (Hospitalization) and B (Physicians' Services) of the law would continue to be available to those eligible for Medicare, with Alternative C—the HMO option—provided as an additional enrollment method. State Medicaid programs also would be permitted to contract with HMOs for services for Medicaid recipients.[7]

The administration's goal in developing Alternative C is stated by Faith Rafkind:

Finch's March 1970 statement focused on use of the Federal Government's contracting authority as a means of improving the purchasing power of Medicare and Medicaid expenditures, and use of such purchasing power to stimulate new financial and organizational realignments of the existent health delivery "system." This initial HMO strategy marked a retreat of the federal programs, as a means of influencing (not mandating) cost consciousness and efficiency of

---

[5]Faith B. Rafkind. *Health Maintenance Organizations: Some Perspectives.* Chicago, Blue Cross Association, 1972, p. 3.

[6]U.S. Department of Health, Education, and Welfare, Office of the Secretary. *HEW News.* Press release. Washington, D.C., March 25, 1970, p. 1.

[7]It is interesting to note that the Social Security Administration has been dealing *directly* with HMO-like organizations since the passage of the Medicare law. The Social Security Administration, for instance, has been "direct dealing" on a capitation basis at Group Health Cooperative of Puget Sound and Community Medical Services of Seattle since 1968. Payment for Part A services is made on a reasonable-cost basis and on a monthly per capita payment for each Part B beneficiary—subject to retroactive adjustments. For a discussion of this subject, see: Jerome L. Schwartz. *Medical Plans and Health Care.* Springfield, Ill., Charles C Thomas, Publisher, 1968, pp. 308–327.

the delivery system. Financial incentives, rather than organizational restructuring, were emphasized as the means by which efficiency, diversity of system and quality of care could be achieved. At the same time, Finch remarked, "the essential point is that the federal government begin to deal with the health industry as a cohesive whole. We will not prescribe the form of health maintenance organization, but we will be concerned that those selling care to the federal government produce a 'quality product.' "

Shortly after the Finch statement was made, it was amplified in a memorandum from Veneman which was disseminated through the Department as an "expression of Departmental policy with respect to . . . purchase of health services." In this document, Veneman presented a series of general concepts that were implicit in the Department's promotion of HMO—one of those being that the term HMO "has a broader meaning than what has been termed prepaid group practice." In this context, he stated that services are to be delivered by a "variety of organizations which meet minimum specifications with respect to organizational characteristics and arrangements. . . . The Department's policy explicitly seeks to avoid interfacing with the internal arrangements of health maintenance organizations such as the form of compensation of physicians or the degree of centralization of personnel and facilities."[8]

Initially, the HMO was proposed as a way to contain the costs of Medicare and Medicaid programs. Upon further review by DHEW of the cost-saving potential, and in recognition of increasing interest in and acceptance of the concept, HMOs assumed a central position in President Nixon's Health Message to Congress, presented on February 18, 1971. The message described the HMO as a *proven* system upon which a national health strategy was to be built. Citizens covered by a national health insurance plan to be developed would be offered the HMO option. "This represented the first major public disclosure of the federal commitment to the establishment of HMOs for *all* segments of the population."[9]

Federal HMO strategy planning continued through 1971, with the development of the HMO Task Force. In May 1971, an HMO office was established in DHEW's Office of the Administrator, Health Services and Mental Health Administration. The Health Maintenance Organization Service (HMOS) (now the Division of Health Maintenance Organizations), established on October 19, 1971, continued the major HMO functions on the federal level, including technical assistance to developing HMOs, backup support for HMO legislation, award and management of planning and development grants, assistance in the development of Title XIX contracts, and evaluation of grants. HMOS operated

[8]Rafkind. *Health Maintenance Organizations*, pp. 4–5.
[9]*Ibid.*, p. 7.

on reprogrammed funds from October 1971 until the passage of the HMO law in December 1973.[10] DHEW support for HMO grants and contracts for fiscal years 1971, 1972, and 1973 totaled nearly $26 million—$16.9 million for direct support of 155 HMO projects.[11] Funds appropriated for fiscal years 1974 and 1975, through June 30, 1976, totaled $97.8 million, of which $61.8 million was obligated for support of 202 organizations.[12]

The administration's support of the HMO concept was reaffirmed in President Nixon's health message in March 1972. It is now obvious that the administration's strategy, which emerged from the 1971 and 1972 health messages and the activities of HMOS/DHEW, was constructed around a program of financing and technical assistance in the planning, development, and expansion of existing HMOs and the planning and development of new HMOs. But, the strategy did *not* include subsidies to cover operating deficits. This was true even though, ultimately, the underwriting of initial operating deficits was to be a part of the strategy—especially for HMOs operating in medically underserved areas. A second aspect of the strategy called for the Federal Government to pay all or part of the premium for specific beneficiary groups, such as Native Americans, Medicare recipients, and the poor. The administration also favored action that would override restrictive state laws that precluded the development of HMOs. Finally, the Federal Government was to develop guidelines to assist in a rigorous review of HMO operations to ensure that the quality of care met professional standards.

The administration established the ambitious goals of developing 450 HMOs by the end of fiscal year 1973 and 1,700 by the end of fiscal year 1976, with an enrollment capacity of 40 million. The ultimate goal was to make the HMO option available to 90 percent of the population by 1980.[13]

[10]There are basically three authorities under which HMOs operated. These include Section 304 of the Public Health Service Act, authorizing grant and contract experimentation with alternative health service delivery forms; Section 314(e) of the Comprehensive Health Planning and Services Act, authorizing health service project grants; and Section 9101(c) of the Regional Medical Programs law.

[11]U.S. Department of Health, Education, and Welfare, Health Services Administration. *Health Maintenance Organization Service: Program Status as of December 1972.* Rockville, Md., 1973, pp. 9, 44.

[12]U.S. Department of Health, Education, and Welfare, Health Services Administration, Division of Health Maintenance Organizations. *Health Maintenance Organizations, 2nd Annual Report to Congress.* (Summary) Rockville, Md., 1976.

[13]U.S. Department of Health, Education, and Welfare. *Towards a Comprehensive Health Policy for the 1970's: A White Paper.* Washington, D.C., U.S. Government Printing Office, 1971, pp. 36–37.

Within this strategy, priority considerations were given to the development of HMOs in underserved areas; however, care was taken to avoid the implication that this was to be a demonstration on a particular segment of society. HMOs were not to be forced on anyone. Rather, they were viewed as an innovation in health care delivery that should be made available to everyone on a free-choice basis.

Prior to 1973, the Nixon administration actively supported legislation that would achieve the goals previously mentioned. A bill prepared by the administration was introduced in March 1971 by Senator Javits (S. 1182) and Congressman Staggers (H.R. 5615) and was joined by other major bills submitted by Senator Kennedy (S. 3327) and Congressman Roy (H.R. 11728). Although all of the bills had the same general goal of stimulating the development of HMOs, they differed considerably in approach, in mechanisms for financing, in types of organizations that could qualify, and in other specific details.

By the beginning of 1973, after numerous HMO bills had been introduced but no law passed, the position of the administration changed substantially from that of the previous two years; the organized medicine lobby, among others, was successful in swaying the administration away from its strong HMO posture of 1971 and 1972. A time-limited demonstration approach was selected as the 1973 HMO strategy. There was, as Casper W. Weinberger, Secretary of the U.S. Department of Health, Education, and Welfare, suggested, no long-term commitment to a federal subsidy for HMO activities. As of March 1973, based on a statement by Frank C. Carlucci, Under Secretary of DHEW, HMOs had been chosen for federal *demonstration* investment because they had proven effective in certain parts of the country; they might improve the effectiveness and efficiency of health services and also might contain, if not reduce, the expenditures that government units as well as individuals and employers must pay for health care; they might encourage and attract the participation of the Federal Government; and they have potential for introducing more competition into the health care field. The administration's bill, however, assumed a *time-limited demonstration approach to HMO assistance.*[14] The overoptimistic goal of making the HMO option available to 90 percent of the population by 1980 was no longer a part of the strategy.

---

[14]"Statement of Frank C. Carlucci Before the Subcommittee on Public Health and Environment, Committee on Interstate and Foreign Commerce. March 6, 1973," pp. 3–4. Mimeographed.

The HMO Enabling and Assistance Laws

Extensive testimony, long debate, and two congressional adjourn-
ments helped to substantially modify the many HMO bills introduced in
Congress (see Table 5). Together with some existing laws, there are
five major laws that enable enrollment in and/or that assist with the
planning, development, and operation of HMOs:

> P.L. 84-569 and P.L. 89-614, Civilian Health and Medical Program of
> the Uniformed Services
> P.L. 86-382, Federal Employees Health Benefits Act of 1959
> P.L. 92-603, Social Security Amendments of 1972
> P.L. 93-82, Veterans Administration
> P.L. 93-222, Health Maintenance Organization Act of 1973, as
> amended by P.L. 94-460, Health Maintenance Organization
> Amendments of 1976

TABLE 5   Major HMO Bills Introduced in Congress Between 1970 and
1973

House		Senate	
	1970		
H.R. 17550	(Mr. Mills)		
	1971		
H.R. 1	(Mr. Mills) 1/22/71	S. 3	(Senator Kennedy) 1/25/71
H.R. 22	(Mrs. Griffiths) 1/22/71	S. 1182	(Senator Javits) 3/10/71
H.R. 5615	(Mr. Staggers) 3/4/71	S. 1354	(Senator Pearson) 3/24/71
H.R. 5766	(Mr. Nelsen) 3/9/71	S. 1623	(Senator Bennett) 4/22/71
H.R. 7764	(Mr. Ford) 4/27/71		
H.R. 7741	(Mr. Byrnes) 4/27/71		
H.R. 9123	(Mr. Frenzel) 6/15/71		
H.R. 11728	(Mr. Roy) 11/11/71		
H.R. 11981	(Mr. Hastings) 12/1/71		
H.R. 12372	(Mr. Ralesback) 12/16/71		
	1972		
H.R. 12936	(Mr. Robinson) 2/3/72	S. 3327	(Senator Kennedy) 3/13/72
H.R. 16782	(Mr. Roy) 9/21/72		
	1973		
H.R. 51	(Mr. Roy) 1/3/73	S. 14	(Senator Kennedy) 1/4/73
H.R. 4871	(Mr. Staggers) 2/27/73	S. 972	(Senator Javits) 2/22/73
H.R. 7627	(Mr. Conyers) 5/9/73		
H.R. 7974	(Mr. Roy) 5/21/73		
H.R. 9975	(Mr. Murphy) 8/3/73		
H.R. 9991	(Mr. Van Deerlin) 8/3/73		

*P.L. 84-569 AND P.L. 89-614—CIVILIAN HEALTH AND MEDICAL
PROGRAM OF THE UNIFORMED SERVICES (CHAMPUS)*

In 1956, legislation was enacted (P.L. 84-569) that authorized the establishment of a civilian health care program for the spouses and children
of active-duty members of the uniformed services. P.L. 84-569 was
intended to equalize health benefits between the dependents of military
personnel who had access to medical care provided by military
facilities and the estimated 40 percent who did not have such access.
The original program was limited essentially to inpatient hospital care.
In 1966, new legislation was enacted (P.L. 89-614), which added outpatient benefits and extended the program to include retired members and
their dependents; the survivors of deceased, retired, and active-duty
members; and other programs.[15]

Approximately six million persons are now covered by the program,
which is more commonly known by its acronym, CHAMPUS. Nearly
one-third are retired persons and their dependents, whose eligibility for
care in military facilities is on a space-available basis. Even in the face
of a reduced active-duty force, the retired military segment, including
dependents, is expected to reach 4.4 million by 1980. In consideration
of the difficulties expected in staffing military facilities in the absence
of compulsory military service, it is reasonable to assume that a
number of these beneficiaries will be transferred to the already strained
civilian medical market. In fact, a large portion of care authorized to all
military beneficiaries is presently obtained in the civilian sector under
the CHAMPUS program. It seems logical to expect that the Department
of Defense and the Committee on Armed Services will explore innovative and cost-containment delivery systems in light of such large expenditures to a relatively mobile beneficiary population.

The CHAMPUS law limits the operation of the program to traditional
health insurance concepts and methods, particularly from the standpoint of including and excluding benefits and cost-sharing arrangements. Under legislation introduced in the House of Representatives in
1972 and reintroduced in the 93rd Congress, the CHAMPUS law would
be amended to allow the Secretary of Defense, after consulting with the
Secretary of Health, Education, and Welfare, to use HMOs for providing benefits under CHAMPUS. This authority, described as H.R. 107 in
the 94th Congress to amend Title 10 of the *Code of Federal Regulations,* would allow the Secretary of Defense to contract with HMOs

---

[15]U.S. Congress, House of Representatives. *Authorizing the Use of Health Maintenance Organizations as an Alternative to the CHAMPUS Program.* 93rd Congress, 1st
session. October 11, 1973, pp. 1–2. Report No. 93-573.

without having to follow the cost-sharing arrangements presently prescribed and without regard for the present law's prohibition of certain types of care, such as immunizations and well-baby care.[16] The bill received strong support from the Department of Defense and passed the House of Representatives on October 23, 1973. Prospects for further legislative action are uncertain; however, in all probability, arrangements for HMO/CHAMPUS will be developed prior to the termination of the current HMO legislation, P.L. 93-222, at the end of fiscal year 1979.

P.L. 86-382—FEDERAL EMPLOYEES HEALTH BENEFITS ACT OF 1959

Federal employees and annuitants have had the option of electing a comprehensive medical plan to cover their health benefits since enactment of P.L. 86-382, the Federal Employees Health Benefits Act of 1959, which became effective after July 1, 1960. Under this act, the Federal Employees Plan (FEP) beneficiaries can choose between a health service benefits plan (Blue Cross/Blue Shield), several indemnity benefit plans (historically, Aetna was the major plan), one of several employee organization plans, or a comprehensive medical plan consisting of either group or individual practice prepayment plans. Generally, an employee must live within the service area of a comprehensive medical plan to be eligible for that option.

The federal employees health benefits program offers inpatient, ambulatory, and supplemental benefits in a high- and low-option format. Only three of the comprehensive plans offer both the high and low options, but their range of benefits and premium structures are competitive with the other options. The government pays 60 percent of the total premium cost, and the beneficiary is responsible for the remainder.

There are approximately 9.5 million federal employees, annuitants, and dependents. As of March 31, 1973, 53,000 federal employees were enrolled in prepaid individual practice plans; 156,000 were enrolled in prepaid group practice plans. Also, because the employee or annuitant in most cases must reside within the target service area of the plan, the comprehensive medical plan option is not available to all beneficiaries.

---

[16]Ibid., p. 2. Known as the Bennett Bill, H.R. 1681, these ideas were introduced before Congress in 1974; the bill would provide free inpatient care for retirees and dependents and allow for a flat 20 percent charge for outpatient medical costs. It would also extend the CHAMPUS coverage to retirees' spouses 65 years of age or older. Mr. Bennett reintroduced the bill, H.R. 748, in the 95th Congress, and it was referred to the Armed Services Committee, Subcommittee on Military Compensation.

Approximately 60 percent of the federal beneficiaries under this program are enrolled in the national "Blues" option, some 20 percent in the indemnity plans, and the remaining 20 percent are divided among the employee-sponsored plans and the comprehensive medical plans.

The program is administered by the Civil Service Commission, which has the authority to contract for and approve the various health plans. As of August 1973, 19 group and 7 individual practice prepayment plans had been approved for participation, including 2 that were added during 1973. By December 1975, 55 health plans, 41 of which were HMOs, were participating with FEP.

Regulations governing the program as it relates to HMOs are found in Part 890 of the *Federal Personnel Manual,* Supplement 890-1. In general, they detail the type of benefits to be provided, enrollment mechanisms, limitations on copayments, minimum standards of financing, and other management aspects. All plans are subject to audit by the Civil Service Commission and the General Accounting Office. According to officials in the Civil Service Commission, there is no foreseeable limit on the number of HMOs that could be awarded contracts under this program so long as there is a level of interest among the beneficiary population and the applicant organization is in compliance with the laws and regulations specified in the *Federal Personnel Manual.*

P.L. 92-603—SOCIAL SECURITY AMENDMENTS OF 1972

Medicare (Title XVIII): Medicare beneficiaries have been eligible to receive certain services from HMO organizations since the original act was passed in 1965. Under Section 1833(a) of the law, a prepayment organization that provides or arranges for the provision of medical and other health services could elect to be reimbursed on a reasonable-charge (fee-for-service) basis or it could deal directly with the Social Security Administration on a capitation basis (i.e., "direct dealing"). It is important to note that this authority was extended only to Part B, Physicians' Services. The original law did not make provision for a capitation payment to cover both physicians' services and hospitalization.

The Social Security Administration established general guidelines for the type of plans it would approve under this program, encouraging the larger, well-established plans with a broad range of benefits to seek this mechanism. A liberal interpretation of prepaid group practice, however, was made to allow great flexibility in payment. In 1973, the Social Security Administration was dealing directly with 34 plans, covering some 300,000 Medicare enrollees. Expenditures under this authority are $37 million annually. As of December 1975, there were 390,000 Medicare beneficiaries enrolled in 39 HMO plans, with approximately $90 million paid for services on their behalf by the Social Security Administration in 1975.

A number of HMO-like organizations provide services to Title XVIII beneficiaries on a fee-for-service basis. These organizations obtain reimbursement through fiscal intermediaries of the Medicare program, and no data are available to indicate the level of HMO involvement.

Several important changes in the administration of Medicare were proposed in Alternative C to Medicare. A bill, H.R. 17550, which incorporated the administration's recommendations concerning Alternative C, was passed by the House, and a similar bill was passed by the Senate. Before a Joint Conference Committee could be designated, however, the 91st Congress adjourned. When the 92nd Congress convened, H.R. 17550 was reintroduced into the House by Representative Wilbur Mills as H.R. 1. On October 30, 1972, the final version of H.R. 1 became P.L. 92-603, when President Nixon signed the measure. Section 226 of the law provides the authority to contract with HMOs for covered services. Under this section, monthly capitation payments are possible for services covered by Parts A and B. Mature HMOs, as defined in the law, are eligible to apply for an incentive reimbursement formula. Developing HMOs (and those in the previous category that do not apply for the risk mechanism) may contract for a combined capitation payment on a cost basis. The law provides a lock-in feature for those who enroll in the incentive plans. Regulations concerning reimbursement and contract appeals procedures under the 1972 amendments for Medicare were published in July and November 1975. Organizations that would like to enroll Medicare recipients can file a plan with the Social Security Administration's Bureau of Health Insurance Regional Offices. Plans will be reviewed to determine the organization's ability to effectively and efficiently provide quality medical care. The HMO, if qualified, will be requested to enter into a Title XVIII contract with the Social Security Administration.

Medicaid (Title XIX): Medicaid is a federal/state public assistance program which has been implemented in all states, territories, and possessions except Arizona. The program is administered at the state and local levels within very broad guidelines established by DHEW's Social and Rehabilitation Service. Section 206(e) of P.L. 92-603 authorizes federal technical and actuarial assistance to the states upon request, to assist them in negotiating and implementing contracts with HMOs to provide an alternative resource for health care services to

Medicaid eligibles. Because states are not restricted from entering into these arrangements, they are free to negotiate Medicaid/HMO contracts as they desire. As of July 1976, only 18 states had capitated contracts with HMOs. There are approximately 65 separate capitated contracts which cover the cost of care for 3 percent of all Medicaid recipients. California has the largest number of contracts (approximately 48) and the largest number enrolled in the program (795,984).

In May 1975, DHEW's Social and Rehabilitation Service did publish final regulations regarding the Social Security Amendments of 1972, which set forth requirements for states wishing to contract for prepaid health services under Title XIX. Since 1973, only two additional states and the District of Columbia have entered into prepaid Title XIX contracts with HMOs to provide Medicaid benefits. Reasons for this lack of participation vary from unfamiliarity on the part of officials responsible for executing the contracts to limited state budgets, indifference, and lack of provider groups considered acceptable by the Title XIX state agency.[17]

There has been a concerted federal effort to encourage states to enter into agreements with HMOs on a prepaid, capitation basis. In support of this effort, a national conference for developing Title XIX HMO contracts was held in September 1973. Sponsored jointly by DHEW's Health Maintenance Organization Service (HMOS) and the Medical Services Administration, Social and Rehabilitation Service, the conference was held for state representatives who are involved in negotiating state Medicaid contracts with HMOs.

P.L. 93-82—VETERANS ADMINISTRATION

More than 29 million veterans are now eligible for health care in varying degrees. The Veterans Administration is responsible for providing or arranging complete care for veterans with service-connected disabilities; others are seen on a space-available basis, subject to certain conditions. Some 225,000 veterans are authorized to receive care from civilian sources, on an outpatient basis, for specific disabilities.

P.L. 93-82, enacted on August 2, 1973, extends eligibility for the first time to dependents and survivors of veterans with 100 percent service-connected disabilities. The mechanism for furnishing health care to this group, estimated to be 275,000 persons, has not yet been established. One possibility under consideration is to "buy into" the

---

[17]U.S. Department of Health, Education, and Welfare, Health Services Administration and Medical Services Administration. *Proceedings of the National Conference for Developing Title XIX-HMO Contracts.* Rockville, Md., 1974, p. A1.

CHAMPUS program for reimbursement and administrative purposes. Although the HMO vehicle would probably be of limited value to veterans with very specific conditions, it might be an appropriate delivery system for the dependents and survivors addressed by P.L. 93-82. The Veterans Administration, however, has no plan for using HMOs for this group.

P.L. 93-222 AND P.L. 94-460—HEALTH MAINTENANCE ORGANIZATION ACT OF 1973 AND AMENDMENTS OF 1976

The present HMO law, P.L. 93-222 (see Appendix 1), was signed by President Nixon on December 29, 1973. It is a reconciliation of Senator Kennedy's bill, S. 14, and the House bill, H.R. 17550, a modified version of the original Roy bill. Built upon numerous versions since the initial introduction of the first HMO bill in 1971 (see Table 5), P.L. 93-222 amends "the Public Health Service Act to provide assistance and encouragement for the establishment and expansion of health maintenance organizations, health care resources, and the establishment of a Quality Health Care Commission, and for other purposes. . . ."[18] The measure commits the Federal Government to a *time-limited demonstration* effort and support of HMO development. It authorizes the expenditure of $375 million over a five-year period from fiscal 1974 through 1978; P.L. 94-460, the Amendments of 1976, extends the act through fiscal 1979. Development assistance is provided to a limited number of demonstration projects, with the intention that they become *self-sufficient* within fixed periods. The law's major purpose is to stimulate interest of consumers and providers in the HMO concept and to help make health care delivery available through HMOs—and to ". . . allow people to select for themselves either a prepaid system for obtaining health services or the more traditional approach. . . ."[19]

Requirements of the Present HMO Laws

Shortly after the passage of P.L. 93-222, numerous groups, including Paul Ellwood's InterStudy, the Group Health Association of America, and the Department of Health, Education, and Welfare, began to push for revisions in the law because of several essentially unworkable re-

[18]U.S. Congress, House of Representatives. *Health Maintenance Organization Act of 1973; Conference Report.* 93rd Congress, 1st session. December 3, 1973, p. 1.

[19]*Statement by the President.* Press Release. San Clemente, Calif., Office of the White House Press Secretary, December 29, 1973, p. 1.

quirements. On July 29, 1975, Representative James F. Hastings introduced legislation that would amend the HMO Act of 1973 (H.R. 9019).
President Ford signed these amendments into law (P.L. 94-460) on
October 8, 1976; they call for organizational and operational changes to
make HMOs more competitive with fee-for-service health plans and to
extend the HMO program for two years, through 1980.

Federal assistance under the HMO legislation is granted to public or
private entities only if the HMO meets the definitional and organizational requirements of the act. The following discussion of these requirements is from a recent edition of DHEW's *Research and Statistical
Notes.*[20]

DEFINITIONAL REQUIREMENTS

Health maintenance organizations are defined as entities that provide
basic health services to their enrollees and, for an additional payment,
supplemental health services. Prepaid enrollment fees for the basic and
supplemental health services must be fixed uniformly under a community-rating system without regard for the medical history of any individual or family. Nominal differentials may be allowed among the several groups to which HMOs market.

According to the HMO Act, the basic health services that must be
provided by the HMO to its enrollees are:

1. Physicians' services (including consultant and referral services by
a physician)
2. Inpatient and outpatient hospital services
3. Medically necessary emergency health services
4. Short-term (not to exceed 20 visits) outpatient evaluative and
crisis-intervention mental health services
5. Medical treatment and referral services (including referral services to appropriate ancillary services) for the abuse of or addiction to
alcohol and drugs
6. Diagnostic laboratory and diagnostic and therapeutic radiologic
services
7. Home health services
8. Preventive health services (including immunizations, well-child
care from birth, periodic health examinations for adults, voluntary fam-

---

[20]U.S. Department of Health, Education, and Welfare, Social Security Administration, Office of Research and Statistics. *Research and Statistical Notes.* Note No. 5.
Washington, D.C., 1974, pp. 1–8.

ily planning services, infertility services, children's ear examinations, and children's eye examinations to determine the need for vision correction)

The HMOs may provide the following supplemental health services—if the necessary health manpower is available and if the member has contracted for such services. These services, at the option of the HMO, may be offered as part of the basic package:

1. Services of intermediate and long-term care facilities
2. Vision care not included as a basic health service
3. Dental services not included as a basic health service
4. Mental health services not included as a basic health service
5. Long-term physical medicine and rehabilitative services, including physical therapy
6. Drugs prescribed in connection with the provision of basic or supplemental health services

The legislation permits an HMO to charge an enrollee nominal payments for these services in addition to the prepaid enrollment fee for basic services. The additional payments, to be made upon receipt of services, must be fixed in accordance with regulations by the Secretary of Health, Education, and Welfare. Such payments would not be required if, as determined under regulations of the secretary, they were a barrier to attainment of health care.

Basic services (and supplementary services when contracted for) must be provided by the HMO staff of professionals under contract or by any combination of staff, that is, medical groups or individual practice associations (IPAs), unless the services of health professionals are determined to be unusual or infrequently used or, because of medical necessity, cannot be provided through the HMO. When basic (and supplementary, if contracted for) services are medically necessary, they must be available and accessible 24 hours a day, seven days a week.

A member must be reimbursed for expenses incurred outside the HMO area if it was medically necessary that services be rendered before the member could return to his HMO. Thus, the HMO enrollee is assured of obtaining services in an appropriate and convenient way whenever they are needed.

ORGANIZATIONAL REQUIREMENTS

Medical groups must be organized as a partnership, association, or other group and must, as part of their total professional activity (no less than 35 percent of all their activities) and as a group responsibility, engage in coordinated practice for an HMO. The medical group must pool its income from the HMO practice and distribute it among themselves in accordance with a prearranged salary or other plan; must share records and substantial portions of major equipment and professional, technical, and administrative staff; and must arrange for and encourage continuing education for its members.

The majority of the physicians in the medical group must be licensed to practice medicine or osteopathy, but may include such other professionals as dentists, optometrists, and podiatrists and may use such other professional, allied health, and other health personnel as are necessary to provide the services for which the group is responsible. Individual practice associations are defined by the HMO Act as a partnership, corporation, association, or other legal entity that has entered into a service arrangement or arrangements with persons licensed in a state to practice medicine, osteopathy, dentistry, podiatry, optometry, or other health professions. The majority of such persons must be doctors of medicine or osteopathy. The arrangement must provide for continuing education of such persons and for their compensation. Requirements for use of additional professional and allied health personnel and for sharing records and staff are similar to those applicable to medical groups.

OTHER REQUIREMENTS

Financial Responsibility: The HMO must have a fiscally sound operation and adequate provisions against the risk of insolvency. It must be at risk, that is, be able to assume full financial risk, on a prospective basis, for the provision of basic health services, with the right to obtain insurance or to make other arrangements for the cost of providing basic health services to any member (the aggregate value of which exceeds $5,000 in any year); the cost of basic health services provided outside of the area because of medical necessity; and not more than 90 percent of the amount by which its costs in any fiscal year exceed 115 percent of fiscal-year income. This arrangement allows the HMO to protect itself against an unpredictably high rate of illness among its members and to still retain financial responsibility for the provision of basic health care services to its enrollees—one of the basic characteristics of a prepaid capitation mechanism of financing health care services.

Open Enrollment and Membership: HMOs are required to enroll persons who are broadly representative of the various age, social, and income groups within the areas they serve, and may not draw more than 75 percent of their enrollment from a medically underserved population unless the area is also a rural area.

The HMO must have annual open enrollment periods. Waivers are permitted, first, if such open enrollment would result in enrollment of a population not broadly representative of the various groups in the service area or, second, if the HMO can demonstrate that it has enrolled or will be compelled to enroll a disproportionate number of high-risk individuals and if enrollment, during an open enrollment period, of an additional number of such individuals will jeopardize its financial stability. An HMO may not refuse to enroll or reenroll members because of health status or needs for health services. Under the HMO amendments, federally qualified HMOs in existence for less than five years and with enrollments under 50,000 or showing a deficit in the most recent fiscal year will be exempt from open enrollment. Other HMOs will be required to openly enroll individual members up to three percent of net new group enrollments.

Consumer Participation: The HMO must be organized to ensure that at least one-third of the members of the policymaking body are enrollees in the HMO and that members from the medically underserved populations it serves will have equitable representation in the policymaking body. Consumers may thus have a role in determining such matters as operating hours, location of satellite facilities, acceptability of health care personnel, and the range of benefits.

Meaningful procedures for hearing and resolving grievances, including malpractice claims between the HMO (and the providers) and the enrollees, also must exist. In this way, consumers have the opportunity to influence the policy of the HMO and to obtain prompt and equitable resolution of their grievances.

Health Education: HMOs are required to provide medical social services for their members and to encourage and actively provide health education services, including education in methods of personal health maintenance and in the use of health services. It is expected that such a program will help patients to recognize and carry out their responsibilities for proper diet, exercise, and use of medications, and, in many cases, to perform certain health services for themselves. Thus, enrollees can contribute to their improved health at lower cost.

Quality Control: An HMO must have an ongoing quality assurance program for its health care services. The program must emphasize health outcomes and provide for review by physicians or other health professionals.

Data Reporting: HMOs must adopt procedures for developing and reporting on data relating to cost of operations, utilization patterns, and the availability, accessibility, and acceptability of their services and on other matters to the Secretary of Health, Education, and Welfare. To the extent practical, information on developments in the health status of HMO members is to be reported.

FINANCIAL ASSISTANCE

To aid in the development of HMOs, the initial legislation authorized a total appropriation of $375 million for a six-year period. Grants and contracts for public or nonprofit private organizations are authorized for surveys or other activities to determine the feasibility of developing and operating, or expanding the operation of, an HMO; planning projects to establish HMOs or to expand the membership of an HMO or the area that it serves; and projects to initially develop HMOs.

For public or nonprofit private HMOs, loans to meet initial operating costs in excess of revenues during the first 36 months of their operation are authorized under the law. Loans also are authorized if there is a significant expansion in the membership or area served.

Aid to private profitmaking entities for planning projects to establish or expand HMOs and for initial operating costs (in the amount and for the period authorized for public and nonprofit private HMOs) is to be limited to loan guarantees. Eligibility for aid is contingent on planned enrollment of medically underserved populations. Priority for grants and contracts for feasibility and planning studies will be given to applicants who can assure that the HMO, at the time it first becomes operational, will enroll at least 30 percent of its members from medically underserved populations.

The aggregate appropriation includes $50 million for research and evaluation studies of quality assurance. Total appropriations authorized by the law are shown in Table 6.

Actual and projected amounts have been substantially lower than the authorized amounts. These reductions are reflected in Table 7, which shows the HMO federal budget for fiscal years 1974 through 1977.

The HMO amendments further modified the HMO authorization by extending the act for two years and providing the following funds for: FY 1976, $40 million; FY 1977, $45 million; FY 1978, $45 million; and FY 1979, $50 million (only for development grants).

TABLE 6   Total Appropriations Authorized Under P.L. 93-222

Purpose	Amounts Authorized in Fiscal Year (in millions)				
	1974	1975	1976	1977	1978
Grants and contracts for					
Feasibility studies, planning, and initial development	$ 25	$55	$85	—	—
Initial development	—	—	—	$85	—
Capitalization of initial operating loan revolving fund	75*	—	—	—	—
Independent study of quality assurance	10†	—	—	—	—
Research and evaluation of quality assurance (DHEW)	4	8	9	9	$10
Totals	$114	$63	$94	$94	$10

*For fiscal years 1974 and 1975.

†The law does not state a fiscal-year limitation. A final report giving the results of the study was to be submitted to the Committee on Interstate and Foreign Commerce of the House of Representatives and the Senate Committee on Labor and Public Welfare by January 31, 1976. Several reports have been submitted including:

Comptroller General of the United States. *Report to the Committee on Finance, United States Senate: Better Controls Needed for Health Maintenance Organizations Under Medicaid in California.* Social and Rehabilitation Service, U.S. Department of Health, Education, and Welfare, September 10, 1974. B-164031(3).

_____. *Report to the Congress, Factors That Impede Progress in Implementing the Health Maintenance Organization Act of 1973.* U.S. Department of Health, Education, and Welfare, September 3, 1976. HRD-76-128.

_____. *Review of Grants to Health Maintenance Organization of South Carolina, Inc.* U.S. Department of Health, Education, and Welfare, May 17, 1974. B-164031(2).

_____. *Relationships Between Nonprofit Prepaid Health Plans With California Medicaid Contracts and For-Profit Entities Affiliated With Them.* U.S. Department of Health, Education, and Welfare, November 1, 1976. HRD 77-4.

OTHER FORMS OF ASSISTANCE

In addition to the limited financial support, the act provides for several other forms of assistance designed to aid HMO development. It was felt by Congress that this kind of encouragement and stimulus was essential if HMOs were to have the opportunity to prove themselves in the competitive health care market.

TABLE 7　Actual and Projected Budget for P.L. 93-222

Purpose	Amounts Authorized in Fiscal Year (in millions)				
	1974*	1975	1976	1977	1978 (projected)
Grants for					
Feasibility, planning, and development	$25.0	$15.0	$15.0	$18.1	$21.1
Program Operations	0.7	3.5	3.6	4.0	5.1†
Total Grants	$25.7	$18.5	$18.6	$22.1	26.2
Loans	35.0	—	—	—	—
Totals	$60.7	$18.5	$18.6	$22.1	$26.2

*Because of a late supplemental appropriation, this amount remained available for use during all of FY 1976. Thus, the total amount used during 1974 was approximately $1 million for program support, and $41 million in 1975 for all purposes. (Karen A. Hunt, ed. *Health Services Information*, 2(3):2, February 10, 1975; and Dr. Frank Seubold [Director, Division of Health Maintenance Organizations, U.S. Department of Health, Education, and Welfare], Personal Conversation. February 22, 1978.)

†This includes the appropriations for the Qualification Office which were not included in the previous year's authorizations.

Restrictive State Laws: First, and probably most important, the federal legislation supersedes certain restrictive state laws to the extent that they impede the development of HMOs in meeting the definitional and organizational requirements of the act. Some existing state legal barriers relate to physician control, open physician participation in HMOs, and the prohibition or restriction of group practice. (Congress had already authorized group practice carriers under the Federal Employees Health Benefits Act to underwrite prepaid group practice without regard to state restrictions.)

Employees' Health Plans: HMOs are given an opportunity to compete in the labor marketplace with other health insurance plans (e.g., dual choice) under a provision of the law that requires employers of 25 or more workers who receive health insurance benefits to give their employees an HMO option to traditional health insurance, if there is an HMO in the area that meets the definitional and organizational requirements of the new law (i.e., is federally qualified). This section of the original law was amended, and now the HMO Act requirement stipulates that

—At least 25 employees must live within the service area of the HMO for the offer to be mandatory; extends mandatory offer of the HMO option to States as a condition of payment of Public Health Service funds (314(d), 317, 318, 1002, 1525, or 1613).

—[An] offer . . . be made first to the recognized bargaining agent if there is one; employer's obligation is satisfied even if the offer is rejected.

—. . . [A] penalty for non-compliance at $10,000 for each 30-day period in which it continues; excludes Federal government, churches.

—On non-compliance of a State or a political subdivision of a State, Secretary is to provide reasonable notice and opportunity for hearing to the State and must withhold PHS funds on continued failure to comply.

—. . . the Civil Service Commission . . . contract with any qualified carrier (5USC 8903 (4)) which is also a qualified HMO.

—. . . HMO qualification and compliance . . . be administered in the Office of the Assistant Secretary for Health.[21]

Regulation for Quality Care Assurance: The assurance of quality care by HMOs is aided by the authority given to the Secretary of Health, Education, and Welfare to continue to regulate HMOs receiving financial assistance under the legislation. Compliance with the provisions of the law may be enforced through a civil action by the secretary in the appropriate U.S. district court.

RELATION TO MEDICARE AND MEDICAID

The law exempts HMOs from the definitional requirements of the act with respect to Medicare and Medicaid enrollees, for whom health care services continue to be those allowed under the two programs. The Social Security Administration, however, through the Medicare program, can contract only with HMOs qualified by the Public Health Service under the HMO Act; those contracts will continue to be under the control of the Social Security Administration. Also, federal participation with HMOs under the Medicaid program is limited to contracts with qualified HMOs, excluding Neighborhood Health Centers, Migrant Projects, Appalachian Regional Commission Projects, and organizations with a contract in effect for several years.

Reimbursement for Medicare is by the capitation method—either through incentive reimbursement or cost reimbursement—as provided in the Social Security Amendments of 1972. For Medicare and

[21]Peter Kirsch. "HMO Update #4" (Memo to Health and Science Community.) Rockville, Md., Bureau of Medical Services, Health Services Administration, U.S. Department of Health, Education, and Welfare, October 25, 1976, p. 4. Mimeographed.

Medicaid purposes, the HMO is not subject to the reinsurance ceilings imposed by the new law but is entitled to insurance against any risk involved in covering Medicare and Medicaid enrollees.

HEALTH SERVICES FOR NATIVE AMERICANS AND MIGRATORY WORKERS

The Secretary of Health, Education, and Welfare is authorized, with the consent of Native Americans served, to contract with private or other nonfederal health agencies or organizations to provide health services to Native Americans on a fee-for-service basis or on a prepayment or other similar basis.

The new legislation also authorizes the secretary to arrange for the provision of health services, through HMOs, for domestic agricultural migratory and seasonal workers who are eligible for health services under already existing authority (except under Section 310 of the Public Health Services Act) and for the families of such workers.

QUALITY CARE ASSURANCE PROGRAMS[22]

P.L. 93-222 calls for research and evaluation programs on the effectiveness, administration, and enforcement of quality assurance programs for health care to be conducted by the Secretary of Health, Education, and Welfare through the Assistant Secretary for Health. Annual reports are to be made to Congress and the president on the quality of health care in the United States, the operation of quality assurance programs, and advances that have been made through research and evaluation of such programs.

The secretary also is directed to contract with an appropriate nonprofit private organization for an independent study of health care quality assurance programs. The study is to include the development of a set of basic principles to be followed by an effective health care quality assurance system that will relate to such matters as the scope of the system, methods for assessing care, data requirements, and specifications for developing criteria and standards concerning desired outcomes of care. The organization selected must have a national reputation for objectivity in the conduct of studies for the Federal Government, expertise, and a history of interest and activity in health policy issues.

---

[22]Evaluations are being performed on a continuing basis by the General Accounting Office. By June 30, 1978, a report will have been submitted to Congress on 14 federally qualified HMOs.

EVALUATION OF HMO PROGRAM [23]

An evaluation of the operation of the HMO program is to be conducted by the Comptroller General of the United States. At least 50 of the HMOs that have been receiving federal funding and have been operational for three years are to be evaluated. The comptroller general will report the results of the evaluation to Congress within 90 days of its completion and will include findings on the ability of the HMOs to operate on a sound fiscal basis without continued federal financial assistance, continue to meet the organizational and operational requirements of the act, provide the required basic and supplemental health services, include indigent and high-risk individuals in their memberships, and provide health services to medically underserved populations.

The comptroller general also is required to conduct a study, and to report to Congress within 36 months after enactment of the legislation, on the economic effects that compliance with the provision on employees' health benefits plans has on employers. He is also directed to evaluate the operations of the HMOs—by category, in comparison with each other, and, as a group, in comparison with other forms of health care delivery—and to evaluate the impact that HMOs individually, by category, and as a group have on the health of the public. The results of this evaluation also are to be reported to Congress not later than 36 months after enactment of the law.

HMO QUALIFICATION

The two HMO laws describe the requirements that an HMO must meet to become a "qualified" HMO—the federal seal of approval. Qualification, or the statement by a new HMO seeking federal funds that it will attempt to become qualified under the HMO law, allows that organization to qualify for federal grant funds, loans, and loan guarantees. Qualification also is required for participation in several of the federally financed health programs such as Medicare and Medicaid. On the other hand, qualification is a long process, requiring complex reporting to the Federal Government as well as meeting the somewhat noncompetitive requirements of the HMO laws.

In order to qualify, application must be made to the federal HMO Qualification Office in Rockville, Maryland. Notification and deficiency letters are then sent to the HMO requesting information on areas needing further clarification or substantiation. Sites are visited by a

[23]*Ibid.*

group of national HMO officials, which include legal, health care, management, marketing, and financial specialists. The team reports its findings to an HMO case officer, who reports his findings to the qualification officer. Ultimately, the DHEW/HMO division administrator approves or disapproves the HMO.

FEDERAL HMO PROGRAM INFORMATION

Information and applications relating to federal financing or qualification can be obtained from the following offices or the DHEW regional offices:

Director
Division of Health Maintenance Organization Development
Public Health Service
U.S. Department of Health, Education, and Welfare
Rockville, Maryland 20857
Telephone: (301)443–4106

Director
Division of HMO Qualification and Compliance
Office of the Administrator
Public Health Service
U.S. Department of Health, Education, and Welfare
Rockville, Maryland 20857
Telephone: (301)443–2778

Director
Office of Health Maintenance Organizations
Office of the Assistant Secretary for Health
U.S. Department of Health, Education, and Welfare
Rockville, Maryland 20857
Telephone: (301)443–4099

Summary

Recent Federal Government interest in the HMO concept is based on a recognition of three major health-related problems that may be partly solved by the use of HMOs. First, it is recognized that there is maldistribution of health resources among geographic areas in the country and among selected socioeconomic groups. A second problem is the escalation in the cost of health care as a result of the increasing demand for services without concurrent increases in supplies of such services or large increases in productivity of present providers. The third general problem is the inability of purchasers of care—the public as well as the Federal Government—to recognize and evaluate the quality of care rendered, as well as the difficulties experienced by providers in controlling the quality of care.

As part of the Nixon Administration's health program, the HMO strategy was developed, following the guidelines envisioned by Paul Ellwood, M.D. In his paper, "The Health Maintenance Strategy," Dr. Ellwood describes several steps that the Federal Government should take to develop a diversified, pluralistic, and competitive health industry. He describes HMOs as organizations providing comprehensive services purchased annually by capitation agreements. The administration's disclosure of the HMO strategy appeared early in 1970, but was more formally described by President Nixon in both his 1971 and 1972 health messages to Congress. Early efforts were directed toward the establishment of Alternative C, an amendment to the Medicare law that would permit the HMO option to be available together with Parts A and B. This was finally achieved with the passage of P.L. 92-603, the Social Security Amendments of 1972. Under Section 226 of the law, the Social Security Administration can contract with HMOs to provide Medicare benefits. In addition, Section 206(e) authorizes federal technical assistance to states to help establish state Medicaid contracts with HMOs.

The HMO concept was described by the Nixon Administration as the keystone of its national health strategy of 1971 and 1972. At that time, HMOs were to be developed not only for federal program recipients but for all Americans. In fact, the ambitious goal was to make HMOs available to 90 percent of the American population by 1980. Steps were taken by the Department of Health, Education, and Welfare to establish first a task force, then an office, and finally an HMO service within the department. Operating on reprogrammed funds, the service obligated $26 million for HMO grants and contracts for 1971 through December 1973.

By the beginning of 1973, with the introduction of numerous bills, none of which were passed, the administration changed its forthright stand for HMOs to a time-limited demonstration approach. No long-term federal commitment was to be made for HMO activities. By December 1973, an HMO bill, S. 14, had been signed into law. P.L. 93-222, the Health Maintenance Organization Act of 1973, authorizes the expenditure of $375 million over a five-year period. P.L. 94-460 extends the authorization for two additional years. Development assistance is provided to a limited number of HMO projects, with the ultimate goal of self-sufficiency. These demonstration projects are designed to help stimulate interest of consumers and providers in the HMO concept and its potential advantages.

The HMO laws authorize a program of financial aid to public and nonprofit organizations through grants, contracts, and loans for the following purposes associated with the development and expansion of HMOs: feasibility and planning studies, initial development costs, and initial operating deficits of HMOs for the first three years. In addition, the laws authorize loan guarantees for profit-making HMOs in medically underserved areas for planning, initial development, and initial operating deficits. Financing of guaranteed loans is accomplished through the establishment of a loan guarantee fund in the U.S. Treasury.

Several other laws and proposed bills to enable HMO enrollment, to assist with HMO planning, development, and operation, or that have the potential to facilitate these HMO activities, have been enacted into law, or are likely to be passed in the near future. P.L. 84-569 and P.L. 89-614 authorize the CHAMPUS program. A bill to amend P.L. 84-569 and P.L. 89-614 is before Congress; it would allow the Secretary of Defense to contract with HMOs for both inpatient and outpatient services, primarily to retired military personnel and their dependents. Federal employees have been eligible for care provided by HMO-like organizations since the passage of P.L. 86-382 in 1959. By March 1973, approximately 53,000 federal employees were enrolled in HMOs. The Social Security Amendments of 1972, P.L. 92-603, strengthened the ties between the Medicare program and the HMOs that provide services to Medicare recipients. Section 226 of the law provides the authority to contract with HMOs to provide covered services for capitation payments for both Parts A and B. Section 206(e) authorizes federal technical assistance and the development of HMO/state Medicaid contracts. Finally, P.L. 93-82, enacted on August 2, 1973, extends the eligibility for health care benefits to the dependents and survivors of veterans with 100 percent service-connected disabilities. Although the use of HMOs for provision of care to this group as well as to veterans has not been determined as yet, such a mechanism for delivery of care is appropriate and may be available in the near future.

One final word concerning the HMO laws. P.L. 93-222 has certainly provided for a far-reaching and innovative approach to traditional health delivery. It is forward looking in that it requires participating HMOs to provide ingenious financing mechanisms for the underserved, it requires employers to provide the HMO option to their employees if a qualified HMO is available in their locality, and it identifies a comprehensive set of treatment and preventive health services. Some experts project that the health industry will not be able to meet these challenges—especially the expanded benefit packages, which they say may not be competitive with the traditional BC/BS and indemnity programs currently available. Only time will tell, but the opportunity is now available for the health industry and the American public to demonstrate that Americans want and can support better health care service. From this point of view, the HMO activity supported by P.L. 93-222 and P.L. 94-460 is certainly an experiment.

References

Dorsey, Joseph L. "The Health Maintenance Organization Act of 1973 (P.L. 93-222) and Prepaid Group Practice Plans." *Medical Care, XIII*(1):1–9, January 1975.

Kress, John R., and Singer, James. *HMO Handbook.* Rockville, Md., Aspen Systems Corporation, 1975, pp. 33–108.

McLeod, Gordon K. "The Federal Role in Health Maintenance Organizations." *In: Health Maintenance Organizations, Proceedings of a Conference, 1972.* Denver, Colo., Medical Group Management Association, 1972, pp. 2–4.

Prussin, Jeffrey A. *HMO Legislation in 1973–74.* The Health Legislation Report Series, Vol. 11. Washington, D.C., Science and Health Publications, Inc., 1974.

Rafkind, Faith B. *Health Maintenance Organizations: Some Perspectives.* Chicago, Blue Cross Association, 1972.

Roy, William R. *The Proposed Health Maintenance Organization Act of 1972.* Washington, D.C., Science and Health Communications Group, 1972, pp. 1–29, 162–257.

"Statement of Frank C. Carlucci Before the Subcommittee on Public Health and Environment, Committee on Interstate and Foreign Commerce. March 6, 1973." Mimeographed.

U.S. Congress, House of Representatives. *Health Maintenance Organization Amendments of 1976.* P.L. 94-460. October 8, 1976.

_____. *Authorizing the Use of Health Maintenance Organizations as an Alternative to the CHAMPUS Program.* 93rd Congress, 1st session. October 11, 1973. Report No. 93-573.

U.S. Congress, Senate. *Health Maintenance Organization Act of 1973.* P.L. 93-222. December 29, 1973.

U.S. Department of Health, Education, and Welfare, Health Resources Administration. *Health Maintenance Organization Service: Program Status as of December 1975.* Rockville, Md., 1975.

_____, Health Services Administration and Medical Services Administration. *Proceedings of the National Conference for Developing Title XIX-HMO Contracts.* Rockville, Md., 1974, pp. 3-1–3-59, 3-101–3-105, A-1–A-31.

_____, Medical Services Administration, Social and Rehabilitation Service. *Medicaid HMO-Type Contracts.* Washington, D.C., 1973.

_____, Social Security Administration, Office of Research and Statistics. *Research and Statistical Notes.* Note No. 5. Washington, D.C., 1974.

4

Organizational Structures

HMOs are characterized by flexibility in both composition and organizational form. This flexibility in organizational structure, in the process of adapting to local viewpoints and requirements, is, in part, the underlying basis for the strength and tenacity of HMOs. As noted in Chapter 3, the law does not dictate an organizational form that must be strictly followed in order to qualify for federal grants, contracts, or loans. On the contrary, the legislation describes only the functions and types of services that should be incorporated in the HMO. The law also allows for some flexibility in the *provider* arrangement; health services may be rendered either by a group of physicians or through an individual practice association (IPA).

Major organizational arrangements that have been successfully used by HMOs are categorized and reviewed in this chapter. Two important issues should be kept in mind. First, although P.L. 93-222 does not specify organizational form, limitations may be imposed by future Office of Health Maintenance Organization Service (HMOs) guidelines and regulations that may be developed after the initial HMO grantees have been evaluated. Regardless of possible federal regulation changes, this discussion, however, will include the major structural models currently in use. Such a discussion is appropriate, because many HMOs that will be developed during the next few years will receive no federal assistance. Second, the successful HMO prototypes have evolved and survive in their own unique settings; to follow one model explicitly, without regard to particular environment, demography, and community needs, would be misleading. Thus, it may be useful to become familiar with the many structural forms available so that, when developing an HMO, one may choose those portions that best suit the individual project.

The term "organizational structure" is defined here as the method by which the HMO component parts can be arranged, established, or ordered to achieve a functioning health-delivery system. The theory of general management suggests that the *purpose* of organization is summarized by two principles—unity of objective and efficiency.

The unity of objective principle suggests that the organizational structure of an HMO is effective if it, as a whole and in all of its parts, facilitates an individual's contribution toward the attainment of the HMO's objectives. Similarly, the principle of efficiency requires that an HMO be structured so as to make possible the accomplishment of organizational objectives by employees with minimum unsought consequences or cost. In addition, two principles associated with the organizational *structure* are necessary for a clear definition—authority and delegation, and departmentalization. Authority is the cement of the organization and the primary line of communication. It is the means by which coordination of HMO units can be promoted. Departmentalization is the framework of the organization in the sense of activity groupings. The organizational structure should reflect a classification of the tasks required of HMO personnel and should assist in their coordination by creating a system of related roles. A discussion of the flow of authority and of departmentalization is included in the following review of organizational models.

Sponsoring Organizations

Like other organizations, HMOs are controlled by a board of trustees (in a nonprofit organization) or board of directors (in a for-profit organization). This primary decision-making body is accountable and responsible for all activities of the HMO. The board usually delegates to a manager—the administrator—the authority for day-to-day management. Although the administrator is held responsible for the activities of the HMO, the board cannot escape the responsibility and accountability for such activities. The discussions that follow describe the several organizational models used by HMOs. The flow of authority residing ultimately with the board is shown, as is the flow of premium dollars.

The differentiation between the *sponsors* of the HMO and its *policymaking body* should be clearly defined. These two groups are

TABLE 8   HMO Sponsors from the June 1975 InterStudy Census

Sponsor	Number of HMOs	Percent of Total* (n = 178 plans)
Community Organization Model	43	24
Carrier Model:		
Blue Cross/Blue Shield	31	17
Private Insurance Company	21	12
Industry/Union Model (all by labor unions)	14	8
Provider Model:		
Physician Groups	93	52
Hospitals	31	17
Other	69	39
TOTAL	302†	

*HMOs reported by sponsorship category divided by 178.

†This figure represents the total universe of 178 HMOs, many of which indicated sponsorship in more than one category.

Source: Karen A. Hunt, ed. "Who Is Sponsoring HMOs?" *Health Services Information,* 2(13):4–5, June 30, 1975.

sometimes thrown together and described as the legal HMO entity. In fact, HMOS has described the sponsoring agency, for grant source purposes, as the HMO prime contractor—that is, the organization that, in its role as prime contractor with DHEW, is held both accountable and responsible.[1] It is necessary that there be an organization that can be held responsible for the developing HMO; this organization is defined as the sponsor. It is just as necessary, however, to identify the decision-making body that is established once the HMO legal entity is formed. The models that follow describe the legal organizational entities, not the sponsoring organizations.

According to a census of HMOs performed by InterStudy, more than half of the plans have been sponsored by physician groups, with consumer groups ranking second. Table 8 presents the results of InterStudy's research, completed in June 1975.

Sponsoring organizations have included a variety of organizations—universities, cities, industries, unions, consumer groups, as-

[1]Faith B. Rafkind. *Health Maintenance Organizations: Some Perspectives.* Chicago, Blue Cross Association, 1972, p. 27.

sociations, insurance companies, hospitals, and neighborhood health centers. Individuals associated with the sponsoring organization as initial advocates may naturally be called on to serve as board members with the newly established HMO entity. The sponsoring organization has, in some cases, co-opted and assumed the functions of the HMO, and has established the HMO as a part of the sponsor's organizational role. Examples of this are the HMOs sponsored and operated by Blue Cross/Blue Shield plans, hospitals, medical schools, and so on. In other cases, the sponsor's role ends when the legal entity is established or, in the case of federal grants, when the grant period expires or the grant or contract is transferred to the new HMO organization.

Initially, in almost every case, the sponsor assumes the risk for the overall performance of the new HMO, influences its contractual arrangements with providers, and is directly involved in the day-to-day management decisions made by the HMO.

Four HMO Models

Examples of four HMO models (legal entities) are identified in Table 9. Included in the discussion of each model are its strengths, weaknesses, and operational format—the channels of authority and cash flow. Examples of each category are provided, and a generalized structure for each model is then developed.

COMMUNITY ORGANIZATION MODEL

Community organization models are established by community groups such as consumer groups, neighborhood health centers, and selected public and private nonprofit organizations, including the consumer associations and cooperatives discussed in Chapter 2. These plans are described as true consumer participative programs. Some characteristics of the community organization model are: it is a nonprofit membership corporation or association; the board of trustees is nominated from and elected by the membership; and membership is open to any person residing within the plan's catchment area. The plan is controlled by the board of trustees, which ultimately is responsible and accountable to the entire plan membership. Active participation in management by the board (decision making and control), however, is guaranteed only when nominations for the board are made by a nominating committee composed of members-at-large or by a general membership vote; a nominating committee composed of present board members

TABLE 9   HMO-like Organization Structures

Category of Organizational Structure	Examples
1. Community Organization	a. Group Health Cooperative of Puget Sound, Seattle, Washington b. Group Health Association, Washington, D.C. c. Watts Extended Health, Los Angeles, California d. Health Insurance Plan of Greater New York, New York City e. Group Health Plan of St. Paul, St. Paul, Minnesota
2. Carrier	a. Columbia Medical Plan, Columbia, Maryland b. Rhode Island Medical Society Physician Service, Providence, Rhode Island c. Metro Health, Inc., Detroit, Michigan d. Genessee Valley Group Health Association, Rochester, New York
3. Industry-Union	a. Kaiser Foundation Health Plan b. Community Health Center, Two Harbors, Minnesota c. Labor Health Institute of St. Louis, St. Louis, Missouri
4. Provider	
Group Practice	a. Ross-Loos Medical Clinic, Los Angeles, California b. Rural Health Associates, Farmington, Maine c. Palo Alto Medical Group, Palo Alto, California
Hospital	a. Geisinger Health Plan, Danville, Pennsylvania b. Ramsey County Hospital, St. Paul, Minnesota
Individual Practice	a. Foundation for Medical Care of San Joaquin County, Stockton, California b. Medical Care Foundation of Sacramento, Sacramento, California c. New Mexico Health Care Corporation, Albuquerque, New Mexico

will most likely foster a self-perpetuating board and an inbreeding of ideas. Election of board members from a slate of nominees by the entire membership or their delegates further ensures and maintains active participation by, or representation from, the entire membership group.

At the present time, community organization models do not follow the aforementioned nomination/election procedure. Consumer participation usually is described as, and limited to, representation on the board of trustees, an advisory group to the board or to the plan administration, or a grievance mechanism. This is true of the community organization model to be discussed—Group Health Association (GHA) of Washington, D.C.[2] The membership of GHA develops the policy of the cooperative by voting on bylaw revisions and by electing nominees presented by the board's nominating committee, composed of board members. Nonboard members can nominate fellow members as candidates for the board upon presentation of a petition signed by 200 members of GHA, usually a somewhat difficult task.

GHA's board of trustees is composed of nine members elected to staggered three-year terms. Approximately 12 standing committees assist the board in carrying out its policymaking function. As shown in Figure 12, an executive director is appointed by the board and is delegated the administrative responsibility for the direction of GHA affairs and the implementation of administrative policies established by the board. The executive director is responsible for all day-to-day operations, implementation of goals and plans, contract negotiations, and coordination of department activities. Although he cannot interfere in the practice of medicine, he receives advice from the health program administrator concerning medically related issues. The health program administrator, also appointed by the board, is responsible for the recruitment of physicians and for the coordination and supervision of the various medical departments.

All medical specialties are represented in the GHA medical group. Paid on a capitation basis, the group contracts with GHA to provide the membership with medical services. The medical group is self-governing; therefore, it determines the salaries of all full-time physicians and pays outside specialists out of its capitation income. Medical group representatives sit on both the executive committee of the medical group and the Joint Conference Committee.

As depicted in Figure 12, the health plan owns and operates outpatient facilities but does not own its own hospital. Area hospitals at which the medical group has staff privileges are used for inpatient hospital care. Hospital claims are processed by Blue Cross of Washington, D.C., which acts as GHA's fiscal agent for both inpatient

---

[2]The discussion of GHA reflects its operational structure prior to 1976. After that period, major changes regarding physician employment and contractual relationships were implemented.

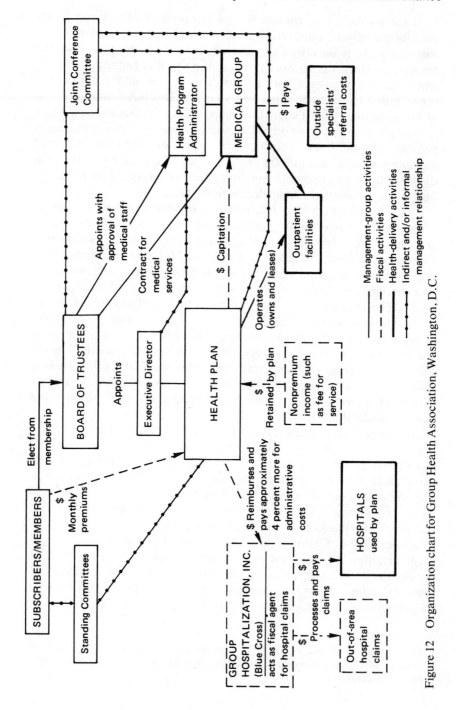

Figure 12   Organization chart for Group Health Association, Washington, D.C.

claims and out-of-area hospital claims. GHA reimburses Blue Cross for these claims, plus an administrative fee of 4.16 percent.

The review of GHA's organizational design suggests an approach for the community organization model. Note that most health plans included in this type of model are based on a cooperative approach (see Figure 13). GHA is representative of the cooperative approach. Subscribers elect a board from among the membership; the membership then appoints an executive director to manage the health plan. Physicians are either employed directly by the plan or are paid on a capitation basis. Hospital coverage is provided by the plan-operated facility or by outside hospitals where plan physicians have staff-admitting privileges. Although the community organization model may retain the insurance function and thus reimburse both physicians and hospitals for medical care by capitation, the GHA model indicates that an outside third party may become the fiscal agent for the plan. Figure 14 shows how Blue Cross of Washington (Group Hospitalization, Inc.) performs the function for in- and out-of-area hospital reimbursement for GHA.

Generally, the following observations can be made concerning the community organization model:

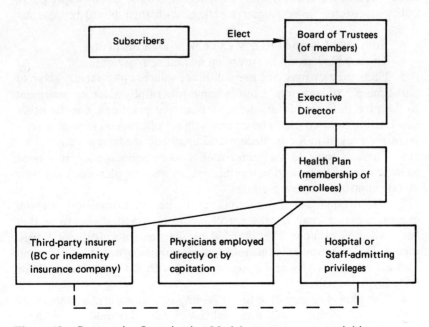

Figure 13   Community Organization Model—management activities.

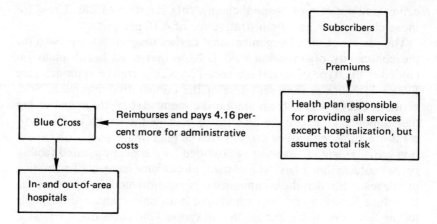

Figure 14   Community Organization Model—fiscal activities.

1. The HMO is developed by consumers, for consumers. Thus, the programs may be tailored to the needs of the enrollees.

2. Subscribers are given a method to actively participate in major policy decisions, either through trustee elections, direct approval of policy decisions, or consumer meetings with their board representatives.

3. Enrollment is open to any catchment-area resident.

4. The medical group is autonomous and self-governing.

5. Plans may or may not use full-time, salaried physicians. (Use of part-time physicians may result in some loss of physician commitment to the plan in favor of outside fee-for-service practices. On the other hand, using salaried plan physicians without offering an incentive payment may result in a complacent and apathetic medical staff.)

6. There is some loss of control of HMO components when outside agencies act as fiscal and marketing agents and the plan does not own and/or control inpatient facilities.

7. Use of staff admitting privileges in lieu of formalized hospital contracts may jeopardize the enrollee/plan contractual guarantee that beds will be available when needed by plan patients. (GHA of Washington, D.C. circumvents this problem by promising only to perform on a "best efforts" basis and by contracting with Doctors' Hospital for beds for its members.)

8. The plan is responsible for providing or making arrangements for services and assumes total financial risk. Under this model, risk sharing with medical groups or fiscal agents is not common.

9. Administrative control of the plan's activities is somewhat more difficult than that of other models' because of loosely affiliated HMO functions—outside hospitals, marketing agents, and fiscal agents—and because of the possibility of board member interference in day-to-day management issues.

CARRIER MODEL

The carrier model is characterized by sponsorship and control by either an indemnity insurance company or a Blue Cross/Blue Shield program. It is only natural that these third-party insurers have become involved with, and are a part of, the HMO programs. In effect, in the carrier model, BC/BS, for example, assumes more responsibility for coordinating and budgeting health care services. This larger role of BC/BS is critical to the success of the HMO movement because of the "Blues" large share of the present health insurance market—in 1972, this was 63 percent of the total number of persons with hospital coverage and 44 percent of the total number of persons with physician insurance coverage.[3] Employers and subscribers are demanding a more effective use of their Blue Cross premiums. Physicians are requesting assistance from Blue Shield plans in developing new financial arrangements, including prepayment programs. Hospitals also have identified the need for restructuring the medical-care delivery system and have requested assistance from Blue Cross. Moreover, beginning with the Nixon Administration, national health insurance proposals looked to private, third-party insurers as the fiscal managers of the federal health programs.

Support for HMOs using the carrier model is derived from the skills and resources currently available from the "Blues" and indemnity carriers. This includes assistance in coordination, marketing, underwriting, and financing—traditional carrier roles. In addition, the HMO, like the carriers, requires benefit rating, professional relations, electronic data processing, and widespread access to purchasers of care, activities that the carriers currently undertake. Some HMOs require financial support from the carriers for capital and start-up costs. A good example of carrier involvement in these management functions is Connecticut General Life Insurance Company's involvement in the development and operation of the Columbia Medical Plan. According to Harold Thalheimer, Connecticut General's former Director of Medi-

---

[3]Health Insurance Institute. *Source Book of Health Insurance Data 1973–74*. New York, 1974, p. 18.

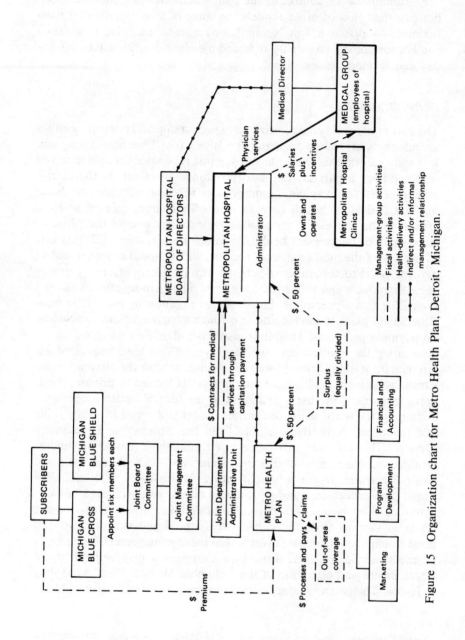

Figure 15   Organization chart for Metro Health Plan, Detroit, Michigan.

cal Programs, there are seven functions that his company performed with the Columbia plan.

1. *Program development*—in cooperation and jointly with The Johns Hopkins University and The Johns Hopkins Hospital
2. *Marketing*—using normal channels on a dual-choice basis, and through its group field force, agents, and brokers
3. *Risk taking*—including the usual fee-for-service, hospital-care risk, underenrollment risk, and operating-deficit risks
4. *Additional benefits*—filling all the gaps in coverage, including out-of-area coverage or special care, such as long-term or psychiatric care and major medical, with indemnity insurance
5. *Administrative*—centralized carrier administration when other carriers sell the plan
6. *Program management*—with Johns Hopkins involved in the management of the medical care, financing, and delivery systems
7. *Financing*—of both the development costs and the facilities capital[4]

The cost to the independent HMO for carrier involvement may be substantial. Some insurance companies are profit-making institutions and, as such, may have interests, goals, and commitments that do not coincide with those of the nonprofit HMO. More important, the use of the carrier in marketing creates a conflict for the insurance company's salesmen; they are now asked to sell two products that compete with one another, one which they have been selling and are very familiar with and one which is foreign and difficult to understand. These and other problems recognized in noncarrier HMOs are not as prevalent in HMOs that are carrier-sponsored and controlled. One such plan, the Metro Health Plan of Detroit, is operated and controlled by Michigan Blue Cross (MBC) and Blue Shield (MBS). Originally sponsored by the United Auto Workers and called the Community Health Association (CHA), it was organized in 1956. On January 1, 1972, the CHA board legally assigned its functions and contracts to MBC and MBS, and the "Blues" assumed total responsibility for CHA coverage. MBC and MBS continue to purchase most medical and health care services from the closely affiliated Metropolitan Hospital and staff through contractual agreements similar to those in operation with CHA. The exceptions are out-of-area and emergency coverage, which are reimbursed to the subscriber directly by the Metro Health Plan. Figure 15 illustrates these arrangements. Subscribers are offered a dual choice between the traditional BC/BS package and the HMO package. The Metro Health Plan,

[4]Harold Thalheimer. (Director of Medical Programs, Connecticut General Life Insurance Company, Hartford, Connecticut.) Internal company memorandum, May 1, 1970.

operating as a broker, contracts on a capitation basis for medical services with area providers—in this case, the Metropolitan Hospital. The Metropolitan Hospital, which is a nonprofit community hospital governed by a board of directors, arranges for medical care by employing a group of physicians. Management activities of the Metro Health Plan are controlled by the boards of MBS and MBC through the use of a Joint Board Committee. The committee is composed of 12 members—6 appointed from each organization—and is responsible for the program and for coordinating policy between MBS and MBC. The Joint Management Committee manages and directs the design, development, and administration of the health plan by supervising the operation of a joint department. Community input is obtained through the two advisory committees—one local and the other statewide. Surpluses are divided equally between the hospital and the plan. The hospital's share cannot exceed 30 cents per member per month; a portion of this surplus is paid to the physician by the hospital as an incentive.

Although the Metro Health Plan appears to be complicated, a general carrier model can be developed, as shown in Figure 16. The model suggests that the health plan is an integral part of the insurance company; subscribers pay their premiums to the company. The company then acts in the capacity of a broker arranging for the provision of health care through contracts with the medical group, hospitals, and other providers. The insurance company provides no medical services itself. Thus, the carrier model has three major characteristics—a dual-choice offering; the broker function, providing most management activities; and little or no incorporation or certificate-of-need problems. The first two characteristics have already been discussed. Because there is no separate and distinct health plan under this model, there is no incorporation problem; all of the components are already incorporated entities—the insurance company, the medical group, and

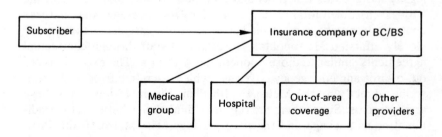

Figure 16   Carrier model.

the hospital. No certificate of need is required unless a new facility or medical group clinic is anticipated. Conversely, because the insurance company is controlling the finances, the company will logically control and even dominate the program with little or no input allowed by the medical group or the hospital. This is even more important for those HMOs that are modeled after noncarrier programs (i.e., consumer, provider, industry models) but have contracted with insurance carriers to provide some management services such as marketing and financing. In these instances, because of control of cash flow, carrier dominance can be very detrimental to the freedom and flexibility of the newly developing plan.

Of special interest is the Columbia Medical Plan in Columbia, Maryland. Although this program is included within the "carrier model" description, it has been described as the "consortium approach."[5] Developed jointly by Connecticut General Life Insurance Company, the Rouse Company builders, and The Johns Hopkins University and Hospital, the plan provides a coordinated management for several independent institutions. The Columbia Hospital and Clinics Foundation—a nonprofit hospital corporation—offers the Columbia Medical Plan to families and groups in the foundation's service area. The foundation contracts with the Columbia Medical Group—a limited partnership—to provide physician services. The partnership reimburses its physicians on a salary basis. In addition, the foundation contracts with the Columbia Hospital, presently a nonprofit community hospital, for inpatient services. The organizational structure of the Columbia Medical Plan, however, is basically that of a triad, composed of the Columbia Hospital and Clinics Foundation, Connecticut General (with provisions for other carriers to participate in the plan), and the partnership of physicians, each unit of which has its own area of responsibility in the overall mixture of finance and delivery of comprehensive health benefits. The consortium approach has the added advantage of a broader management base (i.e., more knowledge and expertise, larger financial reserves, greater management talent to draw from) and greater flexibility. It also may have the problem of longer lines of communication, as well as difficulties in coordinating three strong organizations with possibly conflicting goals. Indeed, these problems have forced the Columbia Plan to terminate the triumvirate approach; currently the hospital is a nonprofit community hospital, and

---

[5]William R. Roy. *The Proposed Health Maintenance Organization Act of 1972.* Washington, D.C., Science and Health Communications Group, 1972, pp. 189–190.

the plan is now wholly owned and operated by Connecticut General with contractual relations with the physician partnership.

INDUSTRY-UNION MODEL

Sometimes referred to as the "Kaiser model," the industry-union model includes the group of HMO-like organizations that are initially developed for employees by their employers or for union members by their unions (e.g., St. Louis Labor Health Institute); for individual, federal, or state employees; or for eligibles of federal, state, or local public-assistance programs. Over time, these plans have opened their doors to all members of their service-area communities. The industry-union model is characterized by the following:

1. The plans are sponsored by and for special-interest groups. Initial sponsorship is by laymen in private industry or in organizations, such as unions, associated with certain large industries.

2. Control of the plan is usually by laymen who may not necessarily represent the subscribers. Control may reside with investors, hospital administrators, unions, employers, or physician-investors.

3. The plans are developed for employees, union members, or government-assistance eligibles; their premiums are paid for by a third party, such as the union, employer, or government. These plans, therefore, are noncontributory or only partly contributory; the latter term is used to describe a group insurance plan under which the employee shares in the cost of the plan with his employer, the policyholder.

4. Both nonprofit and for-profit plans are included in the partly contributory category. Several of the plans are investor-owned, and their major goal is to show a profit from the operation.

5. Many of the plans perform the functions of self-insuring, marketing, enrollment, underwriting, and administration. It is not uncommon, however, for these plans to act simply as brokers—identifying and consummating contracts with providers for health services.

6. As part of the contractual arrangements with the provider, the plan may pass along a part or all of the risk for supplying both inpatient and outpatient services to the providers. The plan, however, is still responsible to the subscriber for the provision of benefit package contractual services.

The most famous example of an industry-union model plan is the Kaiser-Permanente Medical Care Program (KPMCP). This program is not a single legal entity, but a joint endeavor by several Kaiser-developed organizations that together arrange and provide health services to the health plan subscribers. Four entities are included in the KPMCP:[6]

1. The Kaiser Foundation Health Plan, Inc. (KFHP) is composed of six nonprofit corporations—located in California, Oregon, Washington, Colorado, Ohio, and Hawaii. In each of the six regions where the health plan operates, the KFHP functions basically as a contracting and administrative organization whose primary functions consist of entering into medical and hospital service agreements with individuals and groups of members, contracting with the regional Permanente Medical Group to provide medical services to health plan members, and contracting with the Kaiser Foundation Hospitals to provide hospital services to health plan members. The health plan itself does not provide services but arranges for direct medical and hospital services.

2. The Permanente Medical Group (PMG) in each of the six regions previously mentioned provides professional health care services—all are organized as partnerships or professional corporations. Each is an independent medical group that enters into a medical service agreement with the health plan to provide services.

3. Kaiser Foundation Hospitals is a California nonprofit, charitable corporation that owns or operates community hospitals and owns outpatient facilities in several states. These facilities provide both inpatient and outpatient care for health plan members. Overall administrative responsibility for the Kaiser Foundation Hospitals is vested with the 15-member board of directors of the corporation, which is also the board for the Kaiser Foundation Health Plan.

Figure 17 depicts the administrative and fiscal relationships of the Kaiser-Permanente Medical Care Program. The KPMCP is not a centralized organization but is composed of six regional organizations with ties to a central office in Oakland, California. The central office provides a mechanism for coordinating policies on legal and governmental affairs and personnel, as well as assistance in establishing rates and developing benefit packages. All fundamental decisions for a particular region, however, are made through a joint effort between the medical

[6]The following description of the Kaiser-Permanente Medical Care Program is developed from material in Group Health Association of America, Department of Education and Training. *Sample Operating Prepaid Group Practice Medical Care Programs: Organizational and Financial Relationships.* Washington, D.C., 1972, pp. 1–12. Mimeographed.

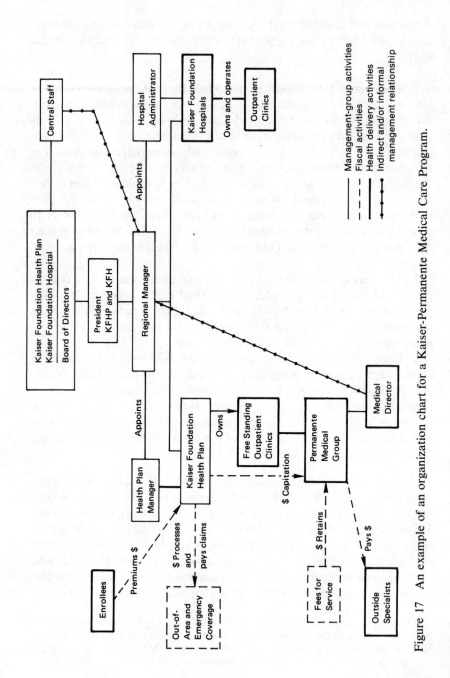

Figure 17   An example of an organization chart for a Kaiser-Permanente Medical Care Program.

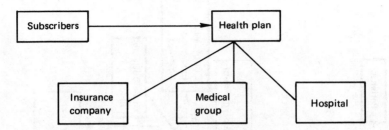

Figure 18   Industry-union HMO model—management activities.

director of the regional Permanente medical group and the regional manager, who has the responsibility for managing the health plan and hospitals of the region. These two individuals and their aides make up the regional management decision-making team.

A generalized industry-union HMO model follows the format shown in Figure 18. The health plan contracts with the medical groups and the hospital for health services. The insurance function also is provided through contractual arrangements with outside organizations, although some plans may retain the insuring function. Based on the Kaiser example, Figure 19 outlines the cash flow and contractual relationships characteristic of the industry-union model.

PROVIDER MODELS

Three provider models are presently exhibited by HMOs—group practice arrangements, individual practice "foundations," and hospital-organized HMOs. Generally, these models are characterized by provider control of the health plan, either directly or through a provider-controlled subsidiary organization. Each will be discussed separately.

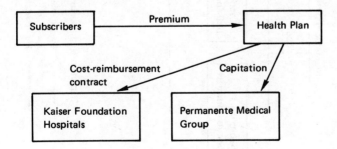

Figure 19   Industry-union HMO model—fiscal activities.

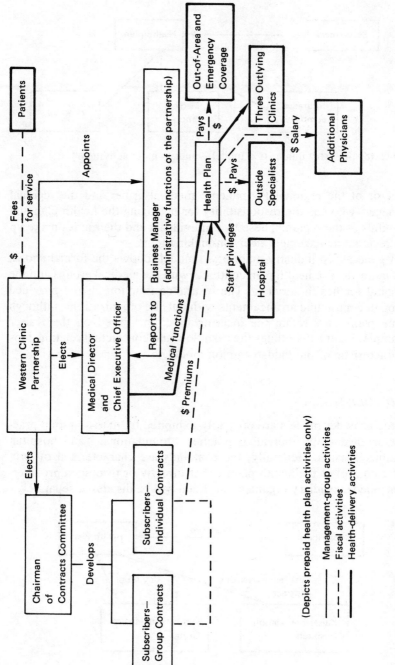

Figure 20 Organization chart for Western Clinic, Tacoma, Washington.

Group Practice "Provider" Model: This type of HMO is sponsored, owned, and operated by a group practice of physicians. The group practice usually is organized as a partnership, a professional corporation, or an unincorporated professional association and, therefore, normally reflects a profit approach. Control of a nonprofit plan is maintained by the physicians if a majority of the plan's board of directors is composed of doctors. Moreover, there may be no need for the plan to establish a separate legal entity since the HMO can be structured within the professional corporation or partnership. In several of the older group practice examples, the physicians have accepted the entire risk of loss for both inpatient and outpatient care; however, most plans developed since 1970 have negotiated stop-loss agreements with outside insurance companies for excessive expenses. Finally, the group practice model may be characterized by a mixture of capitated prepayments and fee-for-service payments in the same setting. Both modes of finance are used by the physicians practicing at the health center, with all income pooled and then distributed according to a prearranged formula.

An example of the group practice model is the Western Clinic in Tacoma, Washington. The clinic is a partnership composed of 14 full-time and 1 part-time physicians, plus 3 physicians employed on a salaried basis. The partners determine all policies of the Western Clinic. The chief executive officer—who is the medical director—is a physician partner elected annually by the partners, who also elect the chairman of the Contract Committee (responsible for conducting contract negotiations with subscriber groups). A lay business manager, appointed by the partnership, manages the business and administrative functions. The clinic is financed by the private resources of the partners; therefore, a return on their investments is expected. After a maximum of three years of service, a physician employed by the clinic is eligible to purchase a share in the partnership. The cost of such a share is equal to 1 percent of the value of a single partnership in the clinic for the previous year. The amount is established by a valuation formula based on the depreciated value of furniture and fixtures, 90 percent of the accounts receivable, and the average earnings of the clinic in the preceding two years. The Western Clinic has found that it is too expensive to obtain underwriters to share the risk involved in prepaid arrangements for overuse and, thus, self-insures. Three area hospitals are used by the clinic for inpatient care; the clinic has no formal contract with these hospitals, but most clinic staff members have staff privileges. These relationships are outlined in Figure 20. Although this figure shows the health plan as a separate unit of the

Western Clinic, it is fully integrated within the partnership. Three out-lying clinics are used by the clinic's membership; these are not owned or controlled by the Western Clinic but are made available through formal working arrangements.

Financial and contractual arrangements, as they existed until 1976, are shown in Figure 21. Clinic income is derived from subscriber premiums, fees for service, and other income from the operation of the clinic's ancillary departments. Disbursement of income is to hospitals, to outside specialists, to other clinics, for out-of-area and emergency coverage, and for salaried physicians, with the remainder divided among the partnership through payment of salaries and a pre-established method for dividing such surplus. In 1976, the Western Clinic decided to end its capitated contracts with union and employer groups and revert to a complete fee-for-service payment system.

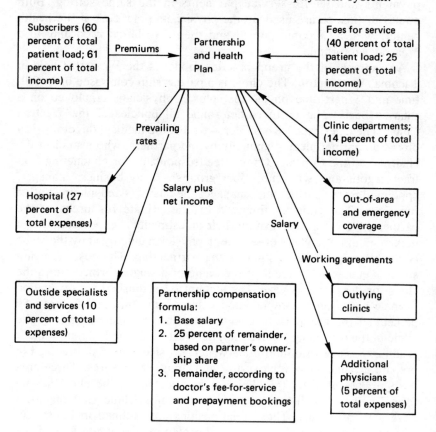

Figure 21   Western Clinic—fiscal activities.

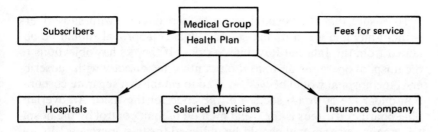

Figure 22   The group practice "provider" model.

Generally, the group practice "provider" model is organized as illustrated in Figure 22. This figure shows salaried physicians and an outside insurance company that provides insurance, marketing, and other functions, although, as with the Western Clinic, an insurance company need not be used. Similarly, the group practice physicians may be able to provide all necessary medical services without the assistance of salaried doctors.

Hospital "Provider" Models: Similar to the group practice approach, the hospital may contract directly with subscribers to provide prepaid health services. It can employ physicians directly, or it may contract, usually on a capitation arrangement, with an outside group practice. Insurance companies may be used to provide marketing and reinsurance, although some hospitals are large enough and have the financial stability to allow the hospital to self-insure.

Although all the models discussed in this chapter, whether nonprofit or for profit, must obtain an Internal Revenue Service (IRS) classification, in almost all instances, nonprofit HMOs have been granted a rating under Section 501(c)(4) of the IRS Code. As 501(c)(4) corporations, the nonprofit plans are exempt from payment of federal income taxes. In the case of the hospital model, this situation becomes more complex. Most hospitals are classified as 501(c)(3) nonprofit corporations, which exempts them from federal income tax and also enables them to receive contributions that are deductible by the contributors, as well as to receive grants from private foundations, which do not have to specify and control the grant expenditures and declare them as qualifying distributions. The 501(c)(3) status, of course, is preferable, because it allows the organization to more readily receive grants and contributions to defray development and start-up costs. This classification however, is not usually granted to HMOs; they normally receive the 501(c)(4) status.

To ensure that the hospital may contract directly with subscribers without any change in its tax status, advance approval should be obtained from the Internal Revenue Service. If the IRS has objections to the hospital operating an HMO (i.e., contracting directly with subscribers), the hospital would be well advised to establish a separate corporation under the 501(c)(4) section of the code for the HMO. An overlapping board of trustees is the usual method of joint control by the hospital. Again, IRS approval should be obtained for this approach.[7] In any event, the hospital's attorney should be asked to handle these legal issues.

Because of the similarity of this model and the group practice model, no example is given. Figure 23 describes the organizational arrangements for hospital "provider" models granted either 501(c)(3) or 501(c)(4) tax exemption status.

Individual Practice "Provider" or Foundation Models: As defined by Carolynn Steinwald,

. . . a Foundation for Medical Care (FMC) is an autonomous corporation sponsored and organized by a local (state or county) medical society concerned with the quality [of medical care]. It is governed by a Board of Directors, nominated and elected by the Board of its sponsoring Medical Society. Membership consists of physicians and sometimes osteopaths, belonging to the Medical Society, who voluntarily apply annually to enlist in the foundation.[8]

Like other HMOs, the Foundation for Medical Care (FMC) develops a package of comprehensive medical-care benefits and guarantees health care by contracting with various physicians in the local medical society and with hospitals and insurance companies. The principal objectives of the FMC are to assure accessibility of care through sponsorship of a prepaid health insurance program and to carefully monitor the quality of services, the appropriateness of delivery point, and the reasonableness of its cost.[9] Broadly, these objectives are implemented through two activities: Utilization Review (of claims processed) and Quality Audits (through peer review of claims).

[7]For an excellent review of this problem, see Robert S. Bromberg. "Tax Statute Problem." *In: Proceedings, Lawyer's Conference on Health Maintenance Organizations, August 20–21, 1971.* Washington, D.C., Group Health Association of America, 1971, pp. 36–53.

[8]Carolynn Steinwald. "Foundations for Medical Care." *In: Blue Cross Reports.* Research Series No. 7. Chicago, Blue Cross Association, 1971.

[9]Roy. *The Proposed Health Maintenance Organization Act of 1972,* p. 221.

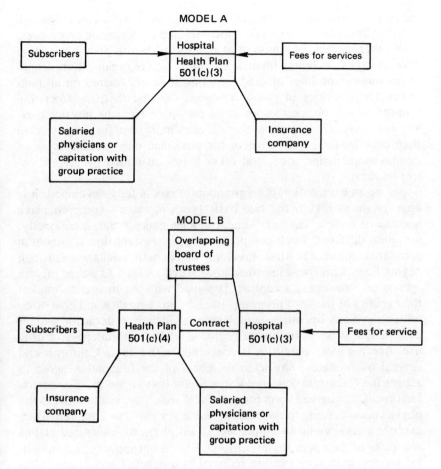

Figure 23   Two hospital "provider" models.

The major characteristic of the FMC is the preservation of the traditional method of health care delivery—solo fee-for-service medical
practice. As noted in Chapter 1, the foundation model is a compromise
between the traditional fee-for-service solo practitioner and the prepaid
group practitioner. The foundation approach was, in fact, first organized in 1954 in the San Joaquin Valley of California to protect the
fee-for-service solo practices threatened by the expansion of the
Kaiser-Permanente Medical Care Program—it incorporates some of
the most attractive features of the prepaid program but still maintains
the private practice of medicine. Another characteristic of the FMC is
that it assumes no risk in the delivery of health care (risk is defined as

the responsibility for covering all costs of the delivery of care). The risk
is either limited by contract or subcontracted to insurance companies.
Like other models, assumption of risk by the health plan is based on
several issues, including financial stability, size of organization, length
of operation, and lines of credit, and must be considered on an individual basis. Critics of FMCs, however, contend that, in effect, the
foundation is a physician-sponsored plan for which the physician assumes no risk. This situation, then, is even more ideal for the physician
than pure fee-for-service, where the physician must assume risks of
nonpayment, malpractice, and other losses sustained by private en-
trepreneurs.

Before an explanation of assumption of risk is fully developed, it is
appropriate to review the two basic types of FMCs—comprehensive
and claims review. Both are similar in legal makeup but, functionally,
are quite different. Each comprehensive FMC establishes a minimum
standards committee that develops the benefit package. Through
negotiations with fiscal intermediaries, such as Blue Cross or private
insurance companies, a contract is signed with the insurer to market
the benefits of the FMC program. In addition, a quality and cost committee develops operating guidelines that include criteria for patient
care: length of stay, treatment routines, and appropriateness of drug
use. Another FMC committee is concerned with fees; in California and
several other states, physician members of the foundation agree to
accept the California Relative Value Study (CRVS) and the conversion
factors that are agreed upon for each local area. Payment is made to the
physicians according to the relative-value system. The comprehensive
FMC then reviews up to 20 percent of all physician-generated claims
according to their peer-review criteria. Claims not approved by an individual physician-reviewer are referred to a panel of physicians. Ultimately, appeals can be made to county or state medical societies.[10]

The comprehensive FMC has the capability of sharing a small portion
of the underwriting risk (with the participating physicians receiving
reduced fees if the capitation does not cover services provided), although the majority of the risk is transferred to the fiscal intermediary.

In contrast to the comprehensive model, the claims-review FMC does
not sponsor a prepaid health plan. It only provides peer review by
physicians to the numerous fiscal intermediaries involved in financing
local health care—Blue Cross, Blue Shield, Medicare, Medicaid, and
so on. In both models, there exists the potential for becoming the
regional Professional Standards Review Organization.

[10]Richard H. Egdahl. "Foundations for Medical Care." *New England Journal of
Medicine, 288:*492, March 8, 1973.

With these concepts in mind, the FMC organizational arrangement can be developed. Figure 24 is based on the organizational arrangement of the San Joaquin Foundation for Medical Care—a comprehensive FMC. The foundation is sponsored by a county or state medical society. The board of directors of the medical society establishes the FMC and nominates and elects its board of trustees, who govern the foundation. Membership of the FMC is composed of physicians who apply voluntarily each year. Committee functions are similar to those previously discussed. In general, both the comprehensive and the claims-review FMCs are structured as illustrated in Figure 25, in which an additional individual practice association model (Model C) is shown—based on regulations contained in P.L. 93-222. Model C provides for the establishment of an HMO that is responsible for providing basic and supplemental health services to its members. The medical society establishes the HMO following a foundation approach (i.e., claims review, quality and peer review, and so on); the HMO assumes full financial risk, ob-

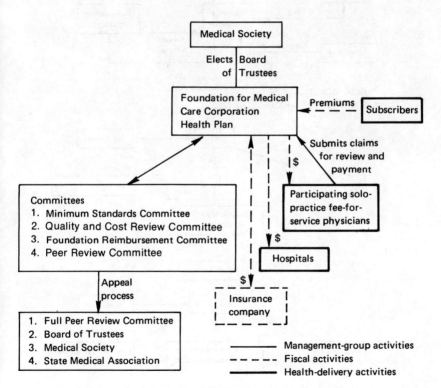

Figure 24   Organization chart for individual practice "provider" or Foundation for Medical Care model.

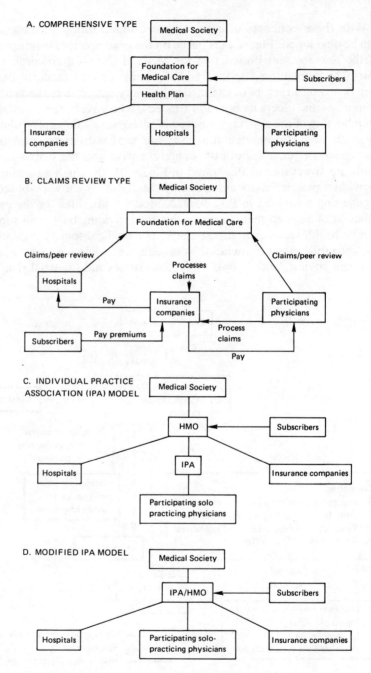

Figure 25 Individual practice "provider" model.

tains insurance, or makes other arrangements to cover risk. The HMO enters into an agreement with an individual practice association (IPA), usually by means of a formal contract, for the provision of health services. The IPA is a medical management organization engaged in arranging for the coordinated delivery of all or part of the health care services to members enrolled in an HMO. The IPA then enters into a service arrangement with individuals licensed to provide health services—persons practicing on a solo basis rather than on a group or salaried basis. An HMO member may reasonably expect the individual practitioner or the IPA to provide all contracted-for benefits, but because the member's agreement is with the HMO, it is the HMO that bears direct responsibility to its members for all benefits covered under the agreement.

A further, more recent modification of the IPA approach is shown as Model D, in which the IPA not only assumes a medical management role, but, in fact, becomes the HMO; thus, it assumes the added role of health plan management (assuring both medical and hospitalization services and underwriting of the benefit [insurance] package).

FMCs: Pro or Con

Traditional HMO managers seriously question the appropriateness of placing the HMO label on FMCs, especially those that are purely claims-review bodies. Certainly, P.L. 93-222 and P.L. 94-460 do allow "individual practice associations" to qualify as HMOs and thus become eligible to receive federal funds. Inclusion of the FMC in a book such as this on HMOs provides some credence to its acceptance by HMO observers. There are, however, many unanswered questions about the legitimacy of FMCs as HMOs—especially concerning their lack of the basic HMO precept of capitation with providers. The issue remains open. To help the student of medical group practice and health maintenance organizations decide, the following list of observations is provided:

1. Most HMOs use closed-panel (i.e., members only) group practice physicians; FMCs use open-panel, solo practice physicians.
2. Most HMOs capitate with providers; FMCs maintain the traditional fee-for-service reimbursement system.
3. Peer review is formalized in FMCs; it usually remains on an informal basis in most other HMOs, although Professional Standards Review Organizations (PSROs), when operational, may require all types of HMOs to develop formal peer-review mechanisms.

4. Patients can choose from among most local participating FMC physicians, while other HMO subscribers must choose from a limited number of physicians.

5. The foundation model is compatible with the present system; it is perhaps easier to move from the traditional delivery system to an FMC than to other HMO models.

6. Physicians' charges under the FMC are set unilaterally, as they are under other HMO models.

7. HMO models, other than FMCs, control both inpatient and outpatient costs; the FMC has not yet found a method for controlling hospital costs.

8. Under the FMC model, most risks are passed on to the insuring agency, while a number of other HMO models underwrite all risks.

9. FMCs are controlled by the local medical society, thereby reducing the chances of physician and other HMO competition.

10. The emphasis on marketing and enrollment in an FMC is directed toward area physicians, while other HMO models market to subscribers.

11. The FMC approach uses existing facilities and delivery systems, while other HMO models quite often build new ones.

12. FMC providers are dispersed, while other HMO models require centralized providers.

13. Salaried doctors may provide too little care, while FMC fee-for-service physicians may provide too much care; both situations are unacceptable.

14. FMCs cannot qualify for 501(c)(4) status because, to qualify, an HMO's medical staff cannot control the organization, and their salaries should be negotiated "at arm's length."

Relative Degree of Organization

The Department of Health, Education, and Welfare has used a classification system designed to show relative degrees of HMO organization. Although this system is no longer used, it does provide another dimension to HMO organizational structure, and it is a useful classification method. It identifies HMOs according to the plan's *control* of its component parts; it shows the relative degree of organization and centralization of the health manpower and facilities. To a lesser degree, the classification system suggests the relative extent of commitment on the part of the HMO to the enrolled population (i.e., exclusive full-time salaried physicians or part-time physicians; control of all facilities and operation of a hospital or use of hospital facilities through plan doctors' staff privileges). The four classifications are *highly centralized, moderately centralized, decentralized,* and *network.*

HIGHLY CENTRALIZED

The plan controls all major components of the HMO delivery system. Facilities are owned or operated by the HMO. Physicians usually are salaried full-time employees. There is minimal, if any, fee-for-service practice. The Kaiser Foundation Health Plans and the Group Health Cooperative of Puget Sound are examples of this classification.

MODERATELY CENTRALIZED

These plans use either full-time or part-time physicians in group practices. There may be contracts with outside facilities for hospital and ancillary services, although staff admitting privileges may be used in lieu of formalized hospital contracts. The Health Insurance Plan of Greater New York and the Group Health Association of Washington, D.C. represent this type of organization.

DECENTRALIZED

These HMOs use individual practicing physicians or groups of affiliated physicians. The plan does not own or operate its own hospitals or other facilities but relies on community health facilities. Fee-for-service remuneration is used. The FMC approach, such as the San Joaquin Foundation, is included in this category.

NETWORK

In the 1977 HMO census completed by the Group Health Association of America, the term "network" was used to describe a type of HMO practice. In effect, the network is another method of describing the relative degree of HMO centralization. This "network of delivery points" was defined in the 1977 census as a "metropolitan, regional, or statewide confederation of independent and separate medical care delivery points, each providing a full range of comprehensive services, and *contractually* linked to a central point of accountability."[11] The census reported a total of 14 network plans in 1977, as shown in Table 10. (Please refer to the glossary for other definitions of network.)

[11]Group Health Association of America. *National HMO Census Survey: 1977 Summary.* Washington, D.C., 1977.

TABLE 10   HMOs—Type of Practice and Membership

Type of Practice	Plans	Membership
Group	106	5,708,130
Foundation/IPA	40	413,852
Network	14	186,044
Other	5	22,650
TOTAL	165	6,330,676

Source: Adapted from Group Health Association of America. *National HMO Census Survey: 1977 Summary.* Washington, D.C., 1977, pp. unnumbered (Table 4).

Legal Issues

In each of the figures presented in this chapter, contractual arrangements among the components of the HMO are outlined. These include contracts between the health plan and subscribers (the policy), the health plan and providers, and the health plan and other outside organizations such as insurance companies. Contracts are agreements between two or more people or organizations; as such the contract sets forth the rights and obligations of the parties. Contracts are enforceable by law and must contain the following elements:

1. A legal purpose
2. Two parties of legal age and legally capable of making a contract
3. Absence of fraud
4. Meeting of the minds
5. An offer and acceptance with consideration
6. A description of the rights and responsibilities of both parties

Individual subscribers consummate contracts between themselves and the HMO by signing an application for enrollment under one of the HMO programs; they are the policyholders. Representatives of groups (i.e., employers, union presidents, and so on) complete the contract for groups of subscribers and, therefore, also are referred to as the policyholders. The application agreement form is the legal document outlining the obligations of both the policyholder and the HMO. It describes the type of coverage to be provided by the HMO and the premium level to be prepaid by the policyholder for services to be provided at a future date. The group subscriber rarely sees a copy of the entire policy between himself or his employer or union and the HMO; he usually receives a verbal description of the benefit package and the premium structure and may receive a brochure that generally describes the benefit package. The brochure and the signed agreement for enrollment, however, refer to a set of benefits and exclusions described in detail elsewhere. Generally, the plan has a list of benefits and exclusions for each program offering, which is available at the plan's administrative or enrollment offices. Problems arise between the plan and the subscribers when this list of benefits is not fully described to the enrollee. As expected, subscribers often feel they have coverage when there may be exclusions, limitations, deductions, or copayments. In some instances, aggressive marketing agents fail to explicitly state the benefits offered and all exclusions. If the subscriber can show proof that the package was not fully explained, he may have a legitimate claim for coverage of those items not described during the marketing activities. It is important, then, to fully describe, explain, and provide, *in writing*, the benefit package, including exclusions, and premium structures. One of the most important selling points of the HMO is its contractual guarantee of 24-hour coverage. A compromising of this posture by lack of appropriate communication of covered services can ultimately weaken the market position of the HMO in the community. In one instance, the Group Health Association of Washington, D.C. (GHA) states in its contract with subscribers that it will put forth its "best efforts" to provide services but does not "guarantee" services. This clause appears to soften the responsibility of the plan to provide care and subsequently may weaken the plan's competitive position. Other HMOs, such as Ross-Loos and Kaiser, write the plan subscriber contracts so that contractual problems initially will go to compulsory arbitration rather than end in a court suit—particularly in cases of possible malpractice. Both the "best efforts" clause and the compulsory arbitration feature have been upheld in court tests, although few, if any, plans other than GHA use the "best efforts" clause. With regard to arbitration, the plan must make certain that it is binding in the state in which it operates. Only in 30 states can contracts be made in anticipation of some possible conflict arising in the future. Then, only if the provider(s) and patient in a malpractice dispute have specifically agreed to do so, may arbitration be used in lieu of traditional litigation.

Thus, three legal issues concerning the policyholder's contract are noteworthy:

1. *Payment:* The subscriber agreement must specify the amount and due date. The specific method of determining the *appropriate* payment should be described.

2. *Benefit package:* The HMO must clearly outline its obligations, as a self-protective measure. Thus, the subscriber should be given the

benefit package in written form, including all exclusions, deductions, and copayments.

3. *Communication mechanism:* There must be a method of ongoing communication between the parties to address such areas as grievance procedures, quality procedures, arbitration, malpractice, and so on.

Contracts with providers, both physicians and hospitals, also are of major importance to guaranteeing the delivery of health services. There are several issues that are of major concern to the HMO when using the resources of a private physician group. For nonprofit HMOs, it is imperative that the proprietary medical group that "profits" from the provision of medical services be separated from the control of the HMO. Accordingly, the determination of the IRS nonprofit tax status will, in part, be based on evidence that the HMO deals with its medical group "at arm's length." The "arm's length" rule applies not only to non-physician group control of the HMO but to the negotiation of the individual physician's salaries. Naturally, a for-profit HMO does not have this problem.

The physician group contract deals with capitation rates, the use of part-time and full-time plan physicians, incentive payments, reporting requirements, contingency payments and sharing the risk of losses, grievance procedures, and use of HMO facilities, staff, and equipment. Again, payment, benefit package, and communication mechanisms should be clearly stated. Contracts with other outside organizations, such as insurance companies, Blue Cross, and hospitals, must precisely describe the services to be provided, payment for these services, and a communication linkage. Because of the importance of these contracts, it is suggested by most HMO administrators that a lawyer be retained to work out the details.

In addition, several outside organizations will need working agreements with the HMO. Such is the case with a hospital that provides inpatient services to the HMO enrollees through the staff-admitting privileges of HMO physicians. Although these agreements may not be legally binding on the parties involved, it is appropriate for the plan's lawyer to review each agreement before its execution.[12]

---

[12]Additional information concerning HMO contracts may be found in U.S. Department of Health, Education, and Welfare, Health Maintenance Organization Service. *Lawyer's Manual on Health Maintenance Organization.* Rockville, Md., n.d. For a further description of the specific elements that should be included in an HMO/IPA foundation model, see Aileen Johnson, Daniel Sheehy, and Richard Sasuly. *Foundations for Medical Care Health Maintenance Organizations: A Planning Manual.* Stockton, Calif., American Association of Foundations for Medical Care, 1974. Other data also can be found in William A. MacColl. *Group Practice and Prepayment of Medical Care.* Washington, D.C., Public Affairs Press, 1966, pp. 106–108.

Summary

This chapter reviewed the organizational structures of four HMO models. HMOs can be sponsored by any number of organizations—hospitals, group practices, local governments. These organizations help establish the HMO and develop its legal entity. The new organization then becomes responsible for HMO activities through its board of trustees, if nonprofit, or its board of directors, if for profit.

The four organizational structures include community organization, carrier, industry-union, and provider models. Community organization models are established and controlled by community groups, such as consumer groups, neighborhood health centers, and so on. Included in this category are the associations and cooperatives discussed in Chapter 2. This model's characteristics include a nonprofit membership corporation, a board of trustees nominated or elected by the membership, and a membership open to any area resident. Ultimate control of the plan resides with the membership. Group Health Association, Inc. of Washington, D.C. is an example of the community organization model.

The carrier model is characterized by sponsorship and control by either an indemnity insurance company or a BC/BS program. Such sponsorship of HMOs is appropriate because of their major role as health care insurers and because of their knowledge and experience in many of the HMO functions—marketing and enrollment, underwriting, financing, and so on. The Metro Health Plan of Detroit, operated jointly by Michigan Blue Cross and Michigan Blue Shield, is an example of this category of HMOs. Another example of the carrier model, the Columbia Medical Plan of Columbia, Maryland, was built around the consortium approach—coordinated management for several independent organizations. This method appears to have the advantage of a broad management base, large financial reserves, a large pool of management talent, and great flexibility; however, other problems may stem from long lines of communication and more complex coordination.

The industry-union, or "Kaiser," model includes HMOs developed initially for employees by their employers or their unions; for individuals; for federal or state employees; or for eligibles of federal, state, or local public-assistance programs. These plans are developed by laymen who may not necessarily represent the subscribers and may be both for profit and nonprofit; several are investor owned. The most prominent example of this model is the Kaiser-Permanente Medical Care Program.

The last category—provider models—are described by three approaches: group practice, hospital, and individual practice. Sponsored and owned by a group of physicians, the group practice approach is organized around a medical group—either a partnership, a professional corporation, or an unincorporated professional association. Control is maintained by the physicians, and the plan may contain a mixture of capitated prepayments and fee-for-service payments in the same setting. The Western Clinic of Tacoma, Washington is an example of the group practice provider model; such plans do not usually own or operate inpatient facilities but do operate outpatient group practice clinics.

The hospital model is similar to the group practice approach, with the hospital acting as the health plan. Because of difficulties encountered in obtaining the I.R.C. 501(c)(3) classification for the health plan, hospitals may be forced to set up a separate corporation under the I.R.C. 501(c)(4) classification. An overlapping board of trustees would ensure control of this plan by the hospital.

The final provider approach is the individual practice model, usually referred to as a Foundation for Medical Care (FMC). FMCs are established by local medical societies to assure accessibility of care through the sponsorship of a prepaid health plan and to provide a careful monitoring of quality through a formal peer-review program. Because the FMC uses solo practitioners and fee-for-service reimbursement, critics have suggested that this model not be considered a full-fledged HMO, although the FMC is recognized by the HMO law as a form of HMO.

Another dimension of HMO organization is provided by reviewing the relative degree of HMO organization. Plans can be categorized as highly centralized (control of all major components of the HMO), moderately centralized (use of full- and/or part-time providers and outside facilities), decentralized (foundation using solo practicing physicians with no ownership of delivery facilities), or networks.

References

Carey, Sarah C., et al. *Health Maintenance Organizations: An Introduction and Survey of Recent Developments.* Washington, D.C., Lawyers' Committee for Civil Rights Under Law, 1972, pp. 60–81.

Egdahl, Richard H. "Foundations for Medical Care." *New England Journal of Medicine, 288:* 491–498, March 8, 1973.

Epstein, Steven B. "HMOs and the Law." *Group Practice, 22*(8): 9–15, August 1973.

Gintzig, Leon, and Shouldice, Robert G. "Prepaid Group Practice—A Comparative Study." Part I. 3 Vols. Washington, D.C., The George Washington University, 1971.

Group Health Association of America, Inc., Department of Education and Training. *Sample Operating Prepaid Group Practice Medical Care Programs: Organizational and Financial Relationships.* Washington, D.C., 1972. Mimeographed.

Gumbiner, Robert. *HMO: Putting It All Together*. St. Louis, Mo., C. V. Mosby Co., 1975, pp. 31–51.

Johnson, Aileen; Sheehy, Daniel; and Sasuly, Richard. *Foundations for Medical Care Health Maintenance Organizations: A Planning Manual*. Stockton, Calif., American Association of Foundations for Medical Care, 1974.

LeCompte, Roger B. *Prepaid Group Practice: A Manual*. Chicago, Blue Cross Association, 1972, pp. 1.14–1.26.

Prussin, Jeffrey A. "Health Maintenance Organizations: Organizational and Financial Models." *Hospital Progress*, 55(4):33–35, April 1974.

Rafkind, Faith B. *Health Maintenance Organizations: Some Perspectives*. Chicago, Blue Cross Association, 1972, pp. 25–46.

Roy, William R. *The Proposed Health Maintenance Organization Act of 1972*. Washington, D.C., Science and Health Communications Group, 1972, pp. 184–190, 220–224, 271–272.

Steinwald, Carolynn. "Foundations for Medical Care." *In: Blue Cross Reports*. Research Series No. 7. Chicago, Blue Cross Association, 1971.

5

The Providers

The HMO brings together providers and consumers, matches health needs with health vendors, and helps fulfill the goals of each group. Without consumer demand for health care and providers to supply scarce health resources, there would be no need for HMOs or any other delivery systems. There is, however, a great demand for health care by consumers and a scarce supply of health resources—manpower, facilities, and equipment. The HMO is one of the best and most efficient ways to match these two components of health-delivery systems.

Chapter 5 discusses providers—physicians and hospitals. Because most HMOs use groups of physicians, the major considerations here will be how they are structured and how they are reimbursed for their services—through both normal income and incentives. The attitudes of the medical groups and control of their activities also will be discussed. Then the relationship of hospitals and HMOs will be reviewed. Chapter 6 considers consumers— their opinions, attitudes, and viewpoints on the methods used to serve urban and rural populations— and the methods used by HMOs to serve consumers in underserved populations.

The Physicians' Group

The medical group practice arrangement began in the 1880s with the formation of the Mayo Clinic in Rochester, Minnesota. Other medical group practices that were formed in the first years of the twentieth century included the Ross-Loos, Western, Palo Alto, and Bridge clinics. The proliferation of medical groups, however, did not occur until the 1930s, with the appearance of specialty boards. With an increasing number of specialty boards and a concurrent increase in the number of physicians who continued their education to qualify for board certification, physicians sought an environment in which they could practice in their limited specialties. They also were seeking a situation where other disciplines of medicine, as well as specialized equipment and diagnostic facilities, would be readily available in the same location. "Other factors which contributed to the rapid growth of medical groups include the surge of definite surgery, with its concomitant need for technical co-workers and team work; the early popularity of spas and sanatoria with their need for specialized staff; the development of large individual practices, with the consequent need for professional associates; and the gradual development of group patterns in clinical teaching."[1]

The number of medical groups has increased dramatically since the 1880s. By 1926, there were 125 groups; in 1932, more than 220. The total number of groups increased from 1,546 in 1959 to 4,289 in 1965, and to 6,371 in 1969.[2] This is an average annual increase of 18.5 percent from 1959 to 1965, and a 10.4 percent increase from 1965 to 1969 (9.5 percent adjusted).[3] The total number of physicians practicing in groups increased from 13,009 in 1959 to 28,381 in 1965, and to an adjusted 38,834 in 1969.[4] Other characteristics of these groups suggest that the largest percentage increase, between 1965 and 1969, was in the category of physicians practicing a single specialty within a group. Full-time group physicians increased at an annual average of 9.4 percent, while part-time physicians increased only 5.4 percent. The sizes of groups, however, have decreased; the average number of physicians was 8.4 in 1959, 6.6 in 1965, and 6.3 in 1969.[5] In 1965, more than 10 percent of the nation's nonfederal physicians were practicing in groups

---

[1]American Association of Medical Clinics, American Medical Association, and Medical Group Management Association. *Group Practice, Guidelines to Joining or Forming a Medical Group*. Chicago, American Medical Association, 1970, pp. 1–2.

[2]B. E. Balfe and Mary E. McNamara. *Survey of Medical Groups in the U.S., 1965.* Special Statistical Series. Chicago, American Medical Association, 1968, p. 2; and Mary E. McNamara and Clifford Todd. "A Survey of Group Practice in the United States, 1969." *American Journal of Public Health*, 60(7):1303, 1311, July 1970.

[3]Adjustments were made in the total number of groups because of changes in the AMA's group definition for 1965 to 1969 and difficulties in reported data on age of the groups.

[4]McNamara and Todd. "Survey of Group Practice," p. 1312.

[5]*Ibid.*

as compared to approximately 17.6 percent in 1969. Some 91 percent of these physicians were engaged full time in group practice. According to the *Profile of Medical Practice,* published by the American Medical Association in 1976, there were 8,483 medical groups in the United States. These groups represented a total of 66,842 physicians or 23.5 percent of all active nonfederal physicians in the United States.

PREPAYMENT

In Balfe and McNamara's 1965 survey, 88 groups were identified as having a significant amount (50 percent or more) of prepayment activity, whereas only 85 groups were so identified in McNamara and Todd's 1969 study (although a total of 396 groups were involved with some prepaid activity). No data concerning prepaid activity were available in AMA's 1976 study. This strongly indicates that groups with more than 50 percent of their activity prepaid did not significantly increase during this period. In 1969, the survey results indicated that approximately 6 percent of the groups, representing 6,540 physicians, were involved with a varying proportion of prepayments and fee-for-service payments.

DEFINITION OF GROUP PRACTICE

The most commonly accepted definition of group practice is that provided by AMA: "Group medical practice is the application of medical services by three or more physicians formally organized to provide medical care, consultation, diagnosis, or treatment, through the joint use of equipment and personnel, and with income from medical practice distributed in accordance with methods previously determined by members of the group."[6]

P.L. 93-222 further describes requirements for "medical groups" and "individual practice associations" that must be met by HMOs receiving federal funds under this statute. Specifically, the federal regulations implementing P.L. 93-222 state:

"Medical group" means a partnership, association, or other group—

1. Which is composed of health professionals licensed to practice medicine or osteopathy and of such other licensed health professionals (including dentists, optometrists, and podiatrists) as are necessary for the provision of health services for which the group is responsible;

[6] American Association of Medical Clinics et al. *Group Practice,* p. 3.

2. A majority of the members of which are licensed to practice medicine or osteopathy; and
3. The members of which

    i. As their principal (over 50 percent) professional activity and as a group responsibility engage in the coordinated practice of their profession for a health maintenance organization or which group presents a time-phased plan, not to exceed three years, to meet this requirement to which they are committed which is acceptable to the Secretary;

    ii. Pool their income from practice as members of the group and distribute it among themselves according to a prearranged salary or drawing account or other plan;

    iii. Share medical and other records and substantial portions of major equipment and of professional, technical, and administrative staff;

    iv. Utilize such additional professional personnel, allied health professions personnel, and other health personnel as are available and appropriate for the efficient delivery of the services of the members of the group; and

    v. Arrange for and encourage continuing education in the field of clinical medicine and related areas for the members of the group.

"Individual practice association" means a partnership, corporation, association, or other legal entity which has as its primary objective the delivery or arrangements for the delivery of health services and which has entered into a written services arrangement or arrangements with persons who are licensed to practice medicine, osteopathy, dentistry, podiatry, optometry, or other health professions in a State and a majority of whom are licensed to practice medicine or osteopathy. Such written service arrangement shall provide:

1. That such persons shall provide their professional services in accordance with a compensation arrangement established by the entity; and
2. To the extent feasible

    i. That such persons shall utilize such additional professional personnel, allied health professions personnel, and other health personnel as are available and appropriate for the effective and efficient delivery of the services of the persons who are parties to the arrangement;

    ii. For the sharing by such persons of medical and other records, equipment, and professional, technical, and administrative staff; and

    iii. For the arrangement and encouragement of the continuing education of such persons in the field of clinical medicine and related areas.[7]

The definitions of both the AMA and federal regulations emphasize the organization of physicians within a formalized, coordinated setting

---

[7]U.S. Department of Health, Education, and Welfare, Public Health Service. "Health Maintenance Organizations, Proposed Rulemaking." *Federal Register,* 39(90):16423, May 8, 1974.

that has become a legal entity—either a partnership, corporation, association, or some other arrangement. Note that even the individual practice association, as defined by the HMO law, requires a formalized joint effort by individual participating physicians. There are advantages and disadvantages to group practice, as described in these definitions.

ADVANTAGES AND DISADVANTAGES OF GROUP PRACTICE

Dr. William A. MacColl identifies 12 advantages of group practice to physicians:

1. Sharing of knowledge and responsibility which allows the physician to apply himself to that part of the practice of medicine for which he is best trained.
2. Best utilization of the skills of the specialist as well as those of the general practitioner. The specialist in a group is not required to function as a generalist, and, conversely, the generalist can act in the capacity of the "manager" of the patient's care by controlling the overall care of the patient.
3. Keeping up with all the developments in medicine more easily than in solo practice because of the free exchange among the specialists and generalists in the group.
4. High standards resulting from this interchange of ideas. Since no one in a group wishes to be associated with a second rater, the net standard tends to be the sum of the high standards of the individuals. Each physician's practice is open to all others through the use of unit medical records—one record for each member, which follows him throughout his enrollment in the HMO.
5. Money and time for study and training, which are usually considered a part of the remuneration of the physician in the group. In fact, group practice physicians normally spend less of their time seeing patients than do doctors in fee-for-service— five hours a week less. This time becomes available for hospital obligations, study, and continuing education and training; group practice physicians are as productive as their counterparts in fee-for-service even with a shorter period set aside to see patients.
6. Regular rotation of hours and a sharing of the after-clinic emergencies. Thus, most of the staff is relatively free in the evenings, on weekends, and on holidays. Scheduling of vacations with the knowledge that several of one's associates are available to care for patients provides for greater continuity of care.
7. Immediate income available to the physician who has just completed the long and costly training period plus a ready-made practice

which can be built upon as the young physician's reputation and skills increase. Starting incomes in group practice are comparable to those in the local community, and continue to parallel community-wide incomes as the physician's practice increases.

8. Additional benefits, including malpractice insurance, time-loss and medical coverage, life insurance, occasionally an automobile, social security and retirement programs, and incentive payments.

9. Relief from the business aspects of the practice of medicine for which most doctors are not trained. The physician does not have to be directly concerned with the billing and collection of fees, the employment of personnel, purchase of supplies and equipment, payment of rent, and so on. He usually is not required to make a large capital contribution to join the group and has a reasonable assurance of a stable income.

10. The ability to present his views concerning policy and programming within the group within a very short period after joining. Most groups are autonomous and self-governing, and the young physician may be granted voting privileges after a short probationary period, usually one to three years.

11. Availability of ancillary services and personnel, and facilities.

12. Cooperative spirit engendered in the "family of doctors for the family of patients." The group practice physician shares in the professional care of the group as his patient shares in the total services the group has to offer. The sense of professionalism is enhanced; group practice is said to offer a check on the possibility of error and a friendly support in adversity.[8]

There are several disadvantages to physician participation in group practice.

1. Physicians may experience some loss of freedom to practice as they wish and some loss of individuality. Because group practice requires a coordinated effort, individual physicians must conform to group patterns, guidelines, and behavior. Work schedules, sharing of patient loads, and questioning by one's peers of treatments provided are a part of group practice.

2. Two aspects of physician income may present a problem—level and method of sharing. Most group practice salaries are based on several factors that are not relevant to solo practice. First, the level of compensation usually follows the median incomes per specialty earned

[8]William A. MacColl. *Group Practice and Prepayment of Medical Care.* Washington, D.C., Public Affairs Press, 1966, pp. 89–91.

by solo practitioners in the community, with a few group practitioners receiving either lower or higher than average salaries. The opportunity for huge solo practice incomes is not available in group practice. Second, the group physicians must arrive at a suitable income-sharing arrangement, usually on a yearly basis. Acceptable arrangements are sometimes difficult to achieve, with the potential for disputes ever present.

3. Physicians have to conform to established levels of practice, quality of care, formulary, and operating procedures. Like all other organized endeavors, the theory of unity of objective places limits on operating procedures and methods, as well as on the establishment of levels of acceptable effort on the part of the organization's personnel. Physicians not familiar with such organization constraints may find such limitations unacceptable.

4. Patients are "plan patients," not a single "physician's patients." As such, the control of the patient's care may reside with a group rather than with one practitioner. Because of office hour scheduling, patients may not always see the same physician each time they come in for medical care. Although most HMOs use the "plan patient" concept, several HMOs have experimented with assigning individual patients to a general practitioner or internist at the time of enrollment. The physician is then responsible for "managing" the patient's care while he is an enrollee in the plan. The "managing physician" is responsible for the total coordination of the enrollee's medical care. Nevertheless, each of the group's physicians shares and suffers to some degree from errors of his associates. Sharing the liability of the group by the individual physicians may be unacceptable to some physicians.

5. Finally, because of the division and departmentalization of effort in group practice, an undesirable degree of overspecialization may result.[9]

PHYSICIAN ATTITUDES CONCERNING MEDICAL GROUP PRACTICE AND HMOs

Ever since the prepaid group practice movement began during the early years of this century, organized medicine has posed a threat for, and has resisted, the closed-panel concept. A closed panel is an arrange-

---

[9]American Association of Medical Clinics et al. *Group Practice*, p. 11. See also, American Association of Medical Clinics, American Medical Association, and Medical Group Management Association. "Advantages and Disadvantages of Group Practice." *Illinois Medical Journal*, 135(4):512–513, April 1969.

ment whereby membership in a physician group is restricted by the present membership to selected individuals. Local medical societies objected to this concept because they felt that prepaid group practice would severely limit the solo practitioner's ability to compete for patients, that prepaid plans and group practice represented a step toward socialized medicine, that there would be lay interference in the doctor-patient relationship, and that the use of advertising by the plan and the potential corporate practice of medicine were unethical. Strong resistance from these local medical societies took the form of "professional isolationism" with plan physicians ostracized, denied hospital privileges, and refused membership in the medical society. Recruitment of physicians by health plans became difficult, and final resolution of the early plans' grievances was achieved only after long legal actions in which the prepaid group practice concepts were upheld.

Today, however, most local medical societies do not openly confront newly developing HMOs. There continues to be some resistance, but usually only on the part of a few members; generally, the local medical societies have reluctantly accepted HMOs as competitors. This change in attitude by the medical societies reflects an important change in the attitudes of individual physicians toward HMOs, as emphasized by the results of a recent (1969) random-sample survey conducted by the American Medical Association (4,500 AMA members and 3,000 non-members). The study results indicated that 30 percent of AMA's members and 47 percent of nonmember respondents preferred some type of prepaid capitation practice over fee-for-service practice. Moreover, a 1972 study of senior medical students, interns, residents, faculty, and full-time staff showed that 50 percent of those responding felt that "working in a prepaid group practice setting is a good way for doctors to practice medicine."[10] The 1969 AMA study, however, identified only 396 group practices in the United States, with 6,540 physicians who provided at least some care on a prepayment basis. Of this number, 85 groups, with 3,900 physicians, had more than 50 percent prepaid activity and approximately one-third were affiliated with the Health Insurance Plan of Greater New York (HIP).[11]

Some additional information concerning physician attitudes is available from a study by D. C. McElrath. Although the study is dated (1958) and deals with a nonrandom selection of medical groups in HIP,

---

[10]U.S. Department of Health, Education, and Welfare, Health Maintenance Organization Service. *Questions Physicians Are Asking About HMOs and the Answers.* Rockville, Md., 1972.

[11]William R. Roy. *The Proposed Health Maintenance Organization Act of 1972.* Washington, D.C., Science and Health Communications Group, 1972, p. 169.

its results are of interest because they identify some major plan operating problems. As reported by Donabedian, the study showed that

> About two-thirds of the physicians felt that prepaid group practice was preferable to the traditional form and permitted them to practice, in association with their colleagues, the kind of medicine carried out at a teaching hospital. But a quarter to a third of physicians were also aware of certain adverse effects that they attributed to this form of organization. They felt that by becoming associated with the type of practice they had lost status in the eyes of medical colleagues as well as of the patients they served. They felt that they did not have time to do a good job. They felt that their patients were demanding, made excessive use of service, complained too much and were lacking in loyalty. For an appreciable number of physicians then, prepaid group practice was seen as having an adverse effect on the patient-physician relationship and a hampering effect on their own careers especially in matters that involved the medical community in general.[12]

In another study, conducted by Gintzig and Shouldice in 1970, the administrators of 15 HMO prototypes were surveyed.[13] The results of the interview surveys showed that a majority of physicians practicing in communities where HMOs were located were skeptical of prepaid health plans for several reasons. First, there was the fear of change from one system to another, and the fear of possible loss of income that change might induce. Physicians feared the unpredictability of growth in this relatively new mode of health care delivery and, in turn, its effect on their current fee-for-service practices. Second, there was the fear that the prepayment propaganda initiated by their medical societies would limit their freedom to practice as individuals and to set their own fees. Finally, there was the fear engendered by some physicians' negative experiences with both military service medicine and actual delivery under a capitation arrangement.

In a 1975 study conducted by David Mechanic, orientations and attitudes of a group of prepaid physicians were compared to those of a group of nonprepaid physicians.[14] He found that doctors have a concept of how much time they should devote to their practice relative to payment received. Capitated physicians feel no financial incentive to

---

[12]Avedis Donabedian. "An Evaluation of Prepaid Group Practice." *Inquiry, VI*(3):10, September 1969.

[13]Leon Gintzig and Robert G. Shouldice. "Prepaid Group Practice: An Analysis as a Delivery System." Washington, D.C., The George Washington University, 1972, p. 12. Mimeographed.

[14]David Mechanic. "The Organization of Medical Practice and Practice Orientations Among Physicians in Prepaid and Nonprepaid Primary Care Settings." *Medical Care, XIII*(3):189, March 1975.

deal with increased patient demand by increasing their work hours, while nonprepaid physicians are more likely to increase their hours to meet high patient demand. Moreover, the study showed that the fee-for-service doctors spend more time in direct patient activity than prepaid doctors, with "patients seen" as the best indicator of income for fee-for-service physicians. Prepaid doctors are more likely to deal with increased patient demand by delaying patient care, using the queue as a rationing device, or allowing patients to see a specially available, urgent-care physician. This practice may result in an assembly-line practice and consequent consumer dissatisfaction with the patient-physician relationship. Thus, there is the tendency in HMOs to limit not only inpatient hospital care but also the resources available for ambulatory medical care relative to demand. This can be resolved by the addition of more ambulatory-care resources, developing better patterns of manpower utilization, using physician surrogates and other paraprofessionals—in other words, by becoming more efficient.

Plan administrators and medical directors should recognize that physicians are concerned with these issues, should confront the issues in physician recruitment efforts, and should develop methods for ensuring that the problems are adequately solved. Informal progress reports should be included in the administrator's conversations with his plan physicians to help pinpoint any issues that have not been resolved or to allay any continuing fear or skepticism on their part.

Another indicator of physician attitudes toward HMOs is turnover rate. In general, turnover rates for physicians who have been with a plan for more than two or three years appear to be very low—from 2 to 3 percent per year. For the Kaiser Foundation Health Plan, Northern California Region, the rates were close to 6 percent for 1970. The reason proffered for the higher than average turnover rate was the lure of higher outside incomes. In three other HMO prototypes, the turnover rate is less than 2 percent—Group Health Cooperative of Puget Sound (Seattle), the Group Health Plan of St. Paul, Minnesota, and the Health Insurance Plan of Greater New York. Rates are somewhat higher during the two- to three-year physician probationary period most plans maintain.[15] It appears that after the physicians are in the program for more than three years, their feelings toward the HMO become more positive.

[15] U.S. Department of Health, Education, and Welfare. *Questions Physicians Are Asking*, pp. 3–4; and Wallace Cook. "Profile of the Permanente Physician." *In: The Kaiser-Permanente Medical Care Program.* Edited by Anne Somers. New York, Commonwealth Fund, 1971, p. 104.

WHY PHYSICIANS JOIN A PREPAID GROUP PRACTICE

The advantages for the physician joining an HMO have been discussed, but what are some of the actual reasons given for joining a group practice prepaid plan? Based on Kaiser-Permanente experience and that of other HMO prototypes, the following list recounts some of the reasons:

1. The growing national reputation for quality prepaid multispecialty HMO practice
2. Personal friends and professional associates practice in the group
3. Ability to practice medicine without immediate financial consideration
4. Time off, colleague availability for consultation, and good coverage for calls
5. Excellent retirement plans
6. A preference for capitated rather than fee-for-service practice
7. Security, convenience, and stability of practice within the group
8. Incomes comparable with those of colleagues in fee-for-service practice

The Structure of Physician Groups

Like the HMO health plan, the HMO medical group must be organized so that medical care can be provided in a coordinated, efficient, and effective manner. The group must maintain an adequate level of professional and paraprofessional staff, as well as adequate facilities for their practices.

STAFFING

Earlier in this chapter, AMA's definition of what constituted a medical group—three or more physicians formally organized—was reviewed. The Medical Group Management Association (MGMA), one of the national group practice associations, also considers medical groups to be the organized practice of three or more physicians. Two other national group practice associations, the American Group Practice Association (AGPA) and the Group Health Association of America (GHAA), include in their medical group standards the specification that medical groups be composed of at least seven full-time physicians with not less than five practicing in different major specialties. Which of these definitions most accurately describes a group practice in the United States? In contrast to the results of AMA's 1969 survey of group practice, McNamara and Todd's survey indicates that the "average size of prepaid groups was 16.5 physicians, but this figure is statistically biased upward by the prepaid giants. It is of greater significance that the medium-size group is 4.8 physicians, and 72 percent have eight or fewer physicians."[16] The same study also revealed that 75 percent of all groups with more than 50 percent prepaid activity are composed of more than seven physicians.

It appears, then, that the average minimum prepaid group is composed of somewhere between five to eight physicians. This does not suggest that there is an optimal size for HMO medical groups; it only suggests that many HMO prototypes have been functioning effectively at these staffing levels. Staffing levels depend on several factors, paramount of which is number of enrollees.

An approach to staffing requires integrated planning, as discussed in Chapter 7—planning based on some generalized HMO guidelines. The staffing of HMOs usually is developed around a staffing ratio of one physician for each 950 to 1,100 enrollees. This ratio is much lower than the national norm (1:700) because of the unified efficiency and effectiveness of HMO operation. Moreover, the ratio varies with the age of the HMO, the demographic characteristics of the population served, and the expectations of the membership population concerning the availability of medical care. Table 11 shows the 1969 staffing ratios of some HMOs; the Columbia Plan's ratio of 1:454 is explained by the fact that Columbia was in the initial stages of operation and had a relatively small enrollment group (approximately 5,000). Approximately 17.5 full-time equivalent physicians serve all Western Clinic patients, 60 percent of whom are prepaid enrollees and the remainder, fee-for-service patients. Generally, there will be a higher ratio of physicians to enrollees during the early months of operation, perhaps as high as one physician to 500 enrollees, because of the normally low number of enrollees at an HMO's onset. After several years of operation, the ratio should drop to a level approximately 1:950 or 1:1,100, as the enrollment increases and as the plan becomes more efficient. It appears that ratios lower than 1:1,200 may be inappropriate, since there may be a greater probability for underutilization of services.

The projected number of enrollees and the physician staffing ratio together guide the HMO administrator in making staffing decisions. Plans that project less than 5,000 initial enrollees probably will use a 1:500 or 1:600 staffing ratio, with internists and generalists providing

[16]McNamara and Todd. "Survey of Group Practice," p. 1309.

TABLE 11   Selected HMO Membership and Staffing, 1969

HMO	Membership	Staff	Staffing Ratio (M.D./Enrollee)
Columbia Medical Plan	5,000 (6/70)	7 full-time 8 part-time	1:454
Community Health Association	71,290	62 full-time 12 part-time	1:1,200
Group Health Association	72,537	45 full-time 73 part-time	1:1,000
Group Health Co-operative of Puget Sound	121,716	102 full-time	1:1,193
Kaiser-Permanente Medical Care Program, Northern California Region	972,000 (12/70)	1,016 full-time equivalents	1:957
Western Clinic, Tacoma, Washington	11,536	17 full-time* 1 part-time	1:1,098

*60 percent of time spent with prepaid patients.

Source: Leon Gintzig and Robert G. Shouldice. "Prepaid Group Practice: An Analysis as a Delivery System." Washington, D.C., The George Washington University, 1972, pp. 102–108, 190–191. Mimeographed.

most of the care. Physicians' time not used to provide care to prepaid patients could then be made available to fee-for-service patients. Eventually, as the prepaid enrollment increases, there can be a corresponding decrease in the number of fee-for-service patients served, until the plan serves only enrolled individuals. Some plans may wish to continue serving both categories of patients, although such an arrangement will lower the efficiency and overall economy of the plan. Smaller plans may supplement their physicians' group with other specialists on a consultant basis, either using a retainer, fee-for-service, or an hourly pay basis.

Physicians are added to the staff on a full-time basis when it has been determined that it is costing the plan more for fees, retainers, or part-time salaries than it would for an equivalent full-time physician. Figure 26 provides a guide for determining at what enrollment level full-time physicians should be added to the staff. This guide is based on the premise that staff is added on a full-time, incremental, and straight-time basis.

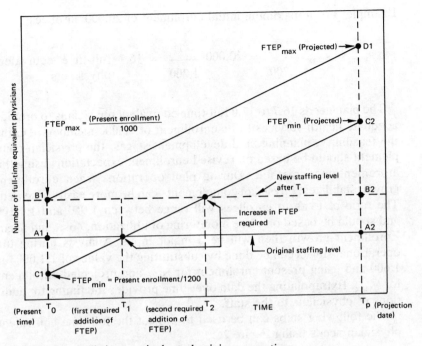

Figure 26   Full-time equivalent physicians over time.

The computation of required full-time equivalent physician (FTEP) complements shown in Figure 26 can be performed as follows: Assuming the initial enrollment will range between N_{min} and N_{max} and the range of full-time equivalent physicians needed is between 1:600 FTEP/enrollees and 1:1,200 FTEP/enrollees, then the maximum physician complement (FTEP$_{max}$) is

$$\text{FTEP}_{max} = N_{min} \frac{(1)}{600} \tag{1}$$

Example: For a minimum initial enrollment of 10,000,

$$\text{FTEP}_{max} = 10,000 \frac{(1)}{600} = 17.0 \text{ full-time equivalent physicians}$$

The minimum physician equivalent requirement (FTEP$_{min}$) is

$$\text{FTEP}_{min} = N_{max} \frac{(1)}{1,200}$$

Example: For a maximum initial enrollment of 20,000 enrollees

$$\text{FTEP}_{min} = N_{max} \frac{(1)}{1,200} = 20,000 \frac{(1)}{1,200} = 16.7 \text{ full-time equivalent physicians}$$

The plan needs 16.7 to 17.0 full-time equivalent physicians to provide adequate health services to its enrollment of 20,000 members. During the feasibility, planning, and development stages, the physician complement should be based on revised enrollment expectations using the aforementioned method. During plan operation, when enrollment growth stabilizes, physician complements can be more easily assessed. The ratio of FTEP to enrollees will range between 1:950 and 1:1,100 and should be based on close monitoring of utilization, cost, and need. Enrollment growth then will be a major input. Analysis during the operational stages can be done by substituting the values of 1:1,000 for 1:600 and using present enrollment for N_{min} and projected enrollment for N_{max}. Extrapolating the data over time provides the timing for additions of physicians to the staff.

The following steps can be used to project the full-time equivalent physician needs using Figure 26:

1. Draw the present FTEP line A_1A_2 for the present number of full-time equivalent physicians.
2. Draw the points B_1 and C_1 representing the maximum and minimum FTEP, based on the present enrollment level at T_0.
3. Draw in the points D_1 and C_2, indicating the maximum and minimum FTEP, based on the present enrollment level at T_0.
4. Connect C_1C_2 and B_1D_1 based on expected growth (i.e., the example assumes a linear growth rate).
5. The time T_1 at the intersection of A_1A_2 and B_1B_2 indicates the time (T_2) at which additional physicians must be added to the HMO.
6. The line C_1C_2 represents the upper limit of physician equivalents that can be added to the staff.

FULL-TIME EQUIVALENT PHYSICIANS BY SPECIALTY

Three further points are important. First, as the size of the membership and medical staff increases, the need for specialists increases. Table 12 provides some guidelines for the appropriate staffing levels of most medical specialists. Second, most specialists will be needed by the HMO on a full-time basis at the 20,000 to 30,000 enrollment level—the

TABLE 12   Specialty Guidelines

Specialty	Physician/Enrollee Ratios
Ear-Nose-Throat	1/32,000–1/30,000
Radiologists	1/40,000–1/30,000
Pathologists	1/60,000–1/50,000
Anesthetists	1/30,000–1/25,000
Psychiatrists	1/75,000
General Surgeons	1/12,000
Chest Surgeons	1/60,000
Dentists	1/1,800–1/1,500
Family Practitioners	1/3,300–1/3,000
Pediatricians	1/8,000–1/7,600
Internists	1/6,200–1/6,000
Obstetrics and Gynecology	1/10,000–1/9,000
Urologists	1/60,000–1/50,000
Orthopedic Surgeons	1/50,000
Ophthalmologists	1/40,000–1/35,000

Source: John E. F. Hastings. *Labor's Plan for a Medicare Program for Toronto*. Washington, D.C., Group Health Association of America, 1962, pp. 21–22.

level that is widely accepted as the breakeven point for an HMO.[17] This breakeven rule of thumb is not sacred, since several HMOs have become financially viable at lower enrollment levels—especially those in rural settings where medical resources may be less available and the use of a mixture of prepaid health plan and fee-for-service patients has helped to successfully control a plan's potential losses. Finally, plans that anticipate an initial enrollment level from 10,000 to 15,000 should include equivalent full-time physicians in the following specialties: general medicine, general practice or internal medicine, obstetrics and gynecology, pediatrics, and surgery. These generalists and specialists should provide 70 to 80 percent of all health services needed by enrollees.

Another method for assessing the number of physicians by specialty can be accomplished by using the maximum and minimum full-time equivalent physicians formula developed in Figure 26. Three steps should be followed.

1. Compute the expected maximum and minimum full-time equivalent physician complement expected for the projected enrollment level.

[17]U.S. Department of Health, Education, and Welfare. *Questions Physicians Are Asking*, p. 1.

2. Compute the maximum and minimum full-time equivalent physicians for each specialty, using the percentage distribution of physicians by specialty (the specialty distribution value provided in Table 13).

3. Adjust the value for variations in plan benefits, operating policy, specific needs, and so on.

Example: Where $\text{FTEP}_{max} = 17.0$ and $\text{FTEP}_{min} = 15.4$

a. General Practitioners and Internal Medicine $= 0.5 \times \text{FTEP}$, maximum $= 8.5$; minimum $= 7.7$

b. Dermatology $= 0.1036 \times \text{FTEP}$, maximum $= 0.612$; minimum $= 0.554$

FULL-TIME AND PART-TIME PHYSICIANS

Based on recent experiences, especially at the Health Insurance Plan of Greater New York, the use of part-time physicians in HMOs has been criticized. Using the definition of full-time physician coverage as 30 to 35 hours of ambulatory office care plus night and weekend coverage, less than 30 hours would constitute part-time physician coverage. The advantage of using part-timers is to fill in when full-time coverage is not required. On the other hand, part-time physicians may not have the same commitment and loyalty to the plan and to its prepaid patients as

TABLE 13   Specialty Distribution × Full-time Equivalent Physician Needs

a.	General Practitioners and Internal Medicine	$= 0.500 \times \text{FTEP}$
b.	Dermatology	$= 0.036 \times \text{FTEP}$
c.	Urology	$= 0.016 \times \text{FTEP}$
d.	Obstetrics and Gynecology	$= 0.093 \times \text{FTEP}$
e.	Allergy	$= 0.007 \times \text{FTEP}$
f.	Pediatrics	$= 0.160 \times \text{FTEP}$
g.	Orthopedist	$= 0.028 \times \text{FTEP}$
h.	General Surgery	$= 0.056 \times \text{FTEP}$
i.	Otolaryngology	$= 0.028 \times \text{FTEP}$
j.	Ophthalmology	$= 0.027 \times \text{FTEP}$
k.	Psychiatry	$= 0.009 \times \text{FTEP}$
l.	Radiology	$= 0.015 \times \text{FTEP}$
m.	Other	$= 0.025 \times \text{FTEP}$

Source: Texas Instruments, Inc. *Development of an Implementation Plan for the Establishment of a Health Maintenance Organization.* Rockville, Md., Health Maintenance Organization Service, U.S. Department of Health, Education, and Welfare, 1971, p. IV–136.

they have to outside fee-for-service patients. The use of part-time physicians creates difficulty in scheduling night and weekend coverage. Thus, the best policy would be to use part-time physicians only when the workload does not demand a full-time physician, or when the cost of the full-time physician is more than that of the part-timer for the same effort. Reimbursement methods for outside physicians vary and include part-time salaries, hourly pay, straight retainers, retainers with membership adjustments, monthly per capita payments, cost-related payments, and fee-for-service.[18]

FACILITIES

Funds for the development of group practice facilities[19] are available from financial institutions; up to 90 percent of the estimated value may be guaranteed by the Federal Housing Authority. Loan guarantees are governed by a $5 million limitation and are available only to nonprofit corporations, associations, foundations, trusts, or other entities. Professionals who wish to develop their own facilities may sponsor an FHA project, but the mortgagor or owner must be completely separate from the group conducting its practice in the facility. In many instances, the owner will lease the facility to the practitioners. Other requirements of the FHA program mandate that the group practice must be composed of at least five physicians or, in isolated or sparsely populated areas, at least three physicians, and that the mortgage bear interest at the current rates but not exceeding that specified in the current FHA regulations. The Department of Housing and Urban Development's handbook concerning group practice facilities (FHA 4465.3) should be consulted for eligibility requirements and appropriate application procedures and forms.

Another possible source of funds for rural programs is the Farmers Home Administration (FMHA). FMHA may make 40-year direct loans at 5 percent to nonprofit facilities in towns of under 10,000 people. In 1973, hospitals and other health facilities, which are considered "Es-

[18]Roger B. LeCompte. *Prepaid Group Practice: A Manual.* Chicago, Blue Cross Association, 1972, p. 5.10.

[19]For a discussion of facilities, see Fred W. Wasserman and Michael C. Miller. *Building a Group Practice.* Springfield, Ill., Charles C Thomas, Publisher, 1973, pp. 72–78; Texas Instruments, Inc. *Development of an Implementation Plan for the Establishment of a Health Maintenance Organization.* Rockville, Md., Health Maintenance Organization Service, U.S. Department of Health, Education, and Welfare, 1971, pp. VII-7–VII-8; and U.S. Department of Health, Education, and Welfare, Office of Health Maintenance Organizations. *The Health Maintenance Organization Facility Development Handbook.* Rockville, Md., 1975.

TABLE 14   Nonphysician Staffing (1968)

Ancillary Personnel per Physician	Size of Clinic (No. of Physicians)					
	1–5	*6–10*	*11–15*	*16–20*	*21–30*	*over 30*
Lab. and X-ray Technicians						
Mean	0.50	0.60	0.43	0.38	0.40	0.60
Median	0.40	0.43	0.35	0.35	0.33	0.55
Range	1.0–0.20	4.33–0.13	1.55–0.13	0.71–0.22	0.73–0.16	1.01–0.38
No. of Clinics	20	33	20	11	9	9
Paramedical Personnel						
Mean	0.99	1.07	1.15	0.95	0.86	1.28
Median	1.0	1.0	0.97	0.92	0.84	1.30
Range	2.0–0.46	2.75–0.30	4.83–0.55	1.39–0.50	1.25–0.43	2.25–0.08
No. of Personnel*	18	34	20	11	9	9
Business and Clerical Personnel						
Mean	1.40	1.69	1.51	1.70	1.71	2.09
Median	1.33	1.56	1.30	1.71	1.80	2.30
Range	2.92–0.70	2.83–0.17	6.55–0.18	2.8–0.78	2.57–0.91	3.07–0.23
No. of Personnel†	19	35	20	11	9	9

*Includes R.N.s, L.P.N.s, nurses aides, therapists, psychologists.
†Includes secretarial and clerical personnel; excludes custodial and housekeeping personnel.

Source: Douglas M. Egan. *Physicians Income, Personnel Utilization, and Physician Productivity: An Analysis of Member Clinics of the Medical Group Management Association.* Corvallis, Oreg., Oregon State University, 1971, p. III–3.

sential Community Facilities," accounted for half of the $50 million loaned in that category. There are no ceilings on individual loans, and construction regulations are minimal. For additional information, the county FMHA office should be contacted.

NONPHYSICIAN STAFFING

The staffing levels of a group practice with nonphysician personnel depend on several factors, the most important of which is the physicians' practice patterns. It has been found that the ratio of prepaid group practice staff is from four to five direct paramedical personnel per physician, with the average usually on the lower side. Table 14 provides the results of a 1969 study of staffing patterns of 33 HMO prototypes. Nonphysician staffing for laboratory and X-ray technicians was found to be from 0.80 to 1.25 per physician; paramedical personnel ranged from 0.50 to 3.0 per physician; and business and clerical, from 1.0 to 5.0 per physician. These ratios are valuable for plans having 16 or more full-time participating physicians.

It is important to note that prepaid group practice plans use physician extenders more frequently than other delivery forms; a description of their economic impact is provided in Chapter 9.

Group Practice Organization and Physician Payment

What is the organizational relationship of a group practice to the HMO? Again, the answer differs with each of the four HMO models because physician groups organize themselves most frequently as profit-making enterprises and many health plans are not for profit. In nonprofit HMOs, the group practice must be "at arm's length" from the health plan in matters concerning HMO operation control and physician compensation. In all HMOs—both nonprofit and investor owned—it is advisable that the medical group be autonomous and free to make decisions concerning medical matters and compensation for physicians. They should be self-governing, although they may rely on the health plan administrator for counsel and advice.

FORMS OF ORGANIZATION

Group practices have four general forms of organization available to them—solo proprietorship, partnership, unincorporated association, or corporation. In the last case, several options are available: regular corporations with stockholders, subchapter S corporations, and professional corporations or professional associations. Obviously, the form chosen depends on many factors, although, based on a 1969 AMA survey, the partnership form was chosen by more than 60 percent of the groups. Other forms and their frequency of use are given in the following listing:[20]

Partnerships 68.7%
Corporations 15.6%
Associations* 9.2%
Proprietorships 2.8%
Other forms 3.7%

*Established in states where professional associations or corporations are prohibited.

Generally, one method is chosen over others because of tax advantages, personal liability of the group members, and retirement funds.[21] Health plan/medical staff organizational relationships can be categorized according to the method of physician compensation. Three methods are prevalent—physician ownership of the HMO, contract, and salary.

For-profit HMOs developed, owned, and operated by the medical group, such as the Ross-Loos, Palo Alto, and Western clinics, control all aspects of the health plan including the method of physician compensation, usually based on salary and bonus.

Medical groups may be under contract with the HMO. The formal contract details the relationship between the two parties, including the duties and obligations of each. Physician compensation may be based on a capitation rate or, for FMCs, on a fee-for-service schedule. The proprietary medical group may take any of the aforementioned forms but must follow the "arm's length" rule with a nonprofit HMO. As an autonomous entity, the medical group negotiates with the HMO concerning capitation rates, number of enrollees to be served, and acceptable utilization ranges. It controls physician membership selection, vacation scheduling, night coverage, and professional standards. In addition, the medical group establishes its own internal payment formula and bonus program. Problem areas that the health plan may encounter in its relationships with contract medical groups may be stand-

[20]Clifford Todd and Mary E. McNamara. *Medical Groups in the U.S., 1969.* Chicago, American Medical Association, 1971.
[21]For a discussion of these organizational forms and issues, see American Association of Medical Clinics et al. *Group Practice,* pp. 23–28.

ards of quality; utilization levels; use of the health plan's facilities, equipment, and personnel; mix of fee-for-service and health plan patients served; and financial remuneration for enrollees served.

The third category is the use of a salaried medical staff. A separate contract is prepared for each physician by the health plan. Payment to physicians can be based on a per capita arrangement, hourly pay, straight retainers, or fee-for-service, although the last method is rare. In some instances, the issue of corporate practice of medicine has been raised with regard to the salaried method of physician payment. To remove any doubt about lay interference in the practice of medicine, plans using a salary payment mechanism point out that the plan's medical director is responsible for all medical aspects of the plan's operation and is the liaison with salaried physicians. Moreover, they note that even though a direct individual payment is made to each physician, the medical staff is still organized as a group practice that is autonomous concerning medical matters and is self-governing. Only on the rarest occasions, and then for the most serious legal or ethical malpractice situations, have there been interventions in medical matters by the medical director, plan administrator, or the board of trustees.

PHYSICIAN COMPENSATION AND PAYMENT FORMULAS

Most HMO physicians are associated with a group practice that pools its income. How, then, is the individual physician's income determined? After expenses are drawn, the net income is distributed on a yearly basis according to a prearranged schedule developed by the physicians themselves. One method of dividing income is for each partner to share equally in the net income, based on the principle that, as a member of the medical team, each is considered to be of equal value to the group. More frequently, the schedule is not an even distribution but is based on a formula that considers a doctor's total bookings (i.e., number of patients served), total collections, length of service, formal training, research efforts, experience, board specialty, standing in the medical community, and other subjective factors. Individual income levels are seldom tied directly to the physician's productivity; however, programs have been established to collect data concerning doctors' bookings—the total number of patients seen and total collecions. Based on these figures, physician productivity can be identified and used to develop salaries.

A point-rating system is used by some groups to determine physician payment levels. Points are assigned to "new patients seen, seniority, group value, professional standing in the community, drawing power, patient volume, patients referred to other clinic physicians, professional changes, publications and research, and administrative ability."[22] Although this system has the advantage of being more objective than one not using a point system, it also has the disadvantage of difficult factor selection and weight determination, as well as difficulty in explaining the system and its justification in physician recruitment.

Other methods include a distribution based precisely on each member's bookings, although such a method maximizes competition among the group practice by introducing an incentive element. Generally, most medical groups use some combination of the aforementioned methods. "Actual figures in one study of over 300 medical groups showed 25% shared income equally, 50% used predominantly an incentive system, 15% used a salary plus other arrangement, and the remaining 10% combined the salary and the incentive distribution."[23]

Agreeing on an acceptable payment formula[24] may be the most troublesome area for the group members. Recognizing this fact, the group practice administrator should build a strategy for the group around the following set of principles:[25]

1. Each member of the medical group is considered equal.

2. Incomes must be competitive with private practice and must be high enough to attract and hold well-trained and competent doctors.

3. Length of training should be recognized only when it increases competency.

4. Although special competencies should be considered, length of service with the group should be the major factor for increasing income.

5. Admission to partnership, where applicable, should bring increased income.

6. Because the physician is concerned with keeping the enrollee well and in increasing his productive years, rather than with sporadic episodes of illness, the physician receives his compensation regardless of fluctuations in load (just as the patient pays a monthly premium whether ill or well).

7. Because of the limited supply of certain specialists, somewhat higher income may be necessary for these physicians.

[22] American Association of Medical Clinics et al. *Group Practice,* pp. 20–21.
[23] *Ibid.,* p. 21.
[24] For a review of several payment formulas and the average physician incomes of several HMO prototypes, see Gintzig and Shouldice "Prepaid Group Practice: An Analysis," pp. 104–108.
[25] MacColl. *Group Practice and Prepayment of Medical Care,* p. 109.

8. Physicians considered for partnership or for purchasing a share of the business, where applicable, should serve a probationary period of from two to three years.

INCENTIVE SYSTEMS AND RISK SHARING

Most of the plans include a quality/quantity incentive system or bonus plan as part of the physician's compensation program. For partnerships and corporations, physicians serving their probationary periods look forward to a somewhat higher income from the group practice after completion of the probationary period, not only because of normal increases due to length of service but because of participation in dividends from investment pools; most partnerships and professional corporations set aside a portion of net income for investment programs. Returns from such programs have been two to three times the initial amount the physician would have shared in had the initial investment been distributed rather than invested.

Direct incentive payments for effective and appropriate utilization also may be part of the system; such incentives can include merit increases, bonuses, and participation in a risk pool—a budgeted amount of money reserved for overutilization contingencies as well as a reserve fund from which bonuses for appropriate utilization are drawn. Such participation by individual physicians is directly related to hospital costs and physician services for outpatient and inpatient medical services.

Most HMO models which have been discussed share the risk of overuse of services by enrollees during a specific period with the providers of care. "Risk sharing," "at risk," and "risk assumption" are terms that refer to the financial risk of providing health services by the plan. *Risk* in this sense is defined as the possibility that revenues will not be sufficient to cover expenditures incurred in the delivery of contracted-for services. *Risk sharing* means that physicians and hospitals have a financial stake in the health plan's operation; their compensation is based, to some degree, on their ability to hold use of services at an appropriate level and to appropriately decrease use of the more expensive source of care, namely, hospitalization. One of the key philosophical issues concerning HMOs is that of risk sharing through provider incentives. The fee-for-service system can be said to encourage inefficient use of medical resources. "In the HMO, where the physician receives an increased compensation for the amount of excess utilization he can control, the risk encourages efficient use of facilities and resources. The most expensive service of the health care system is hospitalization and it is also the area of greatest unnecessary utilization. Thus, incentives for a financially efficient system must include incentives to control unnecessary hospital use.''[26] Operationally, risks that do not affect incentives in the system but are truly unforeseen hazards that cannot be controlled by prudent patients or administrative management should be covered by insurance. Hospital use can be controlled by physicians; therefore, they should be given a financial incentive to control it.

The risk-sharing mechanism using physician incentives is described in the medical group's contract. Simplistically, physicians are placed at risk when the medical group agreement provides for a compensation process that distributes to the individual physicians the surplus (or savings) or loss from the group's operation over a specified period of time. Several risk-sharing models are currently being used; some are described in the discussions that follow. For the clinic manager, it is important to realize that physician risk-sharing models have little in common except that they are a desirable means by which to influence the management of medical-care resources, they must be compatible with the various elements of the health plan, they are seldom permanent, and the more risk that is insured by a private carrier, the greater the cost to the plan.

PHYSICIAN AND HOSPITAL RISK-SHARING MODELS

Stop-loss Model: This model limits the losses of the health plan, medical group, or individual physician after a predetermined level of service has been provided to an individual enrollee. Arranged with an independent insurer, the parties involved are on a complete risk basis (i.e., they will bear the cost of the provision of services) until health care expenditures for any enrollee reach a certain dollar figure or the cost to the plan for their population as a whole reaches a certain dollar amount. The insurer pays the losses above this point. For example, all costs over $5,000 per enrollee per year are paid by the third-party insurer. As such, there is little risk to the physician because he will be compensated by the health plan and the private insurer for total costs of his services.

[26]Paul Kosco and Alan Bloom. ''Risk Sharing Health Maintenance Organizations.'' *In: Development of HMO's Within Existing Group Practices: A Symposium.* Alexandria, Va., American Association of Medical Clinics, 1973, p. A.35.

Complete Risk Arrangement: Premiums paid to the plan first are used to pay hospital charges and other nonphysician expenses incurred by the plan. The remainder is paid to the physicians; the amount of control the physicians exercise over hospital use directly affects this amount.

Capitation Risk Model: Many physician groups assume some risk through the capitation mechanism. In return for the capitation, the medical group agrees to provide all contracted-for physician and hospital services without retrospective adjustment. By doing this, the group takes the risk that the capitation payment may not cover its expenses, especially hospital overuse. The physicians' capitation levels under this model may include budgeted amounts for most of the HMO's operating expenses, including inpatient and outpatient care; ostensibly, premium payments would equal the total yearly physician capitation payments. The HMO's management would then act as a service organization to the physicians' group by coordinating the payments of all operating expenses from the capitation amount.

Band Model: This model calls for "bands" or parameters to be placed around anticipated use rates for hospitalization and/or medical services. The health plan assumes all the risk of use falling within the band. The health plan, physician group, or other third party—such as an indemnity carrier—would assume the risk of overuse (or gain if underuse) if the utilization level fell outside the preestablished "bands." The health plan otherwise would assume small losses or gains if use was contained within the "bands." Note that the health plan and physicians must develop expected levels of use and also must reach an agreement (including an outside insurer, if used) concerning the "bands" and the loss and surplus sharing formula.[27] Table 15 shows an HMO that shares its gains and losses equally with its physician group and with an outside indemnity carrier. The enclosed area represents the "bands" around anticipated utilization. All losses and gains within the "bands" ($\pm$ \$20) are accepted by the health plan. Outside the "bands," gains and losses are shared equally with the physician group and the carrier. In other cases, an insurance carrier may underwrite a portion of the gains or losses outside the "bands" with or without health plan or physician-sharing arrangements; Table 15 is based upon the risk assumption relationship of the Harvard Community Health Plan and the Massachusetts

[27]A discussion of the development of capitated levels of utilization between the HMO and its physician groups is included in Chapter 10.

TABLE 15   Band Model

Actual Use	Percentage of Anticipated Use	Cost Associated with Various Use Levels	Effects
140	140	$140	Insurer assumes loss of $20 and physician loses $20
120	120	120	Plan loses $20
100 Expected level	100	100	—
80	80	80	Plan gains $20
60	60	60	Insurer assumes gain of $20 and physician gains $20

Blue Cross Plan. Currently, however, physicians do not share any risk with Harvard or Massachusetts Blue Cross.

Cooperative Model: Risks are shared on a cooperative level by all HMO components—health plan, physicians, hospital, and insurers. Generally, each component is given a capitation, and a reserve fund is established. At year's end, all expenses are tallied for each component. Those components that show a profit *place* that profit in the reserve fund; those showing losses *draw* the amount of loss from the fund. The remainder is then distributed, in a prearranged manner, to the components. If the fund is depleted, the loss also is distributed according to a prearranged formula.

Nonhospitalization Incentive Model: Incentive programs are sometimes developed which are limited only to the provision of ambulatory-care services; hospital costs are handled separately and are not considered in the capitation payment to physicians. The Group Health Cooperative of Puget Sound has such an incentive built into the capitation payment to the physician group. This incentive is set at a certain physician per enrollee ratio (1:1,053). By operating at a lower ratio (more enrollees per physician, 1:1,200), there is an increased amount of money for the same number of doctors, thereby rewarding increased productivity. Of course, if the ratio increases (e.g., 1:750), the medical group must absorb the cost of the extra staff members, because their load may be lighter.

Examples of Risk-sharing Models Tied to Hospitalization: On the other
hand, incentive payments can be tied directly to hospital use and can
take numerous forms.

The following example illustrates a simple method of determining a
physician's bonus or incentive:

Anticipated hospital days per 1,000 enrollees = 900
Utilized hospital days per 1,000 enrollees = 750
Incentive rate = $50 per day saved
Total incentive payment = $7,500
(900 − 750) × $50 = $7,500

In another example, the incentive model couples the physicians'
share of any surplus to the hospital utilization rate. As the rate decreases, the physicians' share increases to some maximum level (e.g.,
50 percent). To illustrate, the physicians' share of the surplus created
from lower-than-expected hospital use would be computed as follows:

Percentage Rate	if	*Number of Hospital Days per 1,000 Enrollees Is Achieved*
30		700
35		675
40		650
45		625
50		600

This method is used by the Rhode Island Blue Cross and Blue Shield
Program with the Bristol County Medical Group. The medical group's
share of the incentive fund is not allowed to exceed 20 percent of the
total yearly capitation. Table 16 identifies the risk-sharing arrangements used by several health plans.

Group Practice Management

Because most group practices participating with an HMO are autonomous and self-governing, it becomes important for them to have a
governing body—an executive committee having authority and responsibility for the group practice operation. This applies to all group
practices of sufficient size, regardless of the mode of physician compensation, and includes foundation models using individual practice

TABLE 16   Risk-Sharing Arrangements by Type of Service

Plan	Medical Services Utilization	Referrals	Hospitalization	Hospital Use Controls Incentive Plan*
Kaiser-Permanente Oakland, California	Medical Group	Medical Group	Health Plan	Yes
HIP of Greater New York New York City	HIP and Medical Group	Medical Group	Blue Cross	No
Columbia Medical Plan Columbia, Maryland	Hospital-Carrier†	Hospital-Carrier†	Hospital-Carrier†	Yes (but not operative at present)
Harvard Health Plan Cambridge, Massachusetts	Carrier-Plan	Plan	Carrier-Plan	Yes, but physicians do not participate
Ross-Loos Medical Plan Los Angeles, California	Medical Group	Medical Group	Varies‡	Yes
Foundation for Medical Care of San Joaquin County San Joaquin, California	Insures 80 percent with carrier	Insures 80 percent with carrier	Insures 100 percent with carrier	Modified

*Physicians share the savings generated by lower than expected hospital utilization.
†Contract with Connecticut General and other carriers. For the first five years, all losses are insured by carriers; thereafter, Columbia Medical Plan will be responsible for up to 10 percent of losses.
‡Contract with Blue Cross of Southern California.

associations. The executive committee generally appoints a lay administrator who is responsible for all nonmedical aspects of the group practice operation—nonphysician staffing, legal problems, accounting and bookkeeping, plant and equipment, and so on. Depending on the form of organization, the group practice will either elect a physician director or work closely with a director appointed by the health plan. The following discussion concerns the medical administrative leader elected by the group.

It is assumed that this position is not simply an honorific office but that the chief executive officer is the leader of the medical group. The executive officer must be a physician respected by all physicians in the group, because physicians do not easily accept advice, counsel, and direction from lay personnel. This is especially true during physician recruitment efforts, when potential group members reserve their final decision of whether to join the group until after meeting with the group's "physician" representative. Because there are rules of organization and operation, the medical administrative director must determine the degree of compliance with these rules, including peer review and correction of deficiencies through administrative channels—in which instances the medical administrative director plays an important role in maintaining the morale of the group.

Another function of the medical administrative director is that of establishing staffing schedules and making arrangements with community physicians who are not group members but are needed to provide enrollees with certain specialty care. The medical administrative director should be familiar with all health-plan functions—marketing and enrollment, rate setting, financing and cash flow, facilities administration, personnel policies, budgeting, and capitation development, among others. Only with a thorough understanding of these areas will the executive officer be capable of functioning as a medical administrative director and also as a member of the health plan's board of trustees.

FOUNDATION MANAGEMENT

Currently, foundations without an individual practice association arrangement believe that physicians must retain responsibility and leadership in the design, administration, and delivery of medical services. The medical profession must participate in health care planning, influence the benefit package design, monitor the full spectrum of health services, and evaluate existing and emerging health care arrangements. The foundation, sponsored and organized by the local medical society, is governed by a board of directors that is nominated and elected by the board of the sponsoring medical society. The foundation's board of directors appoints a lay executive director, who is responsible to the board and is charged with the operation of four functions—accounting and finance, consumer relations, marketing and enrollment, and that part of the medical service program dealing primarily with the operation of the claims review process. These tasks, except perhaps the last one, are similar to those for which a prepaid group practice administrator is responsible.

In lieu of a medical administrative director, the foundation's board of directors elects a president of the board, who is ultimately responsible for all activities of the foundation—including administrative as well as medical activities. The lay manager reports directly to the president. Medical administrative functions, including establishment of medical standards, fees, and utilization review, are delegated to physician committees that report to the board through the president. All other medical activities are the responsibility of the president. The functions of the president of a foundation can be compared to those of the executive director or the medical director of a prepaid group practice.

THE HOSPITAL

Seldom do HMOs own, control, and operate their own hospitals. Although there are some well-known exceptions, such as the Kaiser programs and the Group Health Cooperative of Puget Sound, most HMOs arrange for the delivery of inpatient care via means other than direct ownership of hospital facilities. The majority of HMO managers agree, however, that they would be in a more favorable position to control use and inpatient costs if their plans owned their own hospitals. Most plans are too small to maintain a hospital, especially one with 250 or more beds (the capacity necessary for efficiency of operation). The least controlled method of obtaining a hospital-bed relationship tends to be the granting of staff-admitting privileges to the plan physicians by the hospital. More formal contracts, in which the hospital guarantees a certain number of beds for which the HMO pays a yearly fee, whether or not they are used, appear to be a more favorable alternative. Working agreements and contracts between the health plan and participating hospitals describe these financial arrangements, which might include a periodic payment similar to a retainer guaranteeing the availability of beds; a prospective payment with or without retrospective adjustments at the end of an accounting period; and retrospective payments. In the

last two approaches, the HMO pays according to a fee-for-service arrangement which may be full or discounted costs or charges.

Control of hospital beds by the HMO raises the question of the plan's
ability to fully meet its contractual obligations to its subscribers—since
all HMO packages include inpatient care when ordered by the physicians. Ownership of the hospital places the HMO in a position of giving
bed preference to plan enrollees; second preference could then be
given to physicians from the community. On the other hand, when
provisions for inpatient care are contingent on staff-admitting
privileges of plan physicians at a nonplan hospital, the enrollees would
have to wait their turn for beds, the same as patients of other staff
physicians from the community. The third alternative—hospital/plan
contracts for beds—although seemingly advantageous for the plan
and, perhaps, the hospital, also can have disadvantages, since such
contracts require that the plan pay for beds when they are not in use,
thereby potentially increasing plan costs or increasing the plan's use
rate if the beds were occupied. This practice may be of value if a
hospital has a low occupancy rate and desires a guaranteed income for
at least some of its beds—which could be a point of contention during
periods of high occupancy when "outside-the-plan physicians" are
competing vigorously for all beds available. The most important point,
however, is the assurance that hospital beds are available to HMO enrollees when required. Any arrangement is satisfactory if it generally
accomplishes this objective.

OTHER PROVIDERS

Benefit packages may require the services of other providers, including
all levels of long-term care facilities; pharmacy, dentistry, and optical
services; home health care; and so on. Plans may wish to own the
facilities and directly control the delivery of these services or they may
find it more advantageous to contract with outside organizations, especially for services that are infrequently used.

Summary

Chapter 5 deals with providers of care—physicians and hospitals. Emphasis is placed on physicians in group practice because of their major
role in the provision of most care to HMO subscribers. The Individual
Practice Association (IPA), as a physician association providing care

under the medical foundation model, is specifically reviewed in Chapter 4, although several issues addressed in this chapter, such as staffing ratios and risk sharing, may be applied to the HMO/IPA model.

Group practice of medicine began in the 1880s with the formation of the Mayo Clinic of Rochester, Minnesota. This provider mode grew in the years that followed to 125 groups in 1926, more than 220 in 1932, 1,546 in 1959, and 4,289 in 1965. By 1969, 38,834 physicians were practicing in 6,371 groups. During this same year, there were 85 prepaid group practices providing services to patients, representing 6,540 physicians. The number of groups had grown to 8,483 by 1976, representing 66,842 physicians—a total of 23.5 percent of all practicing physicians in the United States.

Definitions of group practice describe the number of formally organized, multispecialty physicians, their joint use of facilities and personnel, and a method of sharing income. The American Medical Association and the Medical Group Management Association define a medical group as three or more physicians formally organized and providing care through the joint use of facilities and personnel, and with income distributed according to a prearranged formula. Similar definitions of group practice also are provided by the American Group Practice Association and Group Health Association of America, although they describe the size of a group as seven full-time physicians with not less than five practicing in different major specialities. The aforementioned statistics use the "three or more physicians" definition as the basis for growth trend analysis. Most important, however, is that the median group had 4.8 physicians in 1969, and groups with 50 percent or more prepaid activity were composed of more than seven physicians.

There are advantages and disadvantages to group practice for the physician. Among the major advantages are the sharing of knowledge, talent, responsibility, and the interchange of ideas; regular rotation of hours and coverage for evenings, weekends, and vacations; immediate practice and income for young physicians; salaries comparable to fee-for-service practice; and relief from the business aspects of practice. Disadvantages include loss of freedom and some loss of individuality; problems with the level of individual physician's income and the establishment of an equitable income-sharing arrangement; conformity to the group's standards of practice, conduct, and operating procedures; sharing in the group's liability; and the loss of the "physician's patients" to the "plan."

The attitude of physicians toward medical group practice HMOs and their participation in HMO activities can be traced from outright, vocal, and legal resistance on the part of organized medicine to the present resigned acceptance on the part of most individual physicians. For the most part, physicians are not becoming participants in HMOs because of the relatively small number of such programs. Where HMOs present a competitive threat, some medical societies have developed foundations for medical care—an attempt to retain the fee-for-service, solo practice concept for members. Other individual physicians have joined with HMOs on a full-time or part-time basis. Recent research suggests that physicians of the new generation have a more positive attitude toward practicing in a prepaid group practice setting, although they still have questions concerning such associations. Paramount among these questions are the fear of loss of status in the eyes of medical colleagues and patients, lack of time to do a good job, a breakdown in the patient-physician relationship, possible loss of income, unpredictable growth of HMOs, loss of freedom to practice and set fees, and advancing the socialized medicine concept. One indicator of physician attitudes is the physician turnover rate. Rates of from 2 to 3 percent per year are normal in HMOs, suggesting that physicians like to practice in the HMO setting once they complete the initial probationary period.

What size group is needed for adequate HMO coverage? The staffing of the health plan is based on some generalized guidelines; a staffing ratio of one physician for 950 to 1,100 subscribers for fully operational plans is the national level. The ratio, however, varies with the age of the HMO, its consumers' characteristics, and the level of its membership's medical expectations. Generally, there will be a higher ratio of physicians to subscribers during the early months of operation, even as high as one physician to 500 enrollees, and a lower ratio (as low as 1:1,200) for mature plans.

Physicians are added to the staff on the basis of health-plan administration and board decisions on appropriate physician/subscriber ratios. Both full-time and part-time physicians are used; physicians are added to the staff on a full-time basis when it has been determined that it is costing the plan more for fees, retainers, or part-time salaries than it would for an equivalent full-time physician. Usually, the equivalent full-time physician groups should include the following specialties: general medicine, general practice or internal medicine, obstetrics and gynecology, pediatrics, and surgery. Nonphysician staffing also depends on several factors, most important of which is the physician's practice pattern and the use of physician extenders. Experience shows that HMOs staff at a ratio of four to five direct paramedical personnel per physician.

Group practices follow four general forms of organization—solo proprietorship, partnership, unincorporated association, or corporation. In the past, the partnership form was chosen by more than 60 percent of the groups. The form of the medical group also can be described by its relationship with the HMO health plan—either physician ownership of the plan, contract with the plan, or full-time salaried employees of the plan. The nonprofit HMOs must take care to follow the "arm's length" rule in negotiations with proprietary medical groups, which requires that the physician not be directly involved in matters concerning HMO operation, control, or physician compensation. Failure to follow this rule could result in the loss of the HMO's nonprofit tax status.

Physician compensation and payment formulas normally are developed by the physician group on a yearly basis. Expenses are paid first; net income is then distributed according to a prearranged schedule. The individual physician's share may be based on his total bookings, total collections of fees-for-service, length of service, formal training, research efforts, experience, board specialty, and so on, or partners may share equally in net income. Studies of more than 300 groups show that 25 percent share equally, 50 percent use an incentive system, 15 percent use a salary-plus arrangement, and the remaining 10 percent, a salary and incentive distribution formula. Incentive systems are based on the principle that physicians will be more productive and more satisfied with their lot if their superior service both individually and as a group is tied to additional income. Likewise, inferior service and/or inability to manage the group's time effectively at an acceptable level results in sharing losses sustained by the plan and by the medical group. Thus, many incentive systems and risk-sharing models have been developed. Risk-sharing models include the stop-loss, complete risk, capitation risk, "band," and cooperative models.

Risk sharing through provider incentives is a key philosophical issue of HMOs, because the physician decides whether to use HMO funds and the form of health care services to be administered. To share in the risk that these funds will not be sufficient to cover all health care services places the provider in a position to hold use at an appropriate level and to appropriately decrease utilization of expensive hospitalization. This philosophy is opposite to that of the fee-for-service system, in which the physician, because of the enticement of larger income not regulated by a fixed monthly payment, increases units of services provided.

Although most services are provided by the group practice, other, more expensive, services are provided by hospitals to HMO subscribers. HMOs seldom own, control, or operate their own hospitals. Inpatient hospital services are arranged through several mechanisms— ownership of hospital, staff admitting privileges of plan physicians at a nonplan hospital, contracts between the hospital and plan for beds, or informal working arrangements with staff-admitting privileges. HMOs are in the most favorable position with regard to controlling use and inpatient costs if they have their own hospitals. The least favorable position is the granting of staff-admitting privileges without the advantage of an informal or formal working arrangement. Services other than outpatient and inpatient hospital beds may be provided by the HMO through ownership of facilities, contractual arrangements, or informal working arrangements with outside providers.

References

American Association of Medical Clinics, American Medical Association, and Medical Group Management Association. *Group Practice, Guidelines to Joining or Forming a Medical Group*. Chicago, American Medical Association, 1970.

Gintzig, Leon, and Shouldice, Robert G. "Prepaid Group Practice: An Analysis as a Delivery System." Washington, D.C., The George Washington University, 1972, pp. 43–47, 95–108, 190–193 (Tables 19, 20, 21). Mimeographed.

LeCompte, Roger B. *Prepaid Group Practice: A Manual*. Chicago, Blue Cross Association, 1972, pp. 5.01–5.32(a).

MacColl, William A. *Group Practice and Prepayment of Medical Care*. Washington, D.C., Public Affairs Press, 1966, pp. 88–130.

Mechanic, David. "The Organization of Medical Practice and Practice Orientations Among Physicians in Prepaid and Nonprepaid Primary Care Settings." *Medical Care*, XIII(3):189–204, March 1975.

Newman, Michael A., ed. *The Medical Director in Prepaid Group Practice Health Maintenance Organizations*. Rockville, Md., Health Maintenance Organization Service, U.S. Department of Health, Education, and Welfare, 1973, pp. 1–39.

Roemer, Milton, and Shonick, William. "HMO Performance: The Recent Evidence." *Milbank Memorial Fund Quarterly, Health and Society*, 278–280, Summer 1973.

Schenke, Roger, and Curtis, Spicer, eds. *Development of HMO's Within Existing Group Practices, A Symposium*. Alexandria, Va., American Association of Medical Clinics, 1973, pp. A-30–A-39.

U.S. Department of Health, Education, and Welfare, Health Maintenance Organization Service. *Questions Physicians Are Asking About HMOs and the Answers*. Rockville, Md., 1972. DHEW Publ. No. (HMS) 73–13009.

Vayda, Eugene. "Stability of the Medical Group in a New Prepaid Medical Care Program." *Medical Care*, 161–168. March–April 1970.

Wasserman, Fred W., and Miller, Michael C. *Building a Group Practice*. Springfield, Ill., Charles C Thomas, Publisher, 1973, pp. 60–78, 94–104.

6

The Consumer

The consumer is the third segment of the HMO triumvirate—providers, health plan, and enrollee groups. In this chapter, consumer opinions, attitudes, and roles are appraised; the chapter concludes with a discussion of the one major aspect of HMOs that concerns all members of the triumvirate—the quality of medical care in the HMO setting.

P.L. 93-222 and its guidelines define the HMO consumer as an individual who has entered into a contractual arrangement with an HMO for specified health services for himself or his family, or one for whom such a contractual arrangement has been made, who does not work for the HMO.[1] This definition of a consumer is used here as a synonym for *enrollee, subscriber,* or *member* of the HMO.

The Consumer Voice and Public Expectations

Consumers are demanding an opportunity to participate in matters that concern them—an opportunity to speak out, to generate their own representation, to expand their economic influence, and to keep current with new developments and services. In the health care field, consumer demands include expressions of attitudes and opinions concerning the health care organizations and their providers and the evalu-

[1]U.S. Department of Health, Education, and Welfare, Health Services and Mental Health Administration, Health Maintenance Organization Service. *Proceedings: National HMO Consumer Program Development Workshop.* Rockville, Md., 1973, p. 5.

ation of health services. They feel the latter can be adequately performed not only by professionals but also by the recipients of the
service. This point of view is partly due to the increasing number of
individuals with health insurance; care through the health insurance
mechanism is purchased by the consumer who is not sick but well—
not dependent but resourceful.

The consumer's interest and influence is based not only on his purchasing power but on a number of other factors, including higher education levels, improved communication, higher disposable incomes
and higher standards of living, and the frustrations that develop when
the limited supply of health care service does not match the growing
demand for, and quality of, services desired. Consumers are more
capable of making choices between the alternatives available to them.
Payments for the HMO system now come from companies, unions,
associations, and others who are establishing a new economic relationship with medicine.

The new consumer influence is being felt in the areas of cost and the
methods of financing care and in the adequacy of manpower and the
quality of health care and its organization. Heretofore, such considerations have been solely professional decisions. Although consumers
have had to accept much of what traditional fee-for-service and prepaid
medical care have offered, they are beginning to exercise independent
judgment. In the future, consumers will exert the decisive influence in
medical policy.[2]

Consumer Participation

In a free-market economy, the consumer participates by deciding what
product or service shall be used and for whom it will be available; this
is a distinctive feature of our institutions. In health care, such participation has not always held true; only in recent years has there been a
general consumer awakening, and consumer participation is being
sought to help decide what medical care should include and what it
should accomplish. In fact, most health care observers agree that
greater consumer involvement is required in decision making to overcome deficiencies in the health system. Consumer participation also is
seen as a motivation mechanism; people are more likely to accept
decisions that they help to make. For the health planner, although

[2]John H. Knowles, ed. *Hospital, Doctors, and the Public Interest*. Cambridge, Mass.,
Harvard University Press, 1965, p. 167.

consumer participation is now common in policy formulation, such participation is less common in the more specific operational aspects of facility management. Because consumer participation of necessity redistributes responsibility and power, its use in both planning and health care operations is viewed by some as the first step to a socialized and consumer-controlled health care system.

In a study of six consumer-cooperative HMOs and six private-physician HMOs conducted by Jerome L. Schwartz, 11 aspects of the programs evaluated were compared, including the policymaking processes, the value of consumer participation to the members, the degree of consumer participation, and the amount of influence exerted by consumers, physicians, and administrators in setting health-plan policy.[3] Schwartz found that participation changes with the age of the plan. Newly developing plans have general member participation; most of the initial work is voluntary, and decisions are shared by the entire group. As the organization grows, a staff is hired and functions are delegated. The membership's influence begins to decline when professional or technical services are required, or when specific knowledge, training, or education are needed for making decisions. Thus, three indicators of membership participation are customary. First, early tradition embodied in the cooperative effort can set the mode for participation. Second, membership size affects participation: the larger the organization, the lesser the activity by total membership, because members lose interest as the professionals exert more influence. Third, the complex decisions of large organizations require the input of expert opinion; therefore, the enrollees' influence is diminished.

With regard to consumer participation, Schwartz draws the following generalizations:

1. Individual participation in member organizations, in political as well as community life, is low.

2. Most organizations have an oligarchical structure with an active minority and an inactive apathetic majority.

3. The few members who are active are likely to be from the higher socioeconomic level and to have more education and higher income.

4. Policy is rarely made at the membership level—it is usually set and controlled by boards of officials.[4]

[3]Jerome L. Schwartz. *Medical Plans and Health Care.* Springfield, Ill., Charles C Thomas, Publisher, 1968, p. 219.
[4]*Ibid.,* p. 58.

It appears that when consumers are elected to the governing body, they actively participate in policymaking. Their level of activity is related directly to their personality and to the management style exhibited by the president of the board and the plan's administrator—strong authoritative styles tend to restrict consumer participation. Administrators, physicians, and key staff members often have a more significant voice and influence in deciding policy. Conversely, consumer plans that encourage consumer board participation generally have better programs in the following four areas: individual enrollment practices, eligibility policies, complaint procedures, and medical benefits. This may be due to pressures from large, organized purchasers such as unions or employers to add extra benefits. The policies of consumer plans that Schwartz studied were more favorable to enrollees than were the policies of physician plans.[5]

Following are some other major findings of the Schwartz study:

1. Consumer sponsorship of the HMOs had no greater impact than physician sponsorship on basic and preventive coverages offered by the plans. This generalization also can be extended to group enrollment procedures, health education and information programs, evaluation of the quality of care practiced in the clinic, and assessment of consumer satisfaction.

2. Since some of the consumer-sponsored plans had difficulty attracting specialists (a problem not shared by physician-sponsored plans), consumer sponsorship may have been a deterrent in obtaining specialists.

3. Both consumer and physician governing boards devoted approximately the same amount of attention to various subjects at board meetings.

4. Doctors were the most influential group in policymaking decisions in physician-sponsored plans.

5. General member participation in consumer medical cooperatives was low in terms of attendance at meetings, voting, and other activities.

6. In general, administrators and physicians were more influential in deciding policy in consumer-sponsored plans than were the lay board of trustees.

7. In general, administrators had the most important role in cooperative plans and physicians had the second most important role. In plans

with professional or executive trustees, however, the board had a major voice in policy making.[6]

Most importantly, Schwartz concluded from the study that consumer sponsorship of HMOs and consumer participation in the plans can have a favorable influence on health-plan programs. See Chapter 4 for a discussion of consumer plans and the community organization model.

UNION INFLUENCE

For a variety of reasons, unions have been compelled to seek health care primarily through collective bargaining and then to press for it in the political arena. Progress by unions for health care increased during World War II, when, due to wartime control over wage increases, so-called fringe benefits—including health and welfare—were expanded through collective bargaining. It was during the late 1940s that the first effort toward national health insurance was made by unions and socially oriented and concerned groups, such as cooperatives and consumer organizations. Resistance from health providers defeated this early effort, but unions intensified their bargaining for health care, primarily the financing and levels of benefits. It was this collective bargaining that promoted the tremendous growth of the Blue Cross/ Blue Shield plans as mechanisms for prepaying hospital and surgical fees, as well as the growth of several major prepaid group practice plans.

Year after year, collective bargaining brought forth more monies to pay for spiraling costs. Many times unions had to accept losses in the middle of a contract or had to go to the members for contributions to continue the benefits. Because there were frequent discussions concerning benefits at union meetings, union members were well educated regarding benefit packages and the bargaining process. This transformed the consumer from a passive recipient to an articulate "demander" of all kinds of medical-care services. As the consuming public became more sophisticated and the "mystery" surrounding the practice of medicine continued to be dispelled, greater interest was directed toward the quality of care. Today, most people feel that access to high-quality medical care is a right, not a privilege.

With millions of members and their families supporting them, unions are a considerable force in the development of comprehensive health care programs and in the development of dual-choice agreements with

[6]*Ibid.*, pp. 223–225.

HMOs. Dr. I. S. Falk of Yale University summarizes the union's influence:

The unions' increasing interest in health and their goals in matters of medical care are important not only to their own members but for society as a whole. Many union activities are conducted in the framework of community wide services. Union policies and programs for their own members tend to set patterns for others as well.[7]

Subscriber Viewpoint

Four rather subjective indicators are used by HMO administrators in evaluating the level of consumer acceptance and the extent to which HMOs meet the expectations of their subscribers. These are frequency with which persons who are offered alternative choices (dual or multiple) elect the HMO option, subscriber opinion, frequency with which plan subscribers use services outside the plan as opposed to those services available to them within the plan (leakages), and subscriber turnover rate. Although these indicators provide evidence only of consumer opinion, they do offer some guidance to the HMO administrator on how to improve subscriber satisfaction with the plan. Such indicators of consumer acceptance are described in the following sections.

DUAL CHOICE

HMO prototypes (i.e., older prepaid group practice plans upon which the concepts of currently developing HMOs are based) found that their initial marketing activities with employer groups and unions were enhanced by a dual-choice offering—two alternative health plans. "Dual choice" was the prepaid group practice plan's partial (although somewhat inaccurate) answer to the "free choice of physician" controversy. Opponents of the HMO movement argue that, since the HMO represents a closed-panel practice of medicine, subscribers have no choice among physicians; subscribers may receive care under the plan only through the physician group except in emergencies. This, it is contended, violates the right of free choice and impairs the patient's ability to obtain quality medical care. Thus, older HMOs have provided a dual choice in health plans—between the HMO and another health insurance plan—and, hence, wider physician choice. (The argument is

[7]Douglas M. Haynes, ed. *Louisville Area Conference on the Delivery of Health Care.* Louisville, Ky., University of Louisville, 1971, p. 17.

moot, since many people today cannot locate physicians in the fee-for-service system that will accept them as their patients. Subscribers in the HMO system not only are guaranteed a physician but are assisted in selecting one.)[8]

Dual choice is primarily a method for the developing HMO to gain access to traditionally closed markets. The dual-choice strategy may be developed as follows: employers and unions whose present health insurance coverage is through the "Blues" or an indemnity carrier agree to participate in the HMO program and to offer the HMO option to employees or union members in addition to the health plan presently being offered, thereby allowing the employees a choice of health programs. But more importantly for the HMO manager, the HMO gains access to previously closed market segments, a point that is further refined in Chapter 8, concerning marketing. For the present purposes, an analysis of the choices made between the two or more programs offered a group is one indication of public acceptance of the HMO.

There are three methods of designing and providing dual-choice options. First, the HMO may agree to offer (i.e., actually sell) another indemnity and/or "Blue" plan in addition to its own prepaid health-plan offering. To do this, the HMO completes a contractual arrangement or agreement with the other health plan carriers that describes the responsibilities of each under such an arrangement. The HMO may be responsible for the collection of premiums, not only for its health plan but also for the "Blue" or indemnity health plan. Second, an incumbent plan may agree to market the HMO plan and also to collect premiums and manage the account for the HMO. The third and most widely used method is based on negotiations with subscribing groups such as unions, employers, associations, and others. In these negotiating sessions, the HMO obtains permission from the policyholder of the subscribing group to offer the HMO health plan in addition to a currently offered "Blue" or indemnity plan. The subscribing group, however, agrees to continue its current agreement with the existing health plan and to be responsible for its operation. Thus, the HMO is not involved in the collection of premiums or in the actual operation of the existing plan, but a dual choice is created for the subscribing group. Opportunities must be given in both dual-choice offerings for subscribers to transfer between the two health plans—usually an annual open enrollment period lasting several weeks.

---

[8]Walter P. Dearing. *Developments and Accomplishments of Comprehensive Group Practice Prepayment Programs.* Washington, D.C., Group Health Association of America, Inc., 1963, p. 8.

When two competing health plans are *first* offered to a group, experience shows that the enrollment is approximately equal in both plans. Generally, one of the programs achieves over time a substantially larger enrollment than the other. On the other hand, if dual choice is offered after one plan has been available for some time, the incumbent plan has a definite advantage. It may be some years before the HMO achieves parity in enrollment; it may never reach the level of the incumbent plan's market share.[9]

Several studies concerning dual choice have been undertaken: One compared enrollment levels between Blue Cross and a Kaiser program; another study described enrollment in Group Health Insurance (GHI) (Blue Cross/Blue Shield of New York City) and the Health Insurance Plan of Greater New York (HIP). Avedis Donabedian[10] reports that the results of both studies are similar; basically, people who choose prepaid plans do so because of the greater security these plans offer against the costs of illness. Those who select the alternative plan do so because it offers *greater physician choice*. The GHI-HIP study suggests that previous medical experience, in general, and prior relationships with a regular doctor, in particular, are important factors in the consumer's choice of plans; what friends and associates do or say also appears to be an important factor influencing subscribers. Free choice, especially for physician care, was an important factor among the more educated and higher income families. A symbol of economic and social independence appears to be the ability to afford free choice.

There seems to be no appreciable adverse selection by enrollees in the prepaid group practice plans; families with high medical bills or those that perceive themselves to be poor have the same propensity to choose an HMO as families that are similar in all other aspects.[11]

The Kaiser study showed that people joined the Kaiser program because of lower costs and better coverage. One might expect this in a dual-choice situation when the HMO program offers broader benefits and greater economic security against additional charges. The HMO offering a program in a dual-choice arrangement must take special care: to plan for and manage potentially higher use situations; when enrolling large families whose health care needs may be greater; in those areas of

[9]Avram Yedida. "Dual Choice Programs." *American Journal of Public Health,* 49(11): 1477, November 1959.

[10]Avedis Donabedian. *A Review of Some Experiences with Prepaid Group Practice.* Research Series No. 12. Ann Arbor, Mich., School of Public Health, Bureau of Public Health Economics, University of Michigan, 1965, pp. 4–5.

[11]Clifton R. Gaus, Barbara S. Cooper, and Constance G. Hirschman. "Contrasts in HMO and Fee-for-Service Performance." *Social Security Bulletin,* 39(5):7–8, May 1976.

the country that have greater medical-care needs; and in those areas having a higher percentage of young children or a larger proportion of nonwhites.

Other data suggest that vulnerability to health risks is a basic factor affecting the awareness of a subscriber group to available alternatives when choosing between two or more health insurance plans. Rashid Bashshur and Charles Metzner suggest that persons in younger age groups, single persons, those with no dependents, and lower income groups (measured by family income, home ownership, and neighborhood income levels) may be viewed as having less at stake economically and, therefore, as feeling less vulnerable to serious economic loss in meeting health needs. The opposite appears to be true for older persons, those with higher incomes, and those with dependents. Thus, the latter group is more aware of what the choices between health plans offer. Bashshur and Metzner conclude that "it appears that persons with lower vulnerability or with decreased financial capacity to respond to felt vulnerability, and persons who are less involved in organizational activity, are those who are most likely to be unaware of alternatives available to them in such a situation of dual choice."[12]

Studies show that when federal employees have a dual choice between prepaid group practice and other plans, the prepaid group plans have attracted from 2.5 percent in the North Central states to 44.8 percent on the West Coast. There are several unsubstantiated reasons why employees do not select the HMO option. These include the limited geographical area in which a plan operates, lack of free choice of physicians and hospitals, philosophical opposition to HMOs as being components of a socialized medicine program, and potential gaps in coverage not found in the other choices available.[13] Because of the importance of using dual- and multiple-choice plan offerings in attracting persons to the HMO, further discussion of dual choice as a marketing strategy is provided in Chapter 8.

Generally, choice of plans depends on the knowledge that a choice is available; knowledge of specific health care plan attributes and their

[12]Rashid L. Bashshur and Charles A. Metzner. "Vulnerability of Risks and Awareness of Dual Choice of Health Insurance Plans." *Health Services Research, 5:* 106–113, Spring 1970. See also, Klaus Roghmann et al. "Who Choses Prepaid Medical Care: Survey Results from Two Marketings of Three New Prepayment Plans." *Public Health Reports, 90*(6):516–527, November–December 1975.

[13]Marie Henderson. "Federal Employees Health Benefits Program, II: Role of the Group Practice Prepayment Plans." *American Journal of Public Health, 56:*54–57, January 1966. See also Donald C. Riedel et al. *Federal Employees Health Benefits Program, Utilization Study.* Rockville, Md., Health Resources Administration, U.S. Department of Health, Education, and Welfare, 1975.

ascription to one or other plans; and the degree of the importance of, or valuation placed upon, each attribute to the subscriber's needs. This strongly suggests that evaluating the public health care needs and attitudes must be a major function of the HMO.

SUBSCRIBER OPINIONS

There are several studies that discuss subscriber opinions of the care received in HMOs and conditions under which care is provided. These studies offer a highly subjective, although informative, indication of subscriber viewpoints, and they also support some general conclusions. The general impression is that a large majority of subscribers are satisfied with whatever plan they belong to. Donabedian notes that there was general acceptance of three plans that differed greatly as to sponsorship and benefits.[14] Although most subscribers are satisfied, a small "hard core" of dissatisfied persons—approximately 10 percent of all subscribers—have a negative view of almost all aspects of the plan to which they belong, whether it is a prepaid group practice plan or another health insurance program.

The subscribers who complain do so in almost all areas relating to care. They feel that the physicians are impersonal, that obtaining medical care is inconvenient, and that there is an atmosphere of a charity clinic and poverty medical care. Complaints are received concerning long waits and the difficulty of obtaining home visits. Few complaints, however, are received concerning freedom of physician choice. Although more than 55 percent of HMO complaints relate to certain "intrinsic" features of group practice, the remaining 45 percent are common to medical practice in general.[15] It is important for the HMO manager to realize that a considerable portion of subscriber complaints apply to medical care everywhere, although this should not be an excuse to avoid remedying most subscriber complaints; to do otherwise would be harmful to a program that relies primarily on a "word-of-mouth" marketing strategy. Thus, a mechanism to handle consumer complaints is imperative in an HMO for it to be competitive with the fee-for-service medical-care system.

Another study suggests that subscriber opinions are developed in part through their evaluation of medical care received, using two criteria: personal interest in the patient by the physician and technical

[14]Avedis Donabedian. "An Evaluation of Prepaid Group Practice." *Inquiry, VI*(3):7–8, September 1969.
[15]*Ibid.*, pp. 19–20.

competence. Subscribers view prepaid group practice as promoting the technical quality of care but hampering the establishment of a satisfactory personal relationship with a physician. Subscribers feel that quality is not measured by competent physicians but by the use of the technical, diagnostic, and consultative resources offered by the HMO. "Additionally, subscribers appreciate the absence of financial incentives. Labor Health Institute data indicate that subscribers tend to accept perceived limitations in care, so long as the quality of care is thought to be superior."[16] At the outset, there will always be some who will say they like the plan's quality of care, while, at the same time, will complain that they do not like the physician-patient relationship or the perceived lack of personal attention. Some subscribers will bring into the plan a set of prejudices that predludes acceptance or approval of the plan.[17]

Several reasons have been suggested for the negative perception by subscribers concerning the lack of personal interest and the system's unresponsiveness to their needs. It may be that some people feel that the doctors do not care about the patients because there are no financial, fee-for-service incentives for them to do so. Others state that there appear to be too many people—paraprofessionals, clerks, and others—between the patient and the physician. It may be that a high medical staff turnover and the interchangeability of physicians make it difficult to establish deep physician-patient relationships.[18] These attitudes are summarized by studies which show that only two-thirds of all HMO subscribers consider the HMO physician to be their family or regular physician.

Is consumer acceptance of, and satisfaction with, the HMO directly related to certain characteristics of the population served? Several recent studies have revealed that, when given a choice among health insurance plans, subscriber selections were not strongly associated with demographic variables. Generally, preference for prepaid group practice is greatest among those persons between 30 and 60 years of age, with young children in the family, with generally better than average education, and with average to moderately high income levels. Moreover, prepaid group practice plans win enthusiastic acceptance when continuity and quality of care is emphasized by the group, when obstacles between doctor and patient are removed, and when personal attention is given to the subscriber.

[16]*Ibid.*, p. 8.
[17]*Ibid.*
[18]*Ibid.*

The attitudes of consumers are more than mirrors of accumulated experience; they are strong indicators of the plan's general acceptance and of the degree to which it succeeds. "To some extent consumer acceptance of prepaid group practice plans is an expression of the absence of a prior patient-physician relationship or a breakdown of such relationships."[19]

LEAKAGES FROM THE SYSTEM

Another indicator of consumer satisfaction is the extent to which HMO enrollees use services outside the plan in preference to similar services available within the HMO. HMO managers have long felt that enrollees were receiving an appreciable proportion of their services from outside providers. Donabedian reports that outside physicians are used for 37 percent of HIP's surgical operations, 14 percent of all paid physician services and 33 percent of all home calls in the Kaiser-Permanente programs, and 23 percent of physician and dentist services at the Labor Health Institute.[20] Weinerman reports that 15 percent of a sample of HIP members used nonplan surgeons and obstetricians. At HIP, the heaviest users of outside services were wives of subscribers, members with the longest tenure in the plan, and those with the highest educational attainment. Reasons given by HIP subscribers for using outside services included confidence in a prior personal doctor, easier access and convenience of private care, and dissatisfaction with group service.[21] In a more recent study (1973–1976), completed under contract with the Department of Health, Education, and Welfare, using Group Health Association (Washington, D.C.) enrollees, similar statistics were obtained.[22] The proportion of all services that were obtained "out-of-plan" was 14 percent, and at least 20 percent of all enrollees made at least one visit out-of-plan annually. Reasons provided by enrollees for out-of-plan use included personal convenience, receiving services at work or at school, and preferring to use their own outside physician. Dissatisfaction could be interpreted, at least from this study, as the plan's inability to effectively incorporate the enrollee into the HMO system. Out-of-plan use also differed according to enrollee characteristics. Low-income enrollees and

[19]*Ibid.*, p. 10.

[20]*Ibid.*, p. 12.

[21]Richard Weinerman. "Patients Perceptions of Group Medical Care." *American Journal of Public Health*, 54(6):880–889, June 1964.

[22]Sam Myers. (Bureau of Social Science Research, Washington, D.C.) Personal conversation, November 18, 1976.

blacks had more out-of-plan visits than higher income enrollees and whites. Virtually no out-of-plan use was associated with "single" subscribers—members with individual coverage. Thus, the use of outside services may be related to prior physician-patient relationships, dissatisfaction with plan services, greater convenience, and the type of health services desired, even though the use of outside services requires additional expenditures over the premiums paid to the HMO.

SUBSCRIBER TURNOVER RATE

The last method for evaluating subscriber opinion of HMOs is to review on a periodic basis the number of members electing to disenroll from the program. Such a statistic should indicate general public approval or disapproval of HMO programs and operations. The annual turnover rate also can be compared to annual growth rates of new members— another broad indication of a plan's success. Most HMO prototypes must have had satisfied customers, because they had low turnover rates—from less than 1 percent to a high of 3 percent. The Kaiser programs have experienced current growth rates of up to 16 percent annually, with only a 2 percent disenrollment rate. Group Health Cooperative of Puget Sound has a disenrollment rate of less than 2 percent; the individuals that disenroll are identified as subscribers who are actually dissatisfied with the plan.

Based on this data, HMO managers should continually monitor both enrollment and disenrollment rates to obtain broad estimates of consumer satisfaction with HMO programs. Levels of disenrollment below 3 percent can be considered acceptable. Higher levels suggest that the manager should evaluate programs and services to identify areas for improvement.

Special Consumer Groups

Throughout their history, HMOs have been concerned with the delivery of health services to special consumer groups, be they union or employer groups, groups of federal employees, Medicaid and Medicare recipients, or underserved groups or rural populations. P.L. 93-222 has singled out several of these groups for special treatment, including medically underserved groups, rural groups, Native Americans, and domestic agricultural migratory and seasonal workers. The Secretary of Health, Education, and Welfare is authorized to reimburse qualifying HMOs for services rendered to Native Americans and migratory workers, as well as to set aside funds for and give preference to the development of HMOs in underserved and rural areas. In addition, Sections 206(e) and 226 of P.L. 92-603 address the provision of care to Medicare and Medicaid groups through HMOs. The legislative authorization for these and other programs developed for special groups is discussed in Chapter 3.

Because of the emphasis placed on these special groups, their attitudes and opinions and their special needs and desires must be considered. The following sections discuss two of these groups.

UNDERSERVED AREAS: THE RURAL POPULATION

The health care needs of people in rural areas are similar to those of people in urban areas. Their available health resources, however, are much more limited because of distance from, and lower per capita rates of, physicians. Limitations are most obvious in sparsely settled geographic areas and areas that are low in economic resources. While ninety percent of the nation's land continues to be inhabited by a little less than one-third of the nation's population, within this third are half of the nation's poor. Geographic dispersion can be appreciated only when one considers some examples: In western Colorado, only 15,000 families occupy a land mass of 23,000 square miles; in the state of Nevada, excluding Reno and Las Vegas, only 18,000 families occupy 73,000 square miles. Similarly, poverty levels in rural areas can be better understood when one realizes that, among poor rural families, 70 percent exist on less than $2,000 per year, and one family in four, on less than $1,000 per year. Given the current planning constraints for HMO development, which set breakeven enrollment at a level of 20,000–30,000 subscribers and individual premiums at a level of approximately $40–$70 per month, it appears that HMOs are not the answer to the health problems of the rural poor; even DHEW's Division of Health Maintenance Organizations suggests that new HMO federal grantees should not attempt to market to families with an annual income of less than $10,000 except under special circumstances. There are some examples of rural HMOs, however, that serve the nation's rural nonpoor—the Geisenger HMO of central Pennsylvania, Rural Health Associates of Maine, and the Northern Livingston Health Center in the Genessee Valley of New York, among others.

Many questions remain unanswered concerning HMO development in rural areas, and federal programs that aid in their establishment must deal with the following issues, some of which have been suggested by H. J. Johnston, Rural Health Consultant to the Community Health Service of DHEW.

1. Developing and maintaining comprehensive service without sacrificing accessibility in terms of geographic access and family purchasing power and without denying rural consumers a realistic opportunity to share in decisions about matters that affect their health and their finances.

2. Establishing linkages between large and small centers to provide comprehensive services.

3. Maintaining a constant adequate flow of income from enrollees who get their income in lump sums once or twice a year rather than on a regular basis (weekly, biweekly, semimonthly, monthly, and so on); those who may be employed seasonally, sometimes with long periods of unemployment; those who may be affected by a general crop disaster in their area so that, although fully employed, they have little or no income in a given year; or those who may have subsistence-level incomes.

4. Maintaining an acceptable level of health services in rural areas with diminishing populations.

5. Overcoming professional isolation and the poverty of social and cultural life in many rural areas in order to make them more attractive to professional health workers and their families.

6. Coping with development situations created by Medicare and Medicaid that make some of the present rural health care vendors unacceptable for participation under the program.

7. Developing more state Medicaid/HMO contractual relationships for rural populations.

8. Coping with the recurring threat of medical monopoly in rural areas.

9. Coping with high development and initial operating costs for HMOs serving rural areas which have great needs and which have been greatly underserved.

10. Developing total social programs for rural populations in addition to comprehensive HMO benefit packages, which singly will not bring community health to the area.

HMOs must be modified to be effective in rural areas. During the planning stages, lower start-up enrollment and breakeven levels may be appropriate; initial enrollment levels in rural HMOs have been as low as 2,000–3,000 enrollees, and breakeven levels of operation may approach the 8,000–10,000 enrollment level rather than the urban 20,000–30,000 level. This suggests that the rural HMO must become even more efficient and cost-effective than its urban counterpart. Lower breakeven levels may require the following:

1. A less comprehensive benefit package than that suggested by P.L. 93-222 and P.L. 94-460, with a phase-in of additional benefits as the plan increases its cash reserves.

2. Setting premiums at levels that will provide more funds for lower breakeven operation.

3. HMO catchment areas that will include larger geographic areas and, thus, longer travel distances and times for subscribers. HMOs may consider offering a transportation benefit, although, traditionally, rural families always have had to travel long distances for services.

4. Allowing HMO physicians to supplement either their own salaries or the plan's income by accepting fee-for-service patients. Tough management procedures would be necessary for control and for the phasing out of the fee-for-service practice when the capitated practice was large enough.

5. Planning by HMOs to include educational activities for major subscribers to explain why subscriber outlays for the HMO will be larger than they were before joining the program, to explain the HMO concept and how to use the system, and to explain the efficacy of preventive health benefits.

6. Since the HMO would, in all probability, become the major health center for the region, use of an existing hospital site would be most appropriate. This will require close coordination with the hospital and other local health providers.

7. The rural HMO must use every available federal support program, including funds for construction from the Hill-Burton, Farmers Home Loan Administration, and Housing and Urban Development programs; initial operating grants, loans, and loan guarantees through P.L. 93-222; and funds for servicing federal employees, CHAMPUS recipients, Medicare and Medicaid recipients, migrant workers, and Native Americans. Although such funds are "soft money" that easily disappears, these federal programs may be used as an initial financial base, which can then be supplemented by subscribers not in funded projects. The goal of the rural HMO, however, would be to develop a mix of subscriber groups rather than to depend on an enrollee population composed primarily of federal, state, and local government program recipients.

8. Management would have to use every available fiscal monitoring technique and stringent control procedures. Innovative fiscal programs are now available, such as those described in Chapter 10.

These eight points can be instrumental to the success of rural HMOs.

UNDERSERVED AREAS: THE URBAN POVERTY POPULATION

Are HMOs useful in providing services to poverty populations in major metropolitan areas? Before answering this question, several constraints placed on HMOs, concerning their participation with indigent populations, should be discussed. First, HMOs do not want to be considered poor people's programs or poverty clinics; therefore, they prefer to maintain a mixture of subscriber groups. The level of indigents usually accepted by an HMO should not exceed the level found in the general population. Second, it is assumed that poverty populations have a high need for health care, thus, are high users of health care facilities; they are considered high-risk groups, for which HMOs may not be willing to accept the financial risk. Finally, payments for services (benefits) may be limited, based on negotiations with state and federal assistance agencies.

A review of three plans[23] providing care to Office of Economic Opportunity (OEO) program recipients—the Kaiser Foundation of Oregon, Group Health Cooperative of Puget Sound, and Health Insurance Plan of Greater New York—shows that a full range of health care services can be provided to a selected medically indigent population by an already existing HMO. Each of the three programs emphasizes that such care can be rendered on a one-class basis with no differentiation between OEO plan members and regular plan enrollees. Greater than normal emphasis is placed on various supportive activities, such as an effective outreach program, transportation services, and appointment and reminder systems. Through these, enrollees are made aware of the services available to them and are aided in achieving appropriate utilization of services.

Each of the three plans relies on some mechanism for community participation, usually through an advisory body established specifically for this purpose. Moreover, each of the plans draws some of its membership from the population eligible for Medicaid in the particular area

[23]Leon Gintzig and Robert G. Shouldice. "Prepaid Group Practice: An Analysis as a Delivery System." Washington, D.C., The George Washington University, 1972, pp. 134–147. Mimeographed. See also Theodore J. Colombo, Ernest W. Saward, and Merwyn R. Greenlick. "Group Practice Plans in Governmental Medical Care Programs. IV. The Integration of an O.E.O. Health Program into a Prepaid Comprehensive Group Practice Plan." *American Journal of Public Health,* 59(4):641–650, April 1969; Merwyn R. Greenlick et al. "Comparing the Use of Medical Care Services by a Medically Indigent and a General Membership Population in a Comprehensive Prepaid Group Practice Program." *Medical Care,* X(3):187–200, May–June 1972; and Richard Handschin et al. "Effect of Outreach Support on Medical Care Utilization Patterns of Low Income Enrollees in a Prepaid Group Practice: Group Health Cooperative of Puget Sound." Paper presented at the System Science Evaluation Conference, New Orleans, La., March 19–20, 1975.

to be served. On the basis of certain priority criteria, this population is narrowed to the number that the program is designed to accommodate. Such factors as medical need, transportation availability, and family composition are among the membership criteria considered. Finally, each of the three plans have indicated that, although some specific differences exist, these differences are small and rather insignificant. The utilization of services by the urban indigent does not appear too different from that exhibited by the general population of the HMO. Exceptions were noted in two categories: the no-show rate for the OEO population was generally higher than that for the other health plan members, and OEO populations used more services outside of regular clinic hours. These conclusions also are supported by the results of a study completed by Gaus, Fuller, and Bohannon concerning the utilization rates of 1,000 Medicaid beneficiaries before and after enrollment in the Group Health Association plan in Washington, D.C.[24] As in the three previously mentioned plans, the use of services by the Medicaid population was similar to the general GHA population, although slightly higher during the first year. Hospitalization rates were lower for the Medicaid group after GHA enrollment than before. Further results of these studies are reviewed in Chapter 9, which concerns utilization levels.

It appears, from the results of these programs, that if some restraint is used in the number of indigent persons enrolled in the HMO, there should be little or no added financial risk. Emphasis on underwriting activities certainly will be an important aspect in the decision-making process concerning service to poverty populations, and somewhat greater resources must be made available for educational programs to teach this special group about the use of the system. The HMO should be able to deliver quality, comprehensive health services to indigent populations who are recipients of federal, state, and local government programs. No answer is currently available for provision of services to those individuals who cannot pay premiums and for whom no government program has been established.

Consumer Participation Programs

Informed, knowledgeable, and active consumers can be a major asset for HMOs. They can help considerably in identifying problems and in-

[24]Clifton R. Gaus, Norman A. Fuller, and Carol Bohannon. "HMO Evaluation: Utilization Before and After Enrollment." Paper Presented at the Annual Meeting of the American Public Health Association, Atlantic City, N.J., November 15, 1972.

adequacies in the health programs and in ensuring that the solutions developed by the policymaking bodies are based on awareness of consumer needs. In certain circumstances, consumers may help to determine overall policy and may participate in the development of operational plans. Consumers are called on much less frequently to monitor the delivery of health services, that is, to evaluate the HMO activity in terms of accessibility, acceptability, comprehensiveness, and cost. Most importantly, consumers become spokesmen and salesmen for the HMO plan; they either encourage or discourage their friends to join the HMO.

Consumer participation programs are developed around several basic elements:

1. A means of informing members about the HMO operation, programs, choices, enrollment methods, complaint-handling procedures, and so on.

2. A program of consumer education and training that will lead to appropriate utilization of services and good health maintenance and prevention. Training sessions may be tailored to the orientation of enrollees who will participate on boards, consumer councils, or advisory committees.

3. A method of allowing enrollees to augment their role as consumers in a free-market economy by participating in the decision-making process.

4. A mechanism for lodging and handling consumer complaints.

METHODS OF SUBSCRIBER PARTICIPATION

The first two of the aforementioned elements need little explanation. There are, however, several accepted methods for actual consumer participation and the handling of complaints.[25] The consumer-model HMOs traditionally have been built on direct consumer involvement in the policy- and decision-making processes through board of trustee representation. Although formal membership on a board does not assure significant involvement, it does make the opportunity for participation explicitly clear and direct. HMOs like the Columbia Medical Plan have established a consumer advisory council, which provides input to the policymaking bodies of the plan. The advisory council has been

[25]Sarah C. Carey et al. *Health Maintenance Organizations: An Introduction and Survey of Recent Developments.* Washington, D.C., Lawyers' Committee for Civil Rights Under Law, 1972, pp. 10–11.

successful in restructuring the benefit package as well as some operational aspects of the outpatient facility. Direct representation on internal management committees is another method of consumer participation. This form, used by Group Health Association of Washington, D.C., is probably one of the most effective ways for subscribers to share their insights with those who are directly responsible for the plan's day-to-day operation. It is also a valuable method for training and informing consumers and for providing immediate feedback to the subscriber group.

The OEO neighborhood health center programs recruit staff from the enrollee population. Although one objective of the programs was the training of enrollees as well as service delivery, one of the major outcomes of such recruitment procedures was the modification of the delivery system from within. There is no question that this is an expensive proposition, but an HMO, especially in an underserved area, may find it highly desirable as a method of educating consumers concerning the HMO concept and of helping to achieve acceptance of the HMO by the population. Another, more vigorous, method of consumer participation found in many HMOs has been through negotiated labor union contracts. Union representatives are aggressive in their negotiations with HMOs to obtain the best possible contracts, and they raise questions referred to them by their union members. Also, like all other plan members, the union representative can use the ultimate free-market tool of consumer participation to induce changes—the threat of or actual withdrawal from the program.

THE SUBSCRIBER COMPLAINT AND GRIEVANCE
RESOLUTION MECHANISM

P.L. 93-222, Section 1301(c)7 requires that, to qualify as an HMO, a health plan must be organized to provide meaningful procedures for hearing and resolving grievances between the HMO and members of the participating organization. From this, and also as good management, the development of a complaint mechanism is of great importance to the smooth operation of the health plan. Data concerning the use of complaint mechanisms in HMOs is available in a study completed under a contract with DHEW's Health Maintenance Organization Service by Koba Associates, Inc. of Washington, D.C. The interim and final reports of the study reveal that subscribers voiced concerns or complaints related to all areas of HMO operation. Table 17 shows the areas of subscriber concerns and the percentage of all HMOs contacted whose subscribers voiced such concerns. Note that complaints about medical

TABLE 17   Complaints Voiced by Subscribers as Reported by HMO
Managers (multiple responses were received)

	Percent
Scheduling appointments	50
Medical and physician care received	57
Benefit package	38
Paramedical personnel attitudes	35
Waiting time	31
Business office errors	23
Communication problems	19
Level of cost of plan	8

Source: Koba Associates, Inc. *An Inventory Analysis of HMO Consumer Complaint Mechanisms.*
Washington, D.C., 1974. (Interim Report to Consumer Progress Division, Health Maintenance Organization Service, U.S. Department of Health, Education, and Welfare.)

care, physician and staff attitudes, and adequacy and appropriateness
of medical services received make up more than one-half of all subscriber concerns. Other subscriber complaints relate to coverage—
including confusion about uncovered benefits that result in medical
bills to the member and inappropriate use of medical care outside the
HMO that results in ineligible claims—and to the system—including
the accessibility of health care, waiting time for appointments, telephone communication problems, member identification, and billing
procedures.

Methods for handling complaints are varied. Consumer-oriented
plans openly discuss the complaint-handling mechanism with subscribers. Physician-sponsored programs, having less consumer orientation,
do not directly address or inform their members regarding complaint
mechanisms. The foundation-type HMOs are least likely to discuss
complaint-handling methods. As the size of the plan grows, the initial
point of contact and the method for lodging a complaint become more
specific. The identification of a focal point for handling complaints—
usually a department or individual connected with the membership—is
a standard procedure for larger HMOs.

Table 18 summarizes the complaint-handling mechanisms used by
eight HMOs; none of the HMOs studied uses a grievance committee to
hear and resolve complaints, although several such committees are
planned. None of the HMOs surveyed has an appeals system established exclusively for hearing and resolving all types of member grievances, although there is an informal appeals process in approximately
75 percent of the plans.

In conclusion, the Koba Associates' study suggests four basic points that make up a responsive grievance system:

1. The provision of information to members about the existence and procedures of the complaint mechanism.
2. The identification and broad publication of a primary entry point for complaints.
3. The provision of information to the complainant about each stage of referral undertaken by the complaint department and the availability of additional levels of referral and/or appeal.
4. The existence of a standing grievance committee.

It appears that there is critical need for mandatory arbitration regulations concerning all grievances in the health care industry. Minnesota has taken the lead and requires informal discussions, consultations, or conferences between the enrollee and the HMO within 30 days after the complaint is filed. If the problem is not resolved, mandatory hearings must be scheduled within 90 days after filing, so that grievances may be resolved before they become court cases.

Quality of Care

Although the primary concern of medical-care personnel has always been the delivery of quality medical care, two related forces have pushed the quality issue higher on their lists of priorities. The first is the law and the growing number of malpractice suits. In particular, the Darling and New Bedford cases[26] clearly established the necessity for providing the highest level of care, for all patients, at all times, and that this high level of care must be one of excellence, not merely one of local practice. The second force is the consumers, who are demanding high standards of care. More importantly, consumers can, by dropping out of a plan, register their dissatisfaction with the care rendered or, through formal review procedures, may become involved in evaluating the levels of care provided by a plan. It is natural, then, that a discussion of quality should be included in a chapter concerning HMO consumers.[27]

[26]*Darling v. Charleston Community Hospital,* 33 Ill.2d326, 211 N.E. 2n 253, 1965; and *Brune v. Belinkoff,* 354 Mass. 102, N.E. 2d 793, 1968.

[27]This discussion will not provide a review of the conceptual framework that has evolved in the quality assessment area. For an excellent review of quality-of-care issues, see Mary Helen Shortridge. "Quality of Medical Care in an Outpatient Setting." *Medical Care, XII*(4):283–300, April 1974; and Avedis Donabedian. *A Guide to Medical Care Administration. Vol. 2–Medical Care Appraisal—Quality and Utilization.* New York, American Public Health Association, 1969.

TABLE 18   Complaint-Handling Mechanisms

HMO	Members Advised of Procedures	Requirement for Entry: Focal Point	Referral Procedures	Appeals System	Special Procedures	By-Laws
Plan A (97,000 enrollees) Nonprofit membership corporation; 1 central location, 5 outlying clinics	Monthly newsletter; brochures; annual meeting; literature mentions "complaints"	None; executive director's office receives and refers all complaints	Made on form to department; required written response	Monetary claims to claims review; all member committee	Member request for professional standards review	Member must use claims review before litigation
Plan B (6,000 enrollees; 18,000 plan members) Nonprofit physician sponsored; 1 central business office with 180 member physicians	Benefit brochure; employer or union meetings; literature does not mention "complaints"	None; business office for plan problems; member physicians for medical problems	Plan problems to staff general manager; medical problems to member physicians	Medical society; insurance commissioner	None	Arbitration is an option
Plan C (185,000 enrollees) Nonprofit consumer owned; 1 hospital, 8 health centers	Monthly magazine; district councils; brochure; literature mentions "favorable or unfavorable" concerns	Prefer written entry; member relations department centralized with a staff of three	Copy of written complaint to department or individual for reply through member relations; unresolved complaints to assistant director for medical affairs	Not formalized; may request hearing before board committee	Monthly and quarterly complaint reports; consulting nurse	No mention
Plan D (37,000 enrollees) Foundation sponsored; 860 member physicians; 22 affiliated hospitals	Enrollment information quarterly distributed to enrollees; literature mentions "problems"	None; patient services department central business office with staff of two	Patient services department director handles most of referrals; medical problems back to M.D.	Requires disenrollment hearings	None	See Appeals System

Source: Koba Associates, Inc. *HMO Consumer Complaint Mechanisms.* Rockville, Md., Health Maintenance Organization Service, U.S. Department of Health, Education, and Welfare, 1974, pp. 10–12.

Major criticisms about the quality of care provided by HMOs have concerned the proponents of the health plans. These arguments suggest that HMOs use poorly trained doctors who join an HMO because it offers a safe, comfortable place to make a living; provide less than adequate amounts of care because of the use of capitation payments that reverse the physician's traditional fee-for-service incentive; use mostly moonlighting residents or foreign-trained physicians to provide care; place blocks between the patient and the physician by using deductions, copayments, and the like, and by making subscribers wait for long periods in reception rooms; drop the really tough cases as soon as they become expensive, or prohibit high-risk people from joining the plan; and provide adequate general care but send subscribers with major illnesses to outside-the-plan specialists.

Some of the answers to these criticisms can be found in the literature; other arguments may be valid but the evidence of their proof is not available. It might be stated that, if an organization, whether it is a capitated health plan or some other service-oriented plan, consistently provides a product or service that is perceived by the consumer as being of low quality for high cost, it will lose members to the point where the product must be improved or the organization will fail. For some HMOs, this point has become fatally clear; others have become very conscious of their product's quality. Without becoming enmeshed in the question of what constitutes quality and how it is measured, a review of the current evidence is appropriate. Donabedian suggests that the quality of medical care in a prepaid group practice plan can be evaluated using several dimensions, including the effective use of medical-care services by subscribers, the types and kinds of physicians and hospitals used by the health plan, the physicians' performance, and the effects of the services on the health of the subscribers—or outcome measurements.

The question of whether prepaid group practice subscribers use medical-care services more effectively is answered by a review of several studies. Donabedian concludes from two other studies that relatively few (15–30 percent) of the subscribers to prepaid group practice feel that being a member of such a plan has affected their use of medical-care services. In addition, Donabedian states that "the available evidence indicates that prepaid group practice enjoys no superiority in the establishment of a perceived relationship between patient and physician."[28] Long-term patient-physician relationships are considered to enhance the quality of health care. Another measurement of quality, according to Donabedian, may be the use of preventive serv-

[28]Donabedian. "An Evaluation of Prepaid Group Practice," p. 21.

ices. In the studies reported by Donabedian, there was little evidence to show that the use of preventive services was greater by prepaid group practice subscribers. There is some suggestion, however, that members in prepaid plans are more likely to delay less in seeking medical care when ill (i.e., less than one day after illness strikes). In addition, there is substantial evidence that prepaid group practice plans reduce the disparity between high and low socioeconomic groups in the use of health care services.[29] Delays in seeking medical care and disparity between high and low socioeconomic groups may be considered evidence of a poorly functioning health-delivery system, resulting in lack of appropriate care.

The second dimension of quality reviewed by Donabedian is the type and kind of physicians and hospitals used by prepaid group practice plans. Qualified physicians and accredited hospitals may be considered a proxy indicator of the level of health care quality. The studies reviewed by Donabedian suggest that specialty care used by prepaid group practice subscribers is provided by qualified specialists (diplomate or equivalent). But it appears that prepaid group practice physicians are least likely to use accredited hospitals. Reasons given are that prepaid physicians may have difficulty obtaining privileges in accredited hospitals or that there are few accredited hospitals in the regions where the study plans were operating.

Other nonrefuted accusations have been suggested regarding plan physicians—that the least qualified physicians join the group, that greater numbers of minority physicians provide services, and so on. It is reasonable to assume, however, that group practice physicians must be highly qualified, since each physician's work is open to the scrutiny of other colleagues. Patients are exchanged and frequently are reviewed by other physicians. Group practice physicians accept only well-qualified candidates to join the group practice in order to avoid serious malpractice incidents.

Another proxy method for identifying quality, according to Donabedian, is to review how physicians actually manage cases. He states that evidence shows that prepaid group practice appears to exert some control in reducing unjustified surgery and, to that extent, contributes to the quality of care. ". . . the manner in which a group is organized, staffed, and equipped appears to be fairly closely related to the quality of physician performance as judged by a review of case records sup-

[29]L. S. Rosenfeld, Avedis Donabedian, and J. Katz. "Unmet Need for Medical Care." *New England Journal of Medicine, 258:*369–376, February 20, 1958; Colombo, Saward, and Greenlick. "Group Practice Plans in Governmental Medical Care Programs. IV," pp. 641–650; and Gaus, Fuller, and Bohannon. "HMO Evaluation," pp. 6–11.

plemented by interviews with the managing physicians."[30] Thus, a review of practice patterns by the medical group may be important.

The last dimension of quality described by Donabedian is a measurement of the health and well-being of the subscribers. Results of studies concerning morbidity and mortality of the general population are inconclusive. Donabedian noted, however, that, in two studies comparing the population of the Health Insurance Plan of Greater New York (HIP) with the population of New York City and an Old Age Assistance (OAA) recipient group, prematurity and prenatal mortality rates were significantly lower in HIP, and the mortality for OAA recipients also was lower for those patients in the HIP programs than for the New York City population. These data have not been systematically studied, however, and may not represent what occurs in most prepaid group practice populations, but they do suggest far-ranging effects if these results are validated by future study.

Although an analysis of HMOs by these four dimensions shows a somewhat positive performance for prepaid group practice plans in comparison to other forms of health insurance and delivery, much more research and study is necessary to accurately determine both the positive and negative quality issues in prepayment practices. Positive forces include the use of unit medical records for subscribers throughout their association with the prepaid plan, which allows for continuity of medical care. Unit medical records also provide a mechanism to facilitate peer review—each new physician the patient sees is provided with the record of all preceding physician services rendered. As an informal peer review mechanism, this process tends to provide both a retrospective and prospective check on HMO physician services. It should be supplemented by the development of regular, continuous monitoring of care that includes the formulation of standards and formalized case reviews by a quality assurance committee of the medical staff. The use of a managing primary-care practitioner—the assignment of a subscriber to a physician who will "watch over" all care provided to the patient—is a well-used and appropriate quality control mechanism in prepaid group practice. The concept of the managing physician is akin to the family doctor concept, which was lost to increased specialization by physicians in the United States. This concept is now recognized as the first level in a good personal health care system. In addition to controlling medical delivery, the HMO system also may provide greater control and coordination of the physical health care resources made available to the physician. More appropri-

[30]Donabedian. "An Evaluation of Prepaid Group Practice," p. 23.

ate use of available buildings, equipment, supplies, and even ancillary personnel may make the physician's services a better "product." It is well understood that the coordination effort of the HMO makes availability of an HMO service an advantage of the system and that subscribers have fewer and shorter delays for services when ill or injured. The HMO physician's control of services has reduced to some extent the inappropriate and unjustified use of surgery or other health care services. Finally, control of physician appointments by the group practice favorably affects quality of care.[31]

Alternatively, there are several forces that may lower the quality of HMO care. Herbert Klarman suggests that "Ancillary services may be wasted if ordered by the physician without discrimination. Excessive referrals may lead to a wholesale evasion of responsibility for the care of the patient . . . . Finally, the peer review that actually takes place in the group setting may be overrated."[32] By the use of capitation payment, HMOs change physician incentives from providing more services to controlling or reducing unjustified services. Unfortunately, in its cost-controlling efforts, an HMO, especially an investor-owned HMO, may inadvertently achieve this goal by inappropriately reducing the amount of the quality of services provided, although evidence does not support this potential capitation effect.

Because there are some doubts concerning the control of quality by HMOs, a variety of quality-control devices should be considered by the HMO manager, including some of the following.

PHYSICIAN GROUP CONTRACT

In developing capitation levels between the HMO and the physician group practice, the first step should be the determination of "appropriate" utilization levels of service to be provided. Described as a range, the appropriate utilization of services can be converted to dollars of services. For example, physician group x, associated with the Healthville HMO, determines that an appropriate utilization rate for appendectomy surgery is from 4.2 to 6.8 per 1,000. Group x will be providing services to 1,000 subscribers, and the average cost of an appendectomy

[31]Recent studies have suggested that many of these advantages (control of utilization of services, accessibility of care, equality, satisfaction, and so on) are not the result of a capitation payment alone but that organized multispecialty group practice arrangements with largely salaried physicians may be a more significant variable. See Gaus, Cooper, and Hirschman. "Contrasts in HMO and Fee-for-Service Performance," pp. 3–14.

[32]Herbert E. Klarman. "Economic Research in Group Medicine." *In: New Horizons in Health Care; Proceedings of the First International Congress on Group Medicine, Winnipeg, April 26–30, 1970.* Winnipeg, Canada, the Congress Secretariat, 1970.

in its geographic area is $300. Thus, the range of cost to be built into the capitation rate for this service would be from $12,600 to $20,000 per year. Inappropriate levels of care could then be described as levels above or below this range.

Renegotiation of the physician group contract would take into consideration such matters as the group's ability to work within the appropriate range established, the record of consumer grievances, ombudsman reports, peer evaluations, evaluation of interviews with physicians managing the group practice, local professional standards review organization analyses, and staff admitting privileges at local hospitals. Establishing standards of care and acceptable utilization levels similar to the aforementioned example is very important for those health care delivery programs whose care is reviewed by local professional standards review organizations. To cope with this kind of review, many providers have developed "treatment protocols" or patient-treatment algorithms. The protocols provide a description of the treatment program for all of the specific services provided by the health plan. Each treatment program describes the utilization rate and length of hospital stay, if indicated, and then a description of the step-by-step treatment of the condition. Added to this information is the level of consumption (i.e., the average range of utilization for each service by the HMO's service area population) and an average cost. With this information, capitation rates can be developed quickly. Further discussion of these issues is found in Chapter 10.

FORMAL PEER REVIEW

The HMO's contract with the physician group should define the physician's responsibility for monitoring quality, especially for the establishment of quality standards. Naturally, the unit medical record serves as the written evidence. Observations of how medicine is actually practiced should become a part of the formal peer review process. Advanced quality assurance systems using such programs as the protocol or patient-treatment algorithm also may be used. These systems will be built around formal peer review, medical record review, and observation analysis and may cost approximately 2 percent of the total costs of providing care.

HEALTH OMBUDSMAN

An individual may be appointed to answer or find answers to specific subscriber complaints, to follow through on complaints, to monitor spot checks, and to be generally available to help consumers find their way through the HMO. To be effective, the ombudsman should report to the HMO board of trustees through the administrator.

GRIEVANCE PROCEDURE

The complaint-review mechanism is discussed in detail earlier in this chapter.

REINSURANCE

Congress recognized the need to protect the newly developing HMO from financial disaster caused by large and unusual expenses or losses created by accepting unmanageable risks. New HMOs should use a reinsurance mechanism to avoid the temptation of providing less or lower quality care to protect their reserves. On the other hand, passing on the complete risk for providing health care to an outside insurer may be an indication of the HMO's inability to provide adequate service. Older HMO prototypes, with relatively large reserves, may find that the use of reinsurance is not only unnecessary, because of their ability to cover losses, but can be more costly than self-insuring, because of large reinsurance premium payments to outside insurers. Normally, HMOs purchase reinsurance from indemnity carriers for the costs of care above $5,000 per individual subscriber per year.[33]

ACCREDITATION AND AGPA, GHAA, AND MGMA

Accreditation by the appropriate organization may be an indication of successfully meeting generally accepted minimum standards of organizational effectiveness and operation and is suggested by some as a reliable indicator of high-quality care. This is not always the case, because, unlike the accreditation of hospitals, the accreditation of HMOs or medical group practices lacks the special significance, impact, or sanctioning power usually associated with being an accredited institution. While it is true that accreditation of an HMO or a group practice generally indicates a certain level of competence and quality in medical care, it is also true that a great deal of reputable, outstanding HMOs and group practices, for some reason or other, have not been accredited or have not even applied for accreditation. The general

[33]A discussion of reinsurance in HMOs can be found in Richard T. Burke and George Strumpf. *Sharing the Risk: A Guide for the Young HMO*. Minneapolis, Minn., InterStudy, 1973.

response to a lack of accreditation in group practices and HMOs is "so what?" This was the attitude taken by hospitals 10 to 15 years ago regarding the Joint Commission on Accreditation of Hospitals (JCAH). Due to increased prestige associated with being an accredited institution and to the fact that the Federal Government considers accreditation to be a precondition for Medicare and Medicaid reimbursement, however, the loss of accreditation, or the inability to obtain accreditation, is considered a critical issue for many major hospitals. As a result, a new awareness of accreditation and a corresponding trend toward seriousness in accreditation is occurring in the field of ambulatory health care.

Part of the reason for the apparent apathy concerning accreditation of HMOs and group practices may be the relative newness in organizational forms and the lack of coordination among ambulatory health care providers. Although one organization formerly responsible for accreditation of HMOs, group practices, and outpatient facilities—the American Group Practice Association (AGPA)—had been in existence since 1949, its functions of accreditation were not delineated until 1968—20 years after its inception. Other organizations also have been involved in accreditation and have added to the general confusion, as well as to the splintering of provider organization affiliations; for example, the Group Health Association of America (GHAA) has developed standards for member health plans. The Medical Group Management Association (MGMA) provides managers and administrators of group practice clinics with membership categories. JCAH provides review and possible accreditation guidelines to hospitals that are used, owned, or operated by an HMO.

AGPA's accreditation procedures are far from perfect. The application for membership and accreditation is strictly on a voluntary basis and is internally controlled and regulated (i.e., there are no specific external legislative restrictions or mandates). Moreover, accreditation is not a prerequisite for membership in AGPA, and the program is designed for both fee-for-service and capitated prepaid group practice organizations. Although it has been available since 1968, accredited status has not been obtained by a large percentage of AGPA's members. Of approximately 430 members in 1975, only 123 were accredited, and of those, 10 groups have allowed their accreditation to lapse. This small percentage of accredited members may be attributed to the fact that there are separate procedures for membership and for accreditation. Prospective members of AGPA undergo a survey by its credentials committee, which conducts a cursory investigation of the quality of the group's overall medical care and organizational structure. After a specified period, a member can apply for accreditation. At such time, representative physicians from AGPA's accreditation committee conduct an on-site survey, following a set of standards developed by the AGPA membership and focusing on clinical aspects as well as the medical audit program of the practice. Normal accreditation is for a four-year period, at which time reaccreditation is usually sought.

The AGPA accreditation guidelines can be categorized as follows:

1. Size and type of the organization
2. Clinical aspects of the medical practice
3. Educational activities (in-house)
4. Research activities
5. Technology
6. Staffing and specialty distribution
7. Organization
8. Facilities

During the on-site visit, an overall assessment of a practice's performance and its compliance with the criteria within each of the eight categories is made. To become accredited, a practice must comply with the essential criteria; however, failure to meet one standard does not prohibit accreditation status.

Several recent events have affected both the AGPA and the accreditation of HMOs. The most important is the merger of AGPA's accreditation committee with JCAH to form the Accreditation Council for Ambulatory Health Care (ACAHC), which is an interdisciplinary program to establish and oversee standards for outpatient care. The ramifications of this merger are being felt throughout the country. Although the merger was effective in April 1976, as of December 1976, ACAHC had not fully assumed responsibility for accrediting group practices. ACAHC was in a transitional period until January 1977, at which time it became fully operational. During the transitional period, ACAHC adopted the AGPA guidelines with two major additions: presence of a functional, effective, on-going internal medical audit system and existence of unit medical records. In addition to these changes, ACAHC has stated that future noncompliance with any one of the accreditation guidelines would deter accreditation. Specific requirements for the medical records diagnosis summary and for drug administration also have been established. ACAHC projects increasing influence by professional standards review organization programs and a push toward the achievement of accredited status, a precondition of payment by Medicare and Medicaid; it also plans to broaden its range of those ambulatory-care facilities that might be subject to accreditation (i.e., family-planning clinics, neighborhood health centers). In light of the more stringent guidelines adopted by ACAHC, the accreditation of medical group practices and HMOs, as well as other ambulatory-care services, may become a significant indicator of acceptable operation and of quality medical care.

CONSUMER EVALUATION

There is some evidence that consumers are able to evaluate competing health insuring and delivery mechanisms and to choose the one that best meets their needs. Indeed, Smith and Metzner, in an article in *Medical Care,* suggest that patients may be capable of evaluating the nontechnical aspects of care and could theoretically provide a balance usually not found in the traditional mechanisms of evaluation.[34] It appears, however, that most consumers have insufficient information to make accurate judgments. More information about accreditation, physician certification, use of technicians and physician extenders, HMO financial and administrative records, grievance committee reports, enrollment/disenrollment figures, physician turnover rates, and so on, should be judiciously made available to subscribers if they are to evaluate service.

Summary

HMO consumers are becoming more active in the development of health care policy and the evaluation of the health care product. This is the outcome not only of greater general consumer awareness but also (and more importantly) of the increasing number of individuals with health insurance, higher disposable incomes, higher living standards, and improved communications. Consumer participation is or will be felt in the areas of which health care product will be provided, the cost of care, method of financing, adequacy of manpower, quality of practice, organization of the delivery mechanism, policy formulations, and facility management.

A study conducted by Jerome L. Schwartz in six consumer cooperatives and six private physician health plans concludes that consumer participation changes with the age of the plan. An early tradition of

[34]David Barton Smith and Charles A. Metzner. "Differential Perceptions of Health Care Quality in a Prepaid Group Practice." *Medical Care, VIII*(4):273, July–August 1970.

cooperation can set the mode for participation; the size of the membership affects participation; and the influence of ordinary members is diminished when complex decisions are required to run large organizations. Moreover, Schwartz found that the members who are active are normally from higher socioeconomic levels in the community. Generally, consumer sponsorship of a plan appears to influence the programs of the health plan in favor of the members.

Four somewhat subjective indicators can be used in evaluating the level of consumer acceptance and the extent to which HMOs meet the expectation of subscribers—frequency of electing the HMO option under dual choice, subscriber opinion, frequency of use of outside services, and subscriber turnover rates. Generally, two competing health plans will achieve approximately equal enrollment during the first enrollment period, with one taking a definite lead over the other in the long run. People choose the HMO option because of greater security, lower costs, and better coverage, and the alternative plan because of greater physician choice. There appears to be no appreciable adverse selection by enrollees in prepaid health plans. Choice of plans depends on the knowledge of availability of choice, the attributes and drawbacks of each plan, and the degree to which each attribute is of importance to the subscriber.

Most subscribers are satisfied with the health plan they choose; approximately 10 percent are dissatisfied. Complaints concerning HMOs relate to impersonal care, inconvenience of long waits, difficulty in obtaining home visits, and problems common to medical practice in general. Prepaid group practice is perceived by patients as promoting the technical quality of care but hampering the establishment of a satisfactory personal relationship with the physicians. Use of outside services (i.e., leakages from the system) has been estimated to be from 15 to 37 percent of all services provided to plan subscribers. This outside use may be related to prior physician-patient relationships, dissatisfaction with plan services, greater convenience, and the type of health services desired—especially specialty care. Subscriber opinions concerning the plan also are mirrored in its turnover rate. Levels of disenrollment below 3 percent appear to be acceptable.

Service to underserved rural and urban poverty populations has presented special problems for HMOs. It is apparent that HMOs cannot be the single answer to the health problems of rural and urban poverty populations. HMOs were never developed to exclusively serve the needs of either the very poor or the very wealthy; they are more appropriately suited to provide health care to a cross-section of a community. With much care and planning, HMOs have successfully met the needs of these underserved groups together with other sectors of the community; however, there still is no solution to the problem of providing services to individuals unable to pay the premiums and for whom no governmental programs have been established.

HMO consumer participation programs are developed around four elements—a method of informing consumers of HMO procedures and policies, an education and training program, a method of participation in the decision-making process, and a consumer complaint system. Methods of participation include board of trustee representation, consumer advisory councils, and external management committees. Grievance resolution mechanisms are required by the HMO law. At the present time, various complaint mechanisms are used by HMOs, although use of a grievance committee and mandatory arbitration is limited to very few plans. Mandatory arbitration could be a method to settle grievances and malpractice problems before they become court cases.

HMOs have been criticized about the level of quality of health care services. Most research concerning HMO care shows a favorable quality profile; this is logical, since health plans, whether prepaid or fee-for-service, would cease to exist if care was perceived to be consistently poor by patients. There is insufficient data, however, to rate HMOs in comparison to the traditional health-delivery methods. Forces that may positively affect the quality of care provided by an HMO include the use of a unit medical record, formal and informal peer review, use of the managing primary-care physician, control and coordination of health care resources and more appropriate use of these services, and control by the medical group of the appointment of new physicians to its group. The major force that may negatively affect HMO quality may be the capitation incentive system, although the use of treatment protocols or algorithms to determine appropriate practice patterns and use levels may offset any negative aspects of capitated medicine. Quality-control devices available to the HMO manager should be used and should include a strong HMO physician group contract, formal peer review, a health ombudsman, grievance procedures, use of reinsurance, accreditation of the health plan and its administrators, and the use of consumer evaluations of the program.

References

Carey, Sarah C., et al. *Health Maintenance Organizations: An Introduction and Survey of Recent Developments.* Washington, D.C., Lawyers' Committee for Civil Rights Under Law, 1972.

172   *Medical Group Practice and Health Maintenance*

Donabedian, Avedis. "An Evaluation of Prepaid Group Practice." *Inquiry, VI*(3):3–10, 20–25, September 1969.

Ellwood, Paul M., Jr. "Assuring Quality Health Care through HMOs." *In: Proceedings of the National Conference for Developing Title XIX—HMO Contracts.* Miami, Florida, September 18–20, 1973. Rockville, Md., Bureau of Community Health Services, Health Services Administration, U.S. Department of Health, Education, and Welfare, 1974.

Goldsmith, Seth B. "The Status of Health Status Indicators." *Health Services Reports, 87*(3):212–220, March 1972.

Health Services Research and Development Center. *Survey of Quality Assurance and Utilization Review Mechanisms in Prepaid Group Practice Plans and Medical Care Foundations.* Baltimore, Md., Medical Institute, The Johns Hopkins School of Medicine, 1976.

Koba Associates, Inc. *HMO Consumer Complaint Mechanisms.* Rockville, Md., Health Maintenance Organization Service, U.S. Department of Health, Education, and Welfare, 1974.

Metzner, Charles; Bashshur, Rashid; and Shannon, Gary. "Differential Public Acceptance of Group Medical Practice." *Medical Care, X*(4):279–287, July–August 1972.

Schwartz, Jerome L. *Medical Plans and Health Care.* Springfield, Ill., Charles C Thomas, Publisher, 1968, pp. 1–8, 44–64, 219–252.

Shapiro, Sam. "Utilization Control and Quality Assurance." *In: The Medical Director in Prepaid Group Practice Health Maintenance Organizations.* Edited by Michael A. Newman. Rockville, Md., Health Maintenance Organization Service, Health Services and Mental Health Administration, U.S. Department of Health, Education, and Welfare, 1973, pp. 91–100.

Shortridge, Mary Helen. "Quality of Medical Care in an Outpatient Setting." *Medical Care, XII*(4):283–300, April 1974.

Slee, Vergil. "How To Know If You Have Quality Control." *Hospital Progress, 53*(1):38–43, January 1972.

Smith, David Barton, and Metzner, Charles A. "Differential Perceptions of Health Care Quality in a Prepaid Group Practice." *Medical Care, VIII*(4):264–275, July–August 1970.

U.S. Department of Health, Education, and Welfare, Health Maintenance Organization Service, Office of Consumer Education and Information. "Development of a Consumer Program in Health Maintenance Organizations; A Position Paper." Rockville, Md., 1972. Mimeographed.

——————————. *Selected Papers on Consumerism in the HMO Movement.* Washington, D.C., U.S. Government Printing Office, 1973. DHEW Publ. No. (HSM) 73-13012.

Wolfman, B. "Medical Expenses and Choice of Plan: A Case Study." *Monthly Labor Review, 84*:1186–1190, November 1961.

7

Development Activities

This chapter suggests a framework that brings together the major components of the HMO during its initial stages. Several dimensions of the planning and development process are presented; various states and critical areas are discussed; and the many steps and problem areas faced by most developing HMOs are identified.

Phases in Development: The Federal Model

The Rules and Regulations[1] developed by the Department of Health, Education, and Welfare to implement the Health Maintenance Organization Act delineate the rules by which HMOs can receive federal funding. These rules provide for the funding of HMOs through four phases of development—feasibility, planning, initial development, and initial operation. Although these phases are somewhat artificial divisions of the development process, it is important to discuss them because of the direct relationship of each to stages in federal funding of HMO projects and because of published development manuals following these phases.

---

[1] Appendix 3 contains a copy of the Rules and Regulations. A discussion of P.L. 93-222 regulations and the amendments to the HMO Act (P.L. 94-460) appears in Chapter 3.

FEASIBILITY PHASE

HMOs begin as an idea, a concept, or an attitude on the part of someone in the community that perhaps a new method of providing health care may be better than the present system or may be the most logical way to fulfill a felt need. The feasibility phase in development initiates the somewhat expensive and complex process of establishing a new health-delivery structure using existing components—providers, hospitals, and long-term care facilities. Initial effort should be directed toward the completion of a "feasibility study"—a rational method of providing the planner with information upon which to make a "go" or "no go" decision. The study involves an examination of the critical issues that will determine the probable success or failure of the proposed HMO, and it should provide, ultimately, an analysis of the degree of risk (in monetary terms) that the project must face.

The feasibility study should assess the present and projected health needs of the community, the existing and projected resources in relation to such needs, and the interest in, or receptivity of the consumers and providers to, an HMO. Although it is not anticipated that at this stage the study will be in-depth (with the exception of federal HMO grantees), the thoroughness with which the study is conducted should have a direct impact on the potential success of the HMO. The feasibility study provides the structure and foundation on which each succeeding stage can be built, the basis on which feasible objectives can be set, and the basis on which plans and programs may be determined and funded. It also identifies the target population that may be served, the kind of services to offer, and the potential for competing in the existing market and for achieving the desired enrollment. As described in the following pages, Subsection 110:301 of the Program Guidelines and the Rules and Regulations provide an excellent format for completion of a feasibility study.

Initially, the planner will need private funds to hire staff, to complete the federal application for feasibility assistance, and, possibly, to actually complete the feasibility study if no funds are available from the government. The Federal Government requires extensive data concerning the proposed project and reacts favorably to sharing development costs, whether the planner's resources are from the planner directly or from outside philanthropy.[2] Thus, identification of initial funds, and organization of the development team are the first stages in

---

[2]Federal application requirements for all categories of grants, contracts, and loans are provided in U.S. Department of Health, Education, and Welfare, Office of Health Maintenance Organizations. *Health Maintenance Organizations, Guidelines, Subparts B, C, D, E, and G.* Rockville, Md., 1975.

the feasibility study, as outlined in Figure 27. The team will, in all likelihood, be composed of the HMO advocate and others who have realized the need for such an organization. If possible, this team should be composed of individuals with skills that will be valuable during the feasibility phase—a doctor, a health care administrator, a health planner, a service plan or indemnity insurance company executive, a banker and financier, and so on. The first task facing this team will be outlining the HMO's mission and objectives—its reasons for being. These objectives generally will cover the personal convenience of the providers and consumers, the economies that may be realized in the HMO, the professional development of the health care staff, and the introduction of specific medical services to a particular community; statements regarding the use of fee-for-service and capitation arrangements in physician compensation mechanisms also should be included.

Answers to the following questions also should enter into the development of objectives:

1. Which HMO organizational model has been selected? Why was it chosen?
2. What is the degree of commitment of the local providers of care? Have any contributed time, money, or both to the project?
3. What is the level of the planner's knowledge of the HMO concept? What are the planner's skills concerning management of development activities and operations?
4. Are there sufficient sources of information on which to base development decisions?

By now, the reader has probably recognized that planning and developing a new HMO is more than just the step-by-step process outlined in Figure 27; all of the activities shown must be completely carried out, but will they always occur in the order shown? No; most likely the HMO will have preexisting constraints placed on its development activities—a group practice may be converting to capitation, a neighborhood health center may be converting to an HMO, or the developer may own or have available the facilities to house a health plan. But these preexisting conditions should create few, if any, problems for the HMO planner. Development consists of a circular set of activities; it is an iterative process in which all of the activities must be completed—some concurrently, but always with feedback and always with a review of current activities. Figure 28 indicates that there are three major activities in the development process, each of which may be carried out concurrently, but each having an effect on the others.

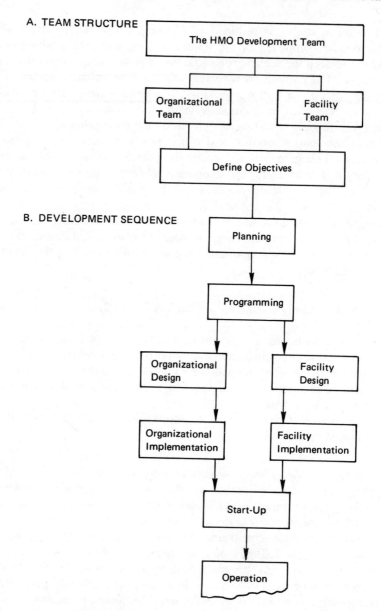

A. TEAM STRUCTURE

B. DEVELOPMENT SEQUENCE

Source: U.S. Department of Health, Education, and Welfare, Health Services Administration, Bureau of Community Health Services. *The Health Maintenance Organization Facility Development Handbook*. Rockville, Md., 1975.

Figure 27   The HMO development process.

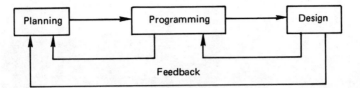

Figure 28   Feedback and interrelationships in the HMO development process.

For the HMO developer with an existing facility, planning, programming, and program design will be directly affected by the size, location, and layout of the facility. The planning and development steps, beginning with team development through implementation and start-up, will be completed and evaluated against the facility constraint.

Because of the importance placed on the feasibility stage, the HMO planner may wish to follow the *HMO Feasibility Study Guide* prepared for the Department of Health, Education, and Welfare by Arthur Young and Company.[3] The *Guide,* based on the requirements of the federal HMO office, describes the completion of five study tasks—management of a feasibility study, legal feasibility, market feasibility, provider-relations feasibility, and financial feasibility. The issues included in each phase are identified in Table 19. Although the developer is advised to use the *Guide* because of its well-structured approach to the feasibility study, each of the main issues included in the *Guide* is reviewed in a chapter of this book; it is suggested that the reader review the planning and development issues in the relevant chapters.[4] Each issue covers an area of risk which requires the planner's evaluation and decision. A "no go" decision in any one of these areas should

[3]Arthur Young and Company. *HMO Feasibility Study Guide.* Rockville, Md., Bureau of Community Health Services, Health Services Administration, U.S. Department of Health, Education, and Welfare, 1974.
[4]The management of a feasibility study addresses the control and coordination activities that the HMO planner must undertake to complete the study in a timely fashion. Legal feasibility allows an evaluation of internal and external legal issues that confront the planner—the HMO must conform to all federal, state, and local laws and regulations; internally, legal organizational issues must be resolved. Available organizational structures are discussed in Chapter 4. Market feasibility is concerned with the analysis of the target catchment area and the probable marketing strategies that will be used. Chapter 8 presents these materials. Provider-relations feasibility allows the planner to evaluate the provider role, relationships, and commitment to the health plan; these issues are addressed in Chapter 5. The financial analysis that brings all development activities together through an identification of demand, capacity, budgeting, and funds flow analysis is presented in Chapter 10.

TABLE 19   Phases in the Creation of an HMO with Selected Characteristics

PHASES	ISSUES	ACTIVITIES	DECISIONS
I. Feasibility 1. Objectives; state of readiness	• Organizational structure • Long-range goals • Objectives	• Initial planning • Funding for feasibility study	Whether to proceed to a formal feasibility study
2. Feasibility Study	• Legal climate • Marketing potential • Provider relationships • Financial capabilities • Need/demand identification	• Management of feasibility study • Data analysis and display of results • Review of analysis by sponsors and funding sources	Whether to proceed with development of an HMO
II. Planning	Same	• Detailed planning • More complete data • Work plan development	How to proceed to initial development phase
III. Initial Development	Same	• Establish HMO as legal entity • Begin marketing and enrollment • Employ or contract with physicians • Complete arrangements for facilities • Complete any insurance contracts	How to proceed to operational phase
IV. Initial Operation 1. Start-up	Same	• Delivery of care to enrollees • Processing of claims • Continue marketing effort • Balance needed services with delivery capability	• Day-to-day policy decisions • Personnel decisions • Whether HMO is self-supporting financially
2. Normal Operations	Same	Same (Also continue evaluation of level of care and services)	• Normal operation decisions • Whether to increase size of HMO, add facilities, increase benefits

Source: Arthur Young and Company. *HMO Feasibility Study Guide.* Rockville, Md.: Bureau of Community Health Services, Health Services Administration, U.S. Department of Health, Education, and Welfare, 1974.

be interpreted as a major impediment to successful development and operation. If a satisfactory solution cannot be devised, the planner should consider terminating the plans for an HMO. Normally, alternate and/or contingency arrangements can be made so that a satisfactory "go" decision will be possible.

One additional critical area of development noted in market analysis but not specifically identified by the *HMO Feasibility Study Guide* is so obvious that it may be overlooked by the planner—evaluation of the health care need and demand in the community. Experience has shown that, where there is a lack of a formalized system of health care delivery and a substantial unmet need, there is a high probability that the HMO will be successful. Another of the study tasks requires that the planner show evidence of unmet need and demand in the service area; there must be a demonstrated lack of adequate primary care. This insufficiency can be measured by four criteria, the first being the primary consideration.

1. *Lack of health care services:* Requires an evaluation of acute and therapeutic services, guaranteed comprehensive care without per-visit financial thresholds, out-of-area coverage, full-time access, preventive services, and annual reviews of benefits per cost.

2. *Lack of facilities:* Requires an evaluation of access to *all* necessary facilities.

3. *Lack of providers of care:* Requires an evaluation of regular hours, removal of nonprofessional administrative functions from physicians, and adequate pay scales to ensure effective specialty practice (primary, secondary, and tertiary care).

4. *Lack of adequate financing mechanisms:* Requires an evaluation of all financing mechanisms, including private third-party coverage (service plans and indemnity companies, employer- and union-sponsored payment mechanisms, and government programs).

The feasibility phase culminates with the completion of the reviews and evaluations of need, legal climate, marketing potential, provider relationships, and financial capabilities. Depending on the availability of initial funding and interest and commitment of the planners and their capabilities, this phase may be completed in as little as four months. Generally, however, it may take one year, and sometimes up to two years, to complete feasibility activities.

Costs of the feasibility stage vary, depending on whether the work is done by in-house staff or whether a consultant is used, on the availability of community data, on the availability of funds to complete the study, and so on. In 1976, costs of the feasibility stage ranged from $30,000 to $150,000.

A quick review of the major issues that must be considered in the first stage follows. Each must be thoroughly evaluated.

Feasibility Checklist

1. Health plan mission statement, goals, and objectives have been identified and clearly stated.

2. A plan of development activities or a work plan has been detailed.

3. The development team has all of the requisite resources (time, money, expertise, experience) to develop the HMO.

4. Funds for feasibility, planning, development, and start-up are available or are forthcoming.

5. The legal review indicates no national or local statutory barriers to the formulation of the HMO (e.g., blue laws, corporate practice of medicine, certificate of need, advertising, tax status).

6. A workable, legal organizational structure has been, or can be, created.

7. There is an unmet need/demand in the catchment area.

8. There is a broad base of support in the community from which enrollment can be drawn.

9. There will be a sufficient level of enrollment (specify level).

10. The prevailing health insurance premiums and benefits are at a level that permits the HMO to be competitive.

11. The demographic, socioeconomic, and epidemiological data necessary to complete underwriting activities are available.

12. The income (or purchasing power) of the target population is high enough to purchase the benefit package.

13. There is provider support in the numbers required to deliver care (including hospitalization).

14. Capitated payment to physicians is acceptable.

15. The preliminary demand, capacity, and funds flow analyses appear to suggest successful breakeven within an acceptable time period.

PLANNING PHASE

The planning stage is essentially an expansion of the activities started during the feasibility study. At the completion of the feasibility study, the planner should briefly evaluate the information collected and decide whether to continue. During the planning phase, the question of how to proceed through development is clearly addressed: the data base for the major development issues listed in Figure 27 is expanded and refined; the decisions that must be addressed prior to actual development are clearly defined; a detailed work plan that describes the tasks to be accomplished and the time sequencing for performing each task is completed; and sources of funding, including both government and private sources, are identified.

Because of substantial study during the feasibility phase (at least for federal grantees), the planning stage needs only to be a refinement of the data and plans for development. The time period allowed for these activities should be short—several months at most. Many HMO planners, however, find that the early stages are critical for identifying development funds and will extend the planning phase, because the search for funds is a slow process and may indicate a general unwillingness of the community to support the HMO; these early fiscal problems should indicate whether or not the HMO will be successful in becoming operational. The planning phase is complete when all activities and plans for development have been delineated and when sufficient funds to continue development have been identified and obtained. In addition to the items on the feasibility checklist, the following elements also should be a part of the development plan at the completion of the planning phase.

Planning Checklist

1. The organizational structure has been developed and is an independent legal entity.

2. Community support and acceptance is neither neutral nor negative; physician and target population attitudes are positive.

3. Highly skilled individuals for top managerial and development positions are employed by the new HMO entity (executive director and medical director).

4. A marketing strategy (membership objectives, marketing and enrollment procedures) for each target population is in draft form.

5. The benefit packages and other structures have been generally described.

6. A guaranteed commitment from providers has been obtained.

7. Guaranteed commitments from groups of enrollees have been obtained.

8. Facility planning is completed.

INITIAL DEVELOPMENT PHASE

Plans formulated during the previous phase now become operational. Actual implementation of the work plan will involve the selection and training of staff, a functional organizational entity, and a facility. According to the example of the Division of Health Maintenance Organizations, DHEW, seven major project areas are identified in the initial development phase.[5] Each of these tasks is shown in Figure 29 and is discussed in the following sections.

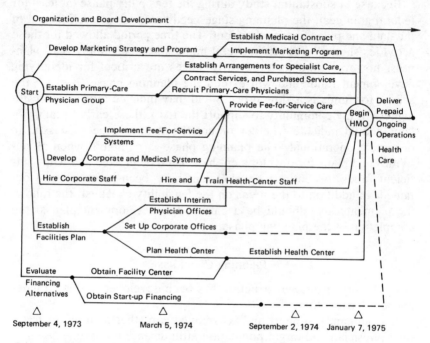

Source: Arthur Young and Company. *HMO Feasibility Study Guide*. Rockville, Md., Bureau of Community Health Services, Health Services Administration, U.S. Department of Health, Education, and Welfare, 1974, p. 96.

Figure 29   HMO development plan.

Organization and Board Development: If the organization's selection of a board of trustees and its institutionalization as a legal entity have not been completed during planning, these matters will be finalized at this time.

[5]This section draws heavily upon the *HMO Feasibility Study Guide* (Arthur Young and Company), pp. 95–99.

Marketing: Activities in this area include the development of benefit packages to match the demands of target populations; creation of a sales strategy; assembly of literature and other sales materials; finalization of dual-choice agreements with employees, unions, and government agencies; and enrollment of members.

Provision of Care: This encompasses all activities necessary to arrange for delivery of care. Thus, a medical-care program at the health plan's center must be designed and implemented. Services of outside providers also must be arranged; contracts with providers for services that the health plan itself cannot provide economically or physically may include medical specialists, pharmacies, hospitals, therapists, and others. Referral relationships also must be facilitated.

Corporate and Medical Systems: These systems include information systems, accounting systems, and personnel management systems, as well as those activities necessary to support, evaluate, and control the quality of medical care delivered to members. Medical systems are internal to the corporation; they support the delivery of care. Examples include evaluation of the quality of care, creation and maintenance of medical records, and procedures to handle member complaints regarding the quality of care.

Personnel: New organizations will require the formulation of hiring, censure, recognition, and termination procedures; these procedures should be used in developing a staff that will perform at a level of productivity required in the organization. This is a major managerial task and requires close coordination with all other development activities.

In the initial development phase, the HMO should include a plan administrator, medical director, nursing director, marketing manager, and financial manager. Each should be hired when their tasks first appear in the development plan. The administrator and medical director will be the first to be hired by the new organization's board of trustees and, generally, will have been active during the feasibility and planning stage, even though they might not have been formally employed by the plan.

Because the most common reason for early HMO failure is the lack of management expertise, the choice of an administrator and medical director is most important. In studies of federally funded HMOs, it has been found that placing the initial HMO planner/advocate in the position of administrator of the formal organization has not been a wise choice.

This position requires an individual with organization, financing, marketing, and control skills, while the initial HMO planner generally is a lobbyist, negotiator, and politician who helps forge and strengthen the relationships between the health plan, its providers, employers, unions, and the population in the service area. Both individuals are essential to the development of the HMO, but they have separate and very distinct tasks to perform. The administrator may come from a sponsoring organization or may be recruited from another health or insurance plan. Additional staffing might follow the ratios provided in Chapter 5.

Administration: Because administration is a continuous function, it is discussed here to emphasize that good management throughout the process of creating the HMO is necessary for its success. The process of management—organizing, directing, staffing, controlling—is the cement that holds all of the organization's activities together so that services can be delivered effectively and efficiently. The administrator must be able to view the entire program's activities from the lowest common denominators—service and the dollar. Evaluating financial alternatives, obtaining required funds for development and start-up, and budgeting are very important activities of this development function and are described in detail in Chapter 10.

Facility Development: This project area provides for the development of necessary facilities to carry out the corporation's activities. Included are all problems associated with site selection, leasing, construction, furnishing, and equipping the offices and medical service facilities to be operated by the HMO. Activities in this project area might include setting up corporate offices, establishing facilities for temporary services, and building and occupying a permanent health center. The following is a checklist for facility development.

Facility Checklist

1. Establish facilities plan
2. Establish interim physician offices
3. Set up corporate offices
4. Plan health center
5. Establish health center

Since most of the development process to this point has concerned the organizational program design and implementation, careful attention must be given to the activities on the righthand side of Figure 27, relating to facility development; the initial cost of a facility has an important and dramatic impact on the operation of the program.[6]

INITIAL OPERATION PHASE

When all development activities are completed, the HMO is ready for the delivery of care to enrollees. Start-up activities should have been well orchestrated prior to the operation phase—with all staff members totally familiar with their duties. During the operation phase, therefore, the HMO manager's major responsibilities are to ensure an even day-to-day operation of the organization and to collect and analyze data to evaluate the level of care being delivered, consumer and provider satisfaction, growth in the organization, and financial and operational stability of the new HMO. This phase ends when the program "breaks even," that is, when the membership grows to a sufficient level so that the cumulative cash flow shows a surplus rather than a deficit. Ordinarily, it takes several years for a new HMO to reach this stage.

Development Guidelines

The preceding discussion of development and the publications suggested in the text define the activities that help lead to successful implementation of the HMO. Discussion of three additional issues may be helpful to the HMO developer—rules of thumb, the critical areas in development, and the major problem areas. In the following two sections of this chapter, "critical" and "problem" areas are presented. The lists that follow are intended to provide the HMO developer with the experience gleaned from the field regarding the rules of thumb generally accepted by HMO administrations. These provide a starting point, but are *not* intended to be used without *modification and caution*. Rules of thumb are merely indicators, guides, and approximations and should not be considered facts. Bearing this in mind, rules of thumb are provided for several HMO activity areas.

---

[6]Additional assistance in facility development may be obtained in U.S. Department of Health, Education, and Welfare, Health Services Administration, Bureau of Community Health Services. *The Health Maintenance Organization Facility Development Handbook.* Rockville, Md., 1975; and Medical Group Management Association. *The Formation and Planning of a Medical Group Practice.* Cambridge, Mass., Ballinger Press, 1976.

HMO Planning Rules of Thumb

Population and Service Area

1. There should be a minimum of 250,000 to 500,000 people in the general population (service area) and the possibility of obtaining at least 1,000 enrollees per physician.

2. A penetration rate of at least 10 percent of total population (250,000) at the breakeven point should be possible.

3. The size of initial service population to be enrolled should be at least 5,000 and likely to reach 20,000 in two to three years (i.e., 5,000 to 6,000 families).

4. At least 50 percent of service population should be below the age of 65.

5. Target population family income should be $10,000 per annum or above.

6. At least 65 percent of the projected service population must live within a 30-minute drive of the facility.

7. No more than 80 to 85 percent of the general population (250,000) should be covered by present insuring mechanisms.

8. The target population should be at least 20 times the service population.

9. The most important population characteristics are age and sex distribution, family size, income level, urban/rural mix, ethnic make-up, and geographic location.

10. Population segmentation may be as follows: by age and sex, by employer or union affiliation, by residency within particular geographic boundaries, by third-party payer representations, or by ethnic, racial, or language characteristics.

Providers

1. The project begins with 5 to 10 equivalent full-time physicians, including the following specialties: general medicine, general practice, family practice or internal medicine, obstetrics and gynecology, pediatrics, and general surgery.

2. Physicians in these specialties will provide 70 to 80 percent of all health services needed.

3. Other specialists will be provided on a referral basis.

4. Each full-time physician will provide 30 to 35 hours of ambulatory office care.

5. Staffing will be according to the following ratios:

Internal medicine—35 physicians per 100,000 enrollees

General medicine—10 physicians per 100,000 enrollees
Pediatrics—15 physicians per 100,000 enrollees
Obstetrics/gynecology—10 physicians per 100,000 enrollees
General surgeons—5 to 8 physicians per 100,000 enrollees

6. Paramedical staffing—4 staff to 1 physician, or 3 paramedical personnel per 1,000 enrollees.

7. Project 1 physician per 1,000 to 1,200 enrollees.

8. Inpatient hospital beds—1.5 to 1.8 beds per 1,000 enrollees per year.

9. Based on 16 full-time equivalent physicians, the following personnel are required:

0.5 to 1.25 laboratory and X-ray technicians
0.5 to 3.0 all other health-delivery personnel
1.0 to 5.0 business and clerical personnel

Marketing and Enrollment

1. Provide multiple or at least dual-choice plans.

2. Provide open enrollment at least annually.

3. There must be a potential market of several good-sized (more than 50 employees) *nonnational* firms, unions, associations, and so on.

4. The HMO should attract at least 25 to 50 enrollees per group, except where the account may grow or has the potential to critically influence other groups.

5. Plan on community rating, but use loading and experience rating for special groups if and when required.

6. Assess the HMO's ability to receive a Medicaid contract within its state and to obtain lists of welfare recipients.

7. If contract marketing is used, a commission rate may be as low as one-tenth of one percent of premiums.

8. To achieve an enrollment rate of 10,000 members, 4 to 8 marketing people will be needed.

9. In 1971, the cost of marketing and enrollment was $200 per family, or $0.17 per month (for marketing-oriented activities and services only, not including overhead).

10. Do not depend on one group for more than 10 percent of health-plan income (except during initial operation). An acceptable initial market penetration for an HMO is the enrollment of 10 percent of one group.

11. Attempt to enroll a population mix that approximates the characteristics of the total community population (balanced enrollment population).

12. In groups, for those given a true dual choice, the expectation of a 5 to 10 percent initial enrollment rate may be appropriate.

13. Penetration-rate studies should be completed by payment mechanism, employer group, age and sex, and so on.

14. An increased deduction of from $8 to $12 per month from an employee's paycheck is the maximum acceptable increase over the present health-plan deduction. Stated somewhat differently, there should be no more than a 10 percent differential between the HMO and the other health insurance plans in the community.

Benefit Package and Utilization of Services

1. Plan at least 90 days in each benefit period for inpatient care.

2. Psychiatric services (if provided): 15 to 20 visits per year, plus 30 to 45 days of hospital treatment.

3. Extended care facilities: at least 100 days per benefit period.

4. Home health services: at least 100 visits per benefit period.

5. When most financial barriers are removed, approximately 25 to 30 percent of persons entitled to service make no visits during the year.

6. Plan from 3.7 to 4.6 outpatient doctor visits per year.

7. Plan five prescriptions per enrollee per year.

8. Plan for approximately 0.5 utilization of other services per enrollee per year (radiology, electrocardiography, electroencephalography, physical therapy, and laboratory).

9. Plan 80 hospital admissions per 1,000 enrollees per year.

10. Plan 465 to 525 hospital days per 1,000 enrollees per year.

11. Plan 616 to 690 X-rays per 1,000 enrollees per year.

12. Plan 2,960 to 3,400 laboratory services per 1,000 enrollees per year.

13. Plan 4.5 to 9.5 of total services per enrollee per year.

14. Approximately 10 to 20 percent of all care received by enrollees will be from out-of-plan services (excluding out-of-area coverage reimbursed by the plan) (i.e., 10 to 20 percent leakage).

15. Increase in present monthly deduction for health care of from $8 to $12 is the critical range; plan rejection, because of cost, may become a critical issue beyond this range.

Financing

1. Construction cost of facilities (clinic for 10 full-time physicians): $5 million.

2. Feasibility, planning, and development costs: $100,000 to $250,000.

3. Start-up costs: $75,000 to $100,000.

4. Add approximately 1.5 percent to these costs for each month that construction, planning, start-up, and operation is delayed.

5. Project a 1- to 2-year planning and development stage prior to operation.

6. Plan not to break even or to make a surplus until at least three years after becoming operational. Return on investment may then average 8 to 9 percent per year and perhaps up to 15 percent per year.

7. Plan on bearing up to $5,000 for costs of care per individual per year prior to reinsurance taking over. A $5,000 stop-loss per person allows the HMO to guarantee approximately 150 percent of the premium.

8. Use the financial ratios and value ranges which can be found in Chapter 10. (Example: current ratio [measure of liquidity] = total sources/total uses.)

9. Sources of revenue for the plan may be from:

Dues	65%
Fees-for-service	5–10%
Copayment	5–10%
Pharmacy and other sales	4– 8%
Other income	8–13%

10. Subscriber costs might be reduced $0.15 to $0.20 per group member each time 2,000 group members are added as subscribers.

11. Average costs of insurance may be:

	% of Total Cost
Nonphysician employee insurance cost (health, disability, life)	0.65
Physician insurance cost (health, disability, life)	0.75
Professional liability	1.1
Other liability	0.25
Stop-loss insurance (reinsurance)	1.0
Total	3.75%

12. Hospitalization will account for 40 percent of the premium dollar.

13. Services contracted with insurance companies (including administrative services—collection of premiums, checking enrollment cards, paying commissions, if used, and so on) may account for 1.5 percent of the premium dollar.

14. The lag time between enrollment and time of premium payment is 45 days.

15. Include in any projected financial plans a 15 percent inflationary factor.

CRITICAL AREAS OF DEVELOPMENT

It is helpful to understand which areas in the development process are considered most critical and to be aware of the problems that occur most frequently. In a study completed by Shouldice in 1974, the Department of Health, Education, and Welfare regional HMO officials and 10 HMO federal grantees were interviewed to identify and rank, by importance, those areas that were considered to be the most critical to development. In analyzing the data obtained during the study, eight major critical development issues were identified, each of which is described in the following sections.

Financing: The funding of HMO operations was considered a major area of concern by all interviewees. Financing was discussed in terms of capital for facilities, underwriting of risks, research and development, start-up costs, and prebreakeven operational costs. Although grant support for these operations was available during the interviewing period, the funds were either insufficient or, for many HMOs, the time was approaching when grant funds could not be used for further development. (For example, DHEW development grant awards can be used only for development activities and cannot be applied toward operational activities.)

Most of the plans described their almost futile efforts to obtain outside financing, especially for risk underwriting. Like other health care organizations, HMO resources and operations do not provide an acceptable form of collateral for obtaining the usual forms of financing. These problems have been recognized by legislators, and the HMO legislation includes provisions for grants and loan guarantees for developing HMOs.

During the interviews, HMO administrators and federal officials were asked to suggest a management approach to indicate financial progress during development (i.e., a financial indicator). Foremost was the measurement of whether or not present or proposed sources of funding were sufficient to support operation until the breakeven point was reached. The indicator may be an inventory of sources and uses of funds. The very existence and use of a financial plan, however, is a strong indication that the plan has its financing under control.

Big Brother: Many new plans are backed by organizations that provide much of the fledgling HMO's support. The "big brother" might be defined as an organization or individual that supports the developing HMO. The support is either formal or informal and can be in the form of experience, knowledge of capitated medical delivery, or essential resources.

It was the opinion of those interviewed that establishing relationships with a big brother substantially increases successful progress in development. This is especially true if the big brother organization is a power base in the community and can help arrange initial marketing contacts with major employers, trade associations, and union representatives. If, on the other hand, the HMO has not established a big brother relationship, it must look elsewhere for its resources—technical assistance, influence in the community, and status may be obtained from consultants, DHEW regional technical-assistance personnel, DHEW regional and national offices, and other local HMOs and state agencies such as the state Medicaid programs.

Providers: The plan directors stated that both hospital and physician relationships with the plan are critical to successful progress in development, with the formation of a physician group being the primary concern and a source for inpatient care being a close second. It was suggested that the latter is not difficult to achieve; hospital working arrangements with the plan can include actual ownership and/or operation of an inpatient facility, contracts with local hospitals for beds, or merely staff-admitting privileges for HMO physicians. Moreover, the hospital may actually be the sponsor of the HMO.

The physician's services are most difficult to obtain, according to the study. To complicate this issue, based on changing enrollment projections and practice patterns, physician needs change. Physician attitudes, which also affect physician participation, are difficult to measure and can quickly change during the development period. Thus, the plan must generate physician interest and a firm, contractual commitment during development. Eliciting the leadership of a well-known and accepted physician is one of the techniques that helps build physician interest.

Data from the interviews suggest that monitoring formal physician-plan contracts may be an acceptable indicator of provider acceptance and commitment in this critical area. Letters of intent, although of limited use, are the first stage in building a solid physician commitment. Formal contracts usually are signed one to two months before operations begin. Contracts, however, should not be signed prior to completion of the delivery components of the system (i.e., before financial arrangements, marketing, and enrollment are well under way).

Legal: Each plan director interviewed agreed that the legal area very often becomes a major stumbling block to HMO progress. Numerous legal restrictions and regulations were mentioned; it is necessary to identify all legal impediments to development and possible alternative legal courses of action. An inventory of legal problems may be useful to the HMO manager to clearly define such problems and their potential solutions.[7] This inventory might include the following:

1. Federal laws and regulations describing participation in federally funded programs such as Medicare, Medicaid, Federal Employees Health Benefit Programs, and IRS classifications concerning profit and nonprofit status.

2. State laws and regulations that may govern professional associations and corporations (Medical Practice acts), HMO enabling legislation,[8] insurance (commissioner) regulations and state attorney general restrictions, liability for negligence and malpractice, health care service corporation acts (blue laws), corporate practice of medicine problems, and so on.

3. Local jurisdictional regulations and laws, including zoning and health-planning regulations, local income tax laws, and property tax laws.

4. Medical society policies concerning advertising, practice ethics, and so on.

The general availability of legal council may be a good indication that the plan is able to cope with most legal restrictions and problems.

Advocacy: Plan managers described the need for support from a community-minded individual to act as the plan's advocate (the person who is the main supporter of the HMO development), one who can lead

---

[7]It is strongly suggested that the new HMO retain a lawyer. A reference that may be helpful to the HMO lawyer is U.S. Department of Health, Education, and Welfare, Health Maintenance Organization Service, Training and Technical Assistance Division. *Lawyer's Manual on Health Maintenance Organization.* Rockville, Md., n.d.

[8]Although there is a federal override of restrictive state laws included in P.L. 93-222, federal officials have been reluctant to use it. Rather, a review of each state's legislation (see InterStudy. *Catalog of 1973 State Health Maintenance Organization Enabling Bills.* Minneapolis, Minn., 1974, for a review of the state laws affecting HMOs) should be undertaken prior to completion of this stage in development.

others to accept the idea and concept of an HMO. Advocates can be either physicians or laymen but usually are not the plan manager or project director. They are important during all phases of activity but especially during the inception stage when the HMO is attempting to obtain grant proposals, private financing, and support from community leaders. Moreover, one of the advocate's most important skills must be the ability to negotiate—the ability to arrange for outside support through loans, employer-employee recognition, and support from organized medicine, if possible. The advocate's standing in the community, personality, drive and tenacity, charm, ability to build relationships, and charisma are some other characteristics that are necessary and important.

Attitude: All plan directors agreed that the attitudes of consumers, providers, and third-party payers were critical to successful development. Negative attitudes toward the HMO must be identified and resolved during the early stages, because such problems can severely limit development. On the other hand, positive attitudes enhance the progress of the developing HMO. The study reported that positive patient-physician relationships under the fee-for-service system suggest that the development of a prepaid, closed-panel group practice may be difficult. These findings are supported by studies completed by other researchers.[9]

Thus, the developing HMO must determine its image in the community, the ties patients have with physicians, and the overall consumer-employer-physician attitude toward the HMO. Measurements that may be used as indicators in this area include the plan's success in attracting physician cooperation and participation and the rate of consumer enrollment. Actual physician participation and consumer enrollment can then be compared with projected levels of physician staffing and subscription. It also may be helpful to perform an informal survey to identify either positive or negative attitudes toward the plan.

Some plans surveyed reported that the reputation of established HMOs in their geographical areas contributed to positive attitudes. When established plans were successful, it was less difficult for the new HMO to generate positive attitudes. If, however, established HMOs were not adequately meeting their contractual relationships or were overselling themselves but not fulfilling all of their promises, the newly developing HMO had difficulties with consumer and physician attitudes.

[9]Avedis Donabedian. *A Review of Some Experiences with Prepaid Group Practice.* Research Series No. 12. Ann Arbor, Mich., School of Public Health, Bureau of Public Health Economics, University of Michigan, 1965, pp. 5–8.

Timing: Another critical issue identified in all of the plans was the timetable for development activities. Timing is one of the basic areas in which many HMO grantees fail in their development attempts; it is obviously a symptom of other major problems being encountered by the HMO. Naturally, the time frame must be tailor-made for each plan and must be flexible enough to compensate for blocks in progress. This suggests the invaluable use of milestone, Gantt, or PERT charts to describe the tasks and the time required to accomplish each task. These management tools have been used irregularly by plans to coordinate developmental activities.

The management guides suggested by plan administrators include an evaluation to determine whether the HMO management has available and is using a timetable. Major emphasis should be placed on frequent updating and explanations of deviations from the timetable. When deviations exist, the plan director should initiate action to correct time sequencing and perhaps to obtain assistance from outside sources.

Management: Generally, plan directors agreed that successful development of an HMO depended, to a large degree, on the managerial ability of the plan director and his assistants. Management includes the basic administrative abilities of planning, coordinating, directing, controlling, and staffing. It also includes the following specific areas: knowledge of the HMO plan objectives (and the federal HMO program objectives, if a federal grantee), negotiating skills, knowledge of the HMO concepts (i.e., prepayment, capitation, insurance, direct service), knowledge of the community characteristics, relationships with community members, marketing, and financing. All plan directors stressed the need for flexibility and adaptability by the HMO and its management. The ability to cope with changes is now recognized as vital to successful development.

PROBLEMS

It is interesting to note that the Department of Health, Education, and Welfare, in June 1976, identified several of the critical issues heretofore reviewed as being key factors in the failure of 23 federally funded HMO feasibility projects. In all but one, the lack of management skills and expertise and of strong commitment to the development of the HMO were identified as the reasons for the failure of the projects. The DHEW study suggested that greater efforts be made to more fully develop the

management skills of HMO administrators and staff. Table 20 lists the
reasons identified by the DHEW study for the 23 failures.[10]

Summary

The activities in the development process of an HMO can be described
by reviewing the various phases or stages involved. The HMO developer can be assisted by identifying the critical areas where major problems may occur. According to federal regulations, development consists of four phases—feasibility, planning, initial development, and
initial operation. The feasibility phase is characterized by the completion of a feasibility study that provides the developer with data and a
rationale for deciding whether to continue or to terminate development
activities. Tasks to be completed in this phase, in addition to the feasibility study, include locating funds to complete the study, organizing a
development team, composing a set of HMO objectives, and establishing a general framework for the new organization.

Development of the HMO includes several activities—setting objectives, planning, programming, initial operation, and implementation. It
is important to note that all developing health plans do not follow a
rigorous step-by-step approach to development, but that preexisting
conditions constrain the process; each development activity must be
completed but, because the process is circular and iterative, tasks may
be completed concurrently and may affect other development activities. Feedback is an important aspect of successful development.
All development activities must, however, be completed before operation of the plan can begin.

The feasibility study requires the completion of five tasks—
development of a management program to control the study, and determination of the plan's legal feasibility, market feasibility, provider-
relations feasibility, and financial feasibility. The Department of
Health, Education, and Welfare's *HMO Feasibility Study Guide* provides a good method for a complete study. An additional study issue,
which is not completely covered in the *Guide,* is the evaluation of

[10]For an excellent article concerning these issues, see George B. Strumpf and Marie A.
Garramone. "Why Some HMOs Develop Slowly." *Public Health Reports, 91*(6): 496–
503, November–December 1976.

TABLE 20   Frequency of Reasons Why 23 Feasibility Projects Did Not Proceed Under HMO Law

Sponsorship	No.	Insufficient Sponsor Commitment	Lack of Understanding of Goals and Objectives of P.L. 93-222	Provider Opposition	Lack of Providers	Failed to Supply Marketing/Financial Feasibility Outputs
Consumer Groups	6	3	6	1	4	6
Hospitals	8	4	7	1	5	7
Physician Groups	8	4	8	2	6	8
Private Organizations	1	—	1	—	1	1
Totals	23	11	22	4	16	22

Source: Karen A. Hunt, ed. *Health Services Information,* 3(25):2, June 28, 1976.

health care need/demand in the service area. High unmet need/demand is justification for additional health care providers and financing mechanisms. Evaluation of the five tasks included in the study provide evidence for a "go" or "no go" decision to be made by the developer.

The next phase, planning, is essentially an expansion of the activities started during the feasibility study and, thus, should include a more complete review of the developmental activities. This phase is concluded when all activities and plans for development have been delineated and when sufficient funds to continue development have been identified.

Plans developed during the planning phase become operational during the initial development period. Initial development activities include the organization of the HMO legal entity, appointment of the board of trustees, marketing, arrangements for the provision of care, corporate medical system development, personnel administration, the process of general administration, and facility development. With the completion of these developmental activities, the plan is ready to "start up," to provide services to its subscribers. This initial operation phase provides a period when the program demonstrates its ability to succeed. During this period, management assesses the HMO's strength in the areas of the level of care delivered, consumer and provider satisfaction, organizational growth, and financial and operational stability. Initial operation ends, usually after several years, at the "break-even" point, when there is a cumulative surplus rather than a cash flow deficit.

To assist the HMO developer, guidelines and rules of thumb are available, as well as an evaluation of critical areas in development. Rules of thumb, although crude, can be used with caution and are available in the areas of population, providers, marketing and enrollment, benefit packages, utilization of services, and financing. Critical areas in development include financing, "big brother" support, providers, legal advocacy, attitudes, and management. The last area, management, appears (from DHEW studies) to be the key factor in the failure of new HMOs. An evaluation mechanism is available to assist developers in gauging their progress toward a successful, operational HMO.

References

Birnbaum, Roger. *Health Maintenance Organizations: A Guide to Planning and Development.* New York, Spectrum Publications, Inc., 1976.
_____ . *Prepayment and Neighborhood Health Centers.* Washington, D.C., Office of Health Affairs, Office of Economic Opportunity, 1972.

Boston Consulting Group, Inc. *Financial Planning in Ambulatory Health Programs.* Rockville, Md., National Center for Health Services Research and Development, Health Services and Mental Health Administration, U.S. Department of Health, Education, and Welfare, 1973. DHEW Publ. No. (HRA) 74-3027.

Kress, John R., and Singer, James. *HMO Handbook.* Rockville, Md., Aspen Systems Corporation, 1975.

Medical Group Management Association. *The Organization and Development of a Medical Group Practice.* Cambridge, Mass., Ballinger Press, 1976.

Shouldice, Robert G. "A Model for Evaluating the Performance of Health Maintenance Organizations." Doctoral Dissertation. Washington, D.C., The George Washington University, 1974.

U.S. Department of Health, Education, and Welfare, Health Services Administration, Bureau of Community Health Services. *The Health Maintenance Organization Facility Development Handbook.* Rockville, Md., 1975. DHEW Publ. No. (HSA) 75-13025.

Arthur Young and Company. *HMO Feasibility Study Guide.* Rockville, Md., Bureau of Community Health Services, Health Services Administration, U.S. Department of Health, Education, and Welfare, 1974. DHEW Publ. No. (HSA) 74-13020.

8

Marketing
Health Services

Conventional (and obsolete) medical-care planning involved the development of health care facilities and programs to be used by physicians and other community providers without any consideration being given to matching the needs of people to services provided. During the last few years, however, medical-care administrators have been forced by increasing costs, feast-or-famine utilization, and government regulations to base their "planning" for services on population "needs"; managers are now studying the long-range demand for services and are building programs to meet that demand. Currently, programs exist for consumers rather than in spite of them.

This logic is extended even further in an HMO. The HMO seeks potential subscribers by creating consumer satisfaction through an integrated marketing program.[1] In an HMO, marketing is defined as the performance of a wide range of activities, including market surveys, designing benefit packages, pricing, promotion and selling, and enrollment. It includes any activity that affects the flow of health care services, the enrollment of members, and ongoing account maintenance; in fact, almost all activities performed by the HMO can be considered marketing activities. Marketing results will be a test of the program's level of

[1]The "new concept" of marketing is provided in Philip Kotler. *Marketing Management: Analysis, Planning, and Control.* Englewood Cliffs, N.J., Prentice-Hall, 1967; see also Robin E. MacStravic. *Marketing Health Care.* Germantown, Md., Aspen Systems Corporation, 1977.

success—its validity as a concept, its ability to educate the public, its ability to meet the needs of the subscribers, its ability to meet its financial obligations, and so on. More than in any other health care delivery mechanism, consumers, through their decisions on whether or not to purchase HMO services, voice their acceptance or rejection of the HMO. It is not an overstatement to suggest that successful marketing is the key to a successful HMO.

The "marketing schema" illustrated in Figure 30 outlines the flow of funds beginning with premiums. Premium income is used to provide services included in the benefit package. Growth and success of the HMO is affected by the free market system, where consumers' attitudes

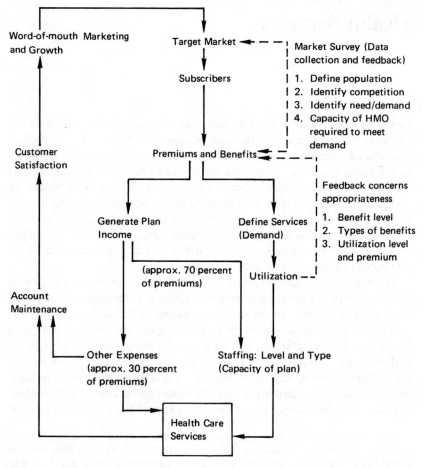

Figure 30 Marketing schema.

and beliefs are important to marketing success. Note that Figure 30 assumes that, once the initial marketing activities are completed, account maintenance by HMO employees and further marketing through word-of-mouth by members are required. In this schema, the orientation of the medical-care delivery system is toward the market, the subscriber, and the potential subscribers instead of toward the products—although service must be competitive or the system will fail.

Marketing Strategy

Marketing HMOs requires both careful planning and developing a strategy that is tailored to the target population. Strategy development demands that substantial funds be available and that experienced marketing personnel be employed if the strategy is to be effective. It is the responsibility of the marketing director to develop the marketing strategy, which is a two-step process.[2] First, the selection of the target population is made through an analysis of particular groups of potential HMO subscribers. The second step is the development of a "marketing mix"—selecting the elements that the HMO intends to bring together in order to meet the needs of the target population. Normally, each target population (e.g., groups of employees, union members, Medicaid and Medicare recipients) may require a separate marketing mix, which is developed around four basic variables: product, place, promotion, and price.[3]

PRODUCT

The "product" under consideration here involves more than deciding which "services" to provide to each target group. Because the product is comprehensive health care or, more accurately, a state of health for subscribers, the HMO product includes an ongoing concern—a monitoring of the membership's health. Considerations that relate to the "product" include demand identification, actuarial analyses and underwriting, and a system of continuing subscriber monitoring. The financial aspects of demand, actuarial analyses, and underwriting are discussed in Chapter 10.

[2]E. Jerome McCarthy. *Basic Marketing.* 4th Edition. Homewood, Ill., Richard D. Irwin, Inc., 1971, pp. 37–38.
[3]*Ibid.*, pp. 44–46.

PLACE

Place in the marketing mix is concerned with the actual delivery of proper services to the target population. HMO services are of little value unless they are available and accessible when and where the subscribers need them; therefore, consideration must be given to the geographic location of the delivery of services, the hours of operation, and the type of provider who will be available (paramedic, technician, physician). The use of outlying satellite clinics is also a consideration.

PROMOTION

Promotion involves the methods by which the HMO communicates with the target population. Issues such as the "hard" or "soft" sell; advertising; public service announcements; the development, training, and utilization of a sales force; one-to-one selling; and group selling are included in this category. All of these promotion activities can add value to the health plan's services.

PRICE

The marketing director, together with the plan administrator, actuaries, and underwriters, must decide on a price that will be attractive to the target groups and that will be competitive with other health insurance programs. Generally, several packages will be made available, with varying prices (e.g., individual membership, family membership, subscriber plus spouse and two or more children). The pricing strategies developed for these categories of membership will be appropriate only if the target groups actually perceive a difference in the benefit packages offered by the HMOs and the coverage now available to them, and if the HMO can effectively appeal to the diverse subgroups within the target population with distinctively different packages. The activities involved with pricing the packages are discussed in the following section; pricing is detailed in Chapter 10.

Marketing Process

Marketing as an HMO-wide set of activities has become the accepted approach; it is a four-step process:[4]

[4]Three of these four steps are suggested in U.S. Department of Health, Education, and Welfare, Health Maintenance Organization Service. *Marketing Pre-Paid Health Care Plans*. Rockville, Md., 1972, p. 2.

1. Market analysis
2. Making choice available
3. Active marketing
4. Account maintenance and growth

MARKET ANALYSIS

The analysis of market feasibility is an important task in planning an HMO; in Chapter 7, the ways to determine market feasibility were described as part of the overall feasibility study. The discussion of the study and analysis that must be accomplished to determine whether a sufficient market exists to support the HMO is continued here. To state this task more precisely, market analysis is undertaken to determine what the consumer demand will be so that HMO services and activities can be adjusted to successfully serve this market. The ultimate objective of such a survey, then, is to provide the HMO with information concerning its competitors and demographic, socioeconomic, and epidemiological characteristics of the area that can guide the decision-making process. Data collected should enable the manager to develop a marketing strategy and, ultimately, to determine if the HMO is feasible, that is, to determine whether there are enough qualified buyers to support the HMO activity. This analysis leads to the other steps in the marketing process—making choices available, active marketing, and continuing market/subscriber relations.

The reader also will realize that market analyses do not end when the initial planning feasibility decision is made. Market study is a continuous process throughout the life of the health plan. Data are required to make decisions concerning new target populations and modifications to marketing strategies for current subscriber groups. Marketing HMOs is a dynamic process that requires continuous feedback of data. It is imperative that the HMO develop systems that will generate a continuous flow of subscriber data without major market analysis studies. When the decision is made to expand the health plan, current subscriber data will be readily available, to which information concerning new groups may be added. Through this method, better marketing strategies can be designed.

Before discussing the market survey itself, it is fundamental to point out that most HMO planners will have a stated set of objectives for their new HMO. These will be accepted or modified by the HMO's board of trustees throughout the planning and development process. Based on the definition of marketing earlier in this chapter, most of these objectives will concern marketing goals. For example, one objective may be the development of a 15-physician, multispecialty group that will provide, on a self-supporting basis, comprehensive health care services to 20,000 enrollees drawn from a population base of 700,000. Although broad, this objective limits the character of the marketing study the HMO administrator should undertake. When the results of the survey are available, a comparison of the population data with the objectives may reveal the need for modification in the HMO's goals to make them realistic and operative. Many new HMOs set marketing objectives that are unrealistic, that are never modified, and that lead to a totally unsuccessful health plan. In a study reported by Shouldice,[5] reviews of 30 HMO grant applications to the Department of Health, Education, and Welfare, and corresponding progress reports submitted to the federal HMO agency, suggested that most HMO grantees overstate their marketing objectives twofold. In very few instances were the marketing objectives modified by the newly developing HMOs upon completion of their market feasibility studies. As a result, impossible marketing goals were established, staffing was based on these goals, and financial projections were made that were totally spurious. The necessity to modify the HMO's objectives after the market feasibility study cannot be overemphasized.

Target Population Identification: Market analysis leads to decisions regarding the target population and the market mix, the two major components of the marketing strategy. The survey provides data concerning the general population—the total population residing in the geographic area to be served—and the target population—those segments of the total population to which benefit packages are to be marketed. The service or beneficiary population is that portion of the target population that is actually enrolled in the health plan.[6] To describe the general population of the catchment area, the market survey identifies broad socioeconomic levels, available insurers, and providers of care. These three areas can be considered as the first cut in the market analysis. Some minimum market conditions concerning these three areas are presented in Table 21.

The market survey also provides information that allows HMO planners to continue refining the general population to the point where

[5]Robert G. Shouldice. "A Model for Evaluating the Performance of Health Maintenance Organizations." Doctoral Dissertation. Washington, D.C., The George Washington University, 1974.

[6]U.S. Department of Health, Education, and Welfare, Health Maintenance Organization Service. *Financial Planning Manual.* Washington, D.C., U.S. Government Printing Office, 1972, p. 4.

TABLE 21 Minimum Market Conditions

Level	Condition
Socioeconomic	
(1) Income	(1) Above $10,000 per family per year
(2) Social	(2) Ability to develop a "balanced" population mix; adequate group structure; accessibility and limited travel times
Insurer	
(1) Market share	(1) 10 to 30 percent of population
(2) Type of insurer	(2) Existing pathfinder HMO
(3) General premium levels	(3) Cost of HMO benefit package similar to existing programs
(4) Coverage	(4) Limited in existing plans
Provider of Medical Care	
(1) Facilities	(1) Existing, modern and attractive facilities
(2) Existing services	(2) Evidence of need
(3) Attitudes	(3) Supportive

target populations surface. The target populations are of more immediate concern than the general population, because they more fully describe the demand that the HMO must meet; this is the population to which the market analysis is directly addressed and for whom the marketing strategies are developed. It is from this group that the HMO seeks enrollment and its service population. During the operational phase, the administrator's primary consideration is the service population, since all operational decisions are made because of and for this enrolled group.

Data Collection—Demography: Data required to identify the target population include demographic, socioeconomic, and epidemiological characteristics.[7] Demography is the study of vital statistics. For HMO purposes, the most important demographic characteristics are age; sex; race; family status; income; employment (or occupation); and population size, density, and distribution. Demography also deals with birth and death rates (mortality statistics) and mobility patterns. These data, together with socioeconomic and epidemiological categories, should be known and understood, for the reasons listed in Table 22.

[7]U.S. Department of Health, Education, and Welfare, Health Maintenance Organization Service. *Marketing of Health Maintenance Organizations.* Vol. I. Rockville, Md., 1972, p. 5.

TABLE 22   Data Requirements in Market Analysis

Factors or Characteristics	Relevance
(1) Size of target population	(1) Population size affects the relative ease in marketing and the nature and size of health resources required
(2) Distribution and density	(2) Location and distance of health facilities influences choice and transportation requirements
(3) Age, sex, race, and so on*	(3) Direct influence on epidemiological characteristics of population that affects desired need for various services (e.g., health needs of an over-65-years-old population differ substantially from an under-10-years-old category)
(4) Birth rates	(4) Pediatric and obstetric sources
(5) Death rates	(5) Age-specific disease and conditions
(6) Mobility information*	(6) Turnover of subscribers
(7) Family status*	(7) Benefit package development and number of programs offered; family size influences overall plan utilization and, therefore, staffing, utilization, and costs
(8) Income*	(8) Ability to pay or contribute toward premium or eligibility for welfare programs; income is also a measure of the potential for episodic illness, bad debt expectation, and an indicator of the effort required to bring population to an acceptable level of health maintenance
(9) Employment*	(9) Group enrollment and possibility of employer contributing toward premiums
(10) Educational level	(10) Direct relation to usage rate
(11) Ethnic make-up	(11) Potential for treatment of special diseases that are prevalent in certain population segments
(12) Housing	(12) Reflects the sociological characteristics of the population, approximate level of income and affluence; housing unit information may indicate individual versus family information
(13) Disease incidence	(13) Required for actuarial and underwriting tasks

*These factors are also important because of consumer-held beliefs and behaviors. For a discussion of these issues, see Chapter 6.

Although collection of the data listed in Table 22 may appear awe-some, the sources are almost limitless. This is true not only for demo-graphic information but also for socioeconomic and epidemiological data. Sources include the Bureau of the Census of the U.S. Department of Commerce; local, county, and state health departments; local and state chambers of commerce; health planning agencies; utility com-panies; tax lists; school enrollments; newspapers; state agencies relat-ing to industry, employment, and trade; voter registration; U.S. De-partment of Labor's *Digest of Health and Insurance Plans;* Blue Cross and Blue Shield plans; Medicare and Medicaid representatives; union representatives; other HMOs; and local hospitals. In addition to these sources, it also may be necessary to survey the target population. An interview guide for such a survey of employees, prepared by Health Systems Research Programs of the Bionetics Research Laboratories, Inc., is provided in Volume VI of *Marketing of Health Maintenance Organizations* listed in the references at the end of this chapter. In addition, Exhibits V–XVII of the *Health Maintenance Organizations Guidelines*[8] provide a method for organizing all data required to com-plete the market feasibility study.

As a part of the demographic review, the health plan manager should prepare general and target population projections for the service area. Future estimates of population size are required for any forecasting by the health plan, whether it concerns enrollment levels, cash flow, staff-ing, or facility development. Various methodologies used to complete forecasts are available from several sources. The method or methods chosen for a given population projection are based on estimates of the availability of data, the type of data required by each projection tech-nique, and the various estimates desired. To develop satisfactory fore-casts, the health plan manager must prepare a description of the re-quirement for a forecast and the specific situation to be projected, and explain how the current situation will evolve into the forecast state.[9] With a perspicuous understanding of the forecast requirements, a fore-casting technique may be chosen. Five approaches to population pro-jections that seem most germane to HMOs are reported in detail by Bergwall, Reeves, and Woodside:[10]

---

[8]U.S. Department of Health, Education, and Welfare, Office of Health Maintenance Organizations. *Health Maintenance Organizations Guidelines.* Rockville, Md., 1975, pp. 125–135.

[9]David F. Bergwall, Philip N. Reeves, and Nina B. Woodside. *Introduction to Health Planning.* Washington, D.C., Information Resources Press, 1974, p. 61.

[10]*Ibid.,* pp. 69–71.

1. Extrapolation
2. Ratio method
3. Correlation method
4. Component method
5. Cohort survival method

Of the five methods, Bergwall et al. suggest that the last approach appears to provide the most accurate projections. They suggest the following steps to be used in the cohort survival method.

a. The population should be broken down into appropriate subgroups. The interval covered by each of the age groups should be equal to the periods of projection; for example, for 5-, 10-, or 20-year projections, use 5-year age groups (10–14, 45–49, etc.).

b. Multiply each subgroup by the appropriate survival rate. The survival rate is the complement of the death rate for the cohort.[11] If the death rate is 10 per 10,000, the survival rate will be 9,990 per 10,000.

c. Multiply female groups (in the 15 to 44 age group) by appropriate birthrates to get the number of births.

d. Multiply the total number of births by the proportion of male births and the proportion of female births to get the number of male and female births.*

e. Multiply male and female births by the appropriate survival rates.

f. Add surviving births to the youngest cohorts.

g. Adjust each group for net migration.

h. Adjust each cohort for the percent who will advance to the next cohort due to age increase during the year.[12]

*Aggregate natality rates should be readily available from vital statistics departments. In the event the state data do not provide a breakdown by sex, one can then apply the national proportion of male to female births to determine how the births should be distributed in the 0–14 cohort.

Examples of the use of the cohort survival method are provided by Bergwall et al.[13] and also in *Marketing of Health Maintenance Organizations*.[14] In the latter, the method is referred to as the "demographic model."

Data Collection—Socioeconomic: Information concerning the economic and sociological dimensions of the population should be added

[11]A cohort is a group of people with similar characteristics born in the same time period. All white women between 15 and 20 years is an example of a race-sex cohort.

[12]Bergwall, Reeves, and Woodside. *Introduction to Health Planning*, p. 71.

[13]*Ibid.*, p. 72.

[14]U.S. Department of Health, Education, and Welfare. *Marketing of Health Maintenance Organizations*, Vol. II, p. 44.

to the demographic data. Socioeconomic data are concerned with income and the distribution of income, the employment pattern of the population, labor-force characteristics, and the economic expansion potential of the community and are important elements in deciding which groups will make up the target populations. The data sources referred to in the preceding section will be generally helpful in obtaining this data, although the HMO manager may find it difficult to obtain access to certain socioeconomic information and, therefore, will be required to be more resourceful in this collection effort. Nonconventional and normally nonaccessible sources may include union and employer employment records, professional association records, state unemployment insurance records, Social Security Administration records for Medicare and Medicaid recipients, local tax records, land developer's projections, and department store and local credit and shopping card programs, among others. Generally, this data should provide the marketing director with an overall view of the local society and its levels of affluence or lack thereof.

Data Collection—Epidemiological: Statistics on the incidence of disease are categorized as epidemiological data. This information is imperative for the completion of the actuarial and underwriting tasks—the calculation of risks and the process by which the HMO determines the basis on which it will accept a group from the target population as subscribers to the health plan. These data are used for generation of the statement of demand for services and thus affect the benefit-package and premium-level development, as well as the level and category of physician and paramedical staffing required to meet the projected demand. Sources of epidemiological data for small communities may not exist. Limited information about infectious diseases will be available on a regional basis because of its reportable nature. Other major sources may be the records of services provided from local hospitals and from outpatient providers such as clinics, group practices, other HMOs, and solo practitioners.

National statistics are being accumulated at present through the efforts of the National Ambulatory Medical Care Survey developed by the National Center for Health Statistics, Scientific and Technical Information Branch;[15] selected statistics are currently available. Care must be exercised in the use of national statistics, because they generally do not reflect accurate local medical practice and usage rates; thus,

---

[15]The center is located at 5600 Fishers Lane, Rockville, Maryland 20851.

these national statistics must be "localized," based on available local information.

The most important source of actuarial information, and typically the most difficult source from which to obtain information, is current insurers. Incidence rates for disease, accident, and injury are maintained by both the indemnity companies and the local Blue Cross and Blue Shield plans. By obtaining such local information, the health plan could reduce considerably the expense of the underwriting activity and may be able to more accurately predict utilization levels. Additional discussion of underwriting is found in Chapter 10.

Data Collection—Existing Delivery System: Identifying the competition provided by the existing medical-care delivery programs and insuring organizations is a more commercialistic issue than gathering data about the target population. All existing providers within the health plan's catchment area need to be identified by type of provider, location, and market share. This information is easily obtained from community medical societies, professional society registers, community health departments, local hospital associations, other professional associations, and the local health planning agency.

Health program insurers, although they can be identified, are more difficult to describe by market share. One rough method of identifying an insurer's market share is through "payment source" studies completed by most hospitals. Although the data relate to payment for inpatient care, the studies, together with information on benefit packages offered by insurers, provide a general indication of the market share of each insurer. In addition, benefit-package and premium-level information is necessary in the development of a competitive HMO package. Some HMO managers have even suggested that a newly developing HMO may assume that the *existing* insurance benefit packages have been constructed to meet the particular needs of the community, and, consequently, an HMO package with comparable benefits will meet the demand of the subscriber population; the HMO manager, by using other insurers' benefit packages, might save considerable effort. This is a risky business practice, because many existing programs are dated, are not based on a market analysis, or are not tailored to the specific target populations to which the HMO will market. Moreover, the HMO will be providing outpatient coverage as its prime benefit and will emphasize preventive medicine; the state-of-the-art in the "Blues" and indemnity programs provides few, if any, benefits in the outpatient and preventive areas.

Information about insurers' market shares and their major accounts is vital to an HMO that plans to use a dual-choice enrollment practice; dual choice suggests that a competitive selection process is operational. As described in Chapter 6, dual choice is an important marketing device that permits the HMO to break into other insurers' accounts and to competitively attract some of their customers. Indeed, if the market has been almost totally consumed by the existing insurers, dual choice is critical to the HMO's marketing strategy and future success. It is also suggested that, because the subscribers under dual choice make up a "noncaptive" membership, those joining are apt to be more satisfied; there is a great deal of intellectual and practical appeal to the dual-choice arrangement. If the health plan is not viewed as a superior system, however, dual choice can operate to the detriment of the HMO. Loss in membership is an indication that changes need to be made in the HMO. The mechanics of establishing a dual-choice program are described on pages 144–147 and 227.

Data Analysis—Target Population: The next stage in the development of a marketing strategy is an analysis of the data concerning the target population and the competition from other insurers. Figure 31 outlines the marketing-financial planning process; this begins with the tasks of population segmentation and estimates of penetration. The process then continues with estimates of demand of the selected target population and, through financial analyses, permits a forecast of the necessary capacity to provide services to meet the demand. The intermediate product of this planning process is the market mix—a definition of the product (the benefit packages), place (geographic location, transportation requirements, hours of operation), promotion (advertising and selling techniques), and price (premium structure). The analysis of population and development of the market mix allow the administrator to decide on the market feasibility—a decision made after the marketing-mix plans are established to continue and to actually offer dual choice and sell the plan's services. Figure 31 is relevant to the remainder of this chapter and also to the issues discussed in Chapters 9 and 10.

Segmentation: If sufficient data have been collected, segmentation can be completed with relative ease. This will accomplish several objectives: First, it makes dividing the total population into discrete segments of users possible, allowing for greater ease in planning. Second, it defines precisely the characteristics of the segments to which the

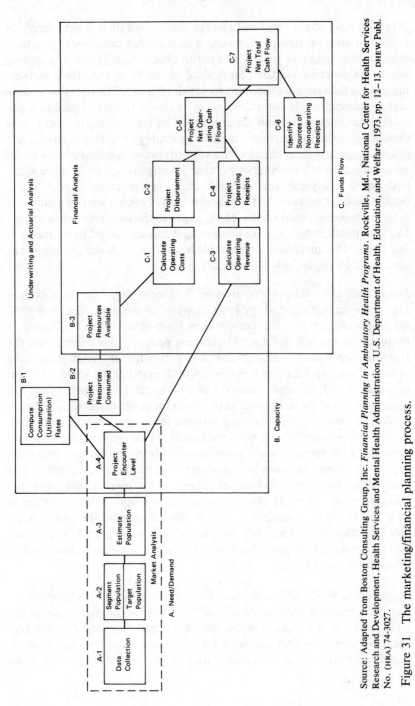

Source: Adapted from Boston Consulting Group, Inc. *Financial Planning in Ambulatory Health Programs.* Rockville, Md., National Center for Health Services Research and Development, Health Services and Mental Health Administration, U.S. Department of Health, Education, and Welfare, 1973, pp. 12–13. DHEW Publ. No. (HRA) 74-3027.

Figure 31   The marketing/financial planning process.

HMO will be providing services and, hence, sets the stage for the underwriting activities that are so very important in this process. Third, because the grouping of people by demographic, socioeconomic, and epidemiological characteristics is inherent in segmentation, the process of identifying groups that might be sources of substantial enrollment is enhanced. Finally, a mistake with one segment will not dramatically affect the total target population.

The segmentation process begins by identifying major groups — groups of 50, 100, 200, 1,000 people, and so on. The following categorization of groups are most important: employer or union affiliation, age, family income, membership, sex, geographic location, third-party payment representation, and ethnic or racial characteristics. Reviews of the data will reveal the most important methods of segmenting the population. It is important in the process, however, to use more than one segmentation method to cross-check the analyses. If geographic location appears to be most important because of a rural location, then the population should be segmented not only by geography but also by one or more of the other groupings. Employment, for example, also may be important. The planning activities delineated in Figure 31 should then be completed, following the methods discussed in Chapter 10. Finally, the results of each segmentation method should be compared with all others, that is, the geographic segmentation should be compared with age, sex, income, and so on, to check for accuracy of demand and capacity forecasts.

Of greater importance will be the listing of large- and medium-sized companies, unions, associations, and government agencies. Because they represent the largest assemblies of potential subscribers, great effort should be expended in their description and analysis. It is obvious that, if success is encountered with these large groups, the success of the HMO will be assured — and at a minimum of cost and time. Consequently, at least segmentation by employment or union membership is essential. Seasoned HMO marketers also realize that the employer or the union representative typically controls the health insurance programs that are offered to employees or to union members. It is imperative that the HMO marketer work with the key employer and union representatives who are responsible for the establishment of dual-choice arrangements for employees or union membership.

Another important segmentation is by third-party payment — a description of the current insurance company's market shares. The service, direct service, indemnity, and government programs should be listed, together with their subscribers, membership, or recipient levels. Again, it is necessary to determine which third-party segments the

TABLE 23   Segmentation by Payment Mechanism

Health Insurer	Health Care Market by Insurer and Market Share			
	A Current Number of Persons Covered	B Insurer (percent of total)	C HMO Projected Market Share of Insurer (percentage)	D Projected Number of HMO Enrollees (A × C)	HMO Enrollees (percent of total)
Blue Cross/Blue Shield	170,000	13.0	1.0	1,700	34.0
Private Insurance	700,000	54.4	0.4	2,800	56.0
Health Maintenance Organization	95,000	7.3	—	—	—
Medicare	150,000	11.6	0.08	120	2.4
Medicaid	80,000	6.2	0.006	5	0.1
Armed Forces/Other Noncivilian	24,000	1.9	—	—	—
Noncovered or Self-insured	75,000	5.8	0.5	375	7.5
Total	1,294,000	100.0	1.986	5,000	100.0

marketing effort will address and which other segments a marketing effort would be ineffective in addressing. As many market segmentations should be undertaken as are necessary to completely describe the major characteristics of the population.

The next logical task is the completion of a market penetration-rate study—an analysis of the target segments that describe the level of the projected market share of each group in each segment. The objective of the penetration study is to precisely identify to whom the HMO will market and to best estimate the membership level from each segment. Table 23 provides data for a hypothetic penetration-rate study, by payment mechanism, for a city of 1,294,000 citizens.

Based on the objectives established by the board of directors or trustees and the data available about the community, the first estimate of market share is made. In Table 23, the board set its first-year enrollment level at 5,000 members (see Column D) with the greatest number being drawn from the present private insurance and Blue Cross/Blue Shield programs. It appears that little hope was given to attracting any subscribers from existing HMO plans. On the other hand, the figure suggests that the board does have a commitment, although low, to provide care to recipients of Medicare and Medicaid programs. In the latter, the HMO will need to negotiate a Medicaid contract with the state in order to serve these individuals. Because the priority appears to be low (five enrollees), and extensive effort is necessary to consummate a state contract, it might be wise to defer activities in the Medicaid area until the HMO is more established; the Medicaid program now requires a successful "track record" before contracts are awarded, therefore, in all likelihood, this will not be a successful effort by the HMO at the present time.

In Table 24, the same market is hypothetically segmented by employment group. Initially, only large employers are included; note that in this example the assumption is made that the HMO will be marketing to employees only and not their families. Again, the HMO administrator follows the objectives established by the board, but is also guided by the reality of the current employment situation—the current carriers, the ability for dual choice, the existence of union contracts, and the length of time the present health plans have been in effect, among other things. In comparing the first segmentation with that in Table 24, the manager identifies some contradictory projections, as noted in Table 25. Although the segmentation and projections by payment mechanism suggest that 34 percent of the enrollees will come from the present BC/BS programs and 56 percent from the private insurance companies, the segmentation by employment suggests that 70 percent of enroll-

TABLE 24 Segmentation by Employment Group

| | Health Care Market by Employment | | | | | |
| | A | B | C | D | E | F |
Company by Type	Number of Employees	Percent Eligible	Carrier	Projected Market Share of Total (percentage)	Projected Number of HMO Enrollees (A × B × D)	HMO Enrollees (percent of total)
Local Government A						
Professional	15,000	100	BC/BS	10.00	1,500	30.0
Blue Collar	7,000	100	BC/BS	100.00	700	14.0
Electronics M	1,020	100	Western Life	—	—	—
Hotel/Motel	4,300	20	Metropolitan Life	—	—	—
Electronics N	2,400	100	BC/BS	24.00	600	12.0
Service X	3,000	100	HMO	—	—	—
Publisher	1,200	65	Self-Insured	6.00	47	0.9
Construction	1,500	90	BC/BS	—	—	—
Research and Development	600	100	Travelers	—	—	—
Engineering	1,100	100	—	—	—	—
Association	500	100	Travelers	20.00	100	2.0
Service Y	1,200	90	Lincoln National	80.00	864	17.3
Manufacturing	7,000	100	BC/BS	10.00	700	14.0
Light Industrial	2,300	93	Conn. General	17.00	364	7.3
Local Government B	6,000	100	Equitable Life	—	—	—
Printer	600	100	Conn. General	—	—	—
Unemployed (7 percent of population)	90,580	20	Medicare/Medicaid	0.69	125	2.5
Totals	145,300				5,000	100.0

TABLE 25   Comparison of Payment Mechanisms and Employment
Group Segmentations

Company	BC/BS	Private Insurer	Medicare and Medicaid	Noncovered or Self-Insured
Local Government A	2,200			
Electronics	600			
Publisher				47
Association		100		
Service Y		864		
Manufacturing	700			
Light Industrial		364		
Unemployed			125	
Company Total (Table 23)	3,500 (70%)	1,328 (26.6%)	125 (2.5%)	(0.9%)
Insurer Total (Table 24)	1,700 (34%)	2,800 (56.0%)	125 (2.5%)	(7.5%)

ment will be from employers now covering their employees by BC/BS
and only 26.6 percent from private insurance companies. Estimates of
Medicare and Medicaid by both methods, however, are very close. The
HMO manager must continue his study in order to come up with acceptable penetration projections.

A decision must be based on the projected market share estimates in
both Tables 23 (Column C) and 24 (Column D). Market share estimates
must be compatible with the organization's objectives, but they also
must be in the realm of reality, based on data collected and alliances
formed with community groups—employers, unions, associations, and
so on. They are critical projections that must be based on solid information and assurance from key community group leaders. The inability
to make these estimates and, thus, realistic decisions suggests incom-
plete information and lack of understanding of the community and its
social and economic order. It indicates that more work will be required
before the discrepancies among the several penetration-rate studies
come close together.

These in-house studies will help to accurately project the service or
beneficiary population—a critical step that must be completed prior to
development of benefit packages and the subsidiary activity of premium formulation. But, even though all of these activities are completed with care and are reasonable, the HMO manager may bungle the
marketing program if personal contact is not established with those key
community individuals in the large employee groups and unions who
control the health benefits for their organizations. The HMO manager
should initiate meetings with group leaders early in the marketing activ-

ity: They should be asked to participate in the development of benefit packages; their assistance should be requested in other plan activities; and their personal commitment to the HMO, especially as plan subscribers, should be obtained. Naturally, close alliances will be easier to achieve if the plan administrator, medical director, and marketing manager are long-standing members of the community and are well known and liked. In other instances, contacts will be on a purely professional level; key group leaders will ask for a cost-and-benefit proposal from the health plan. The HMO manager should prepare a briefing on the goals and objectives of the HMO, its potential ability to contain costs, and a possible benefit package and premium schedules—the manager should take the opportunity to sell the concept as well as the insurance package.

The final products of the segmentation and penetration studies are a list of membership sources and a projection of the level of subscribers from each source. Each source can then be completely described and a marketing mix prepared. Descriptions of employer, union, and association groups and government agencies should include the following:

1. Name of organization and size of group
2. Size of eligible population in group
3. Average wage or family income
4. Residence (geographical distribution)
5. Male/female categorization
6. Current insurance carrier and coverage
7. Insurance coverage—local or national decision
8. Date of last insurance carrier, benefit, or premium change
9. Premium and contribution of individual member
10. Existence of dual choice
11. Family size (distribution)
12. Experience rating or community rating

Additional data elements will be required for the actuarial activities. The health plan is now able to decide to which of the groups to market.[16] In effect, this decision is the first part of the market feasibility decision—there are sufficient groups from which enough subscribers can be enrolled to meet the membership-size objective.

The first phase of the market analysis—population identification—will now have been completed. As outlined in Figure 32, the output of the population analysis is a statement of need/demand.

[16]Group contract marketing is amplified through examples in U.S. Department of Health, Education, and Welfare. *Marketing of Health Maintenance Organizations*, Vol. IV.

Process	Product

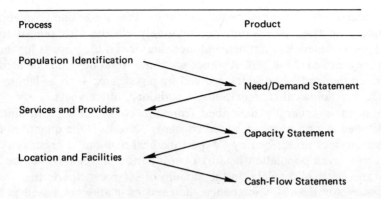

Population Identification

Need/Demand Statement

Services and Providers

Capacity Statement

Location and Facilities

Cash-Flow Statements

Figure 32   The marketing/financial planning process by products.

Demand levels help to determine the size of the organization (facility and staff) needed; the product of this analysis is a statement of capacity. These two products are finally evaluated through a cash flow study; descriptions of financial needs for the year can then be completed. The following section deals with demand statements.

Data Analysis—Market Mix and Demand Statement: The market mix is described as product, place, promotion, and price—a unique mix that is developed for each target group to meet the consumers' needs. The process of market-mix development requires analysis of the demographic, socioeconomic, and epidemiological data to describe a statement of demand, followed by design of the preliminary benefit package.

Although the area of need/demand theory in health care cannot be fully addressed here, some basic concepts are important.[17] Planning for services, the size of the facility, location, types of providers, and ability to break even financially is based on the determination of the target groups' needs and demands.

Demand is defined as that quantity of health service "wanted" by a consumer constrained by limited financial resources. Patients will demand only that amount of service that it is economically rational for them to buy. But, in medical-care delivery, the level of demand also is related to the type of service demanded. The demand for acute or emergency services is inelastic with regard to price—consumers do not consider the long-term economic loss from receiving such services

[17]For an excellent description of need/demand theory, see Bergwall, Reeves, and Woodside. *Introduction to Health Planning,* pp. 90–93, 161–163.

now, because they want immediate attention. Preventive and cosmetic services, on the other hand, are relatively elastic with regard to price—consumers will not demand these services if the price is higher than they can easily afford. Another portion of total demand is called "derived demand"—services ordered by physicians, such as laboratory and radiological examinations or additional office visits.

Demand is generally described from the consumer's viewpoint, while need is a physician-oriented concept. "Need" is the quantity of health services prescribed by "expert medical opinion" as necessary to keep a given population healthy over a period of time. While need estimates are based solely on the amount of services experts feel are necessary for health maintenance, demand estimates are based not only on need but also on other factors, including out-of-pocket costs of care and consumer perceptions of need. Consequently, it is easy to envision several problems in demand identification—individuals may not agree with professional determinations of what the needs might be; the professional does not consider economic factors in his need statement; the limited supply of services may not be sufficient to meet the demand level of care, even without considering need.

How then shall the HMO administrator develop a statement of need/demand that will be appropriate for the target populations? The process requires estimates of both demand and need, and an adjustment of the combined estimates based on the HMO objectives described by the governing body and the medical staff. First, demand estimates are developed on estimates of use; it is here that "ambulatory visit" data becomes useful. This method uses a standard visit-to-population ratio. Second, estimates of need are based primarily on studies of epidemiological, morbidity, and mortality data. The need approach is considered to be within the realm of the actuary and the underwriter. Statements using both methods should be developed as a check in the accuracy of the projections. (See Chapter 10 for a review of both demand and need methods.) The results of need/demand studies will forecast the type and number of services (encounters or visits) that will be demanded by the target population. Thus, through the process of projecting demand, the first part of the market mix is developed—the product or benefit package. A second part of the mix also is addressed—that of the estimated price—but final pricing is deferred until the cash flow analyses are completed. Moreover, the stage is set for the development of a capacity statement—the size of the staff and facility to meet the need/demand.

Decision to Buy—A Value Choice: The decision to buy the HMO product that is offered through the benefit package is viewed by the consumer as a value choice. The decision to buy the HMO services, service plan, or indemnity coverage, or to remain a self-paying patient (not buy at all) is based on how well the values the consumer perceives in the product match his own needs and desires—the use to him. The decision to buy can also be viewed as an "exchange of values," where the consumer believes that he is receiving service equal to or worth more than the charges for the services. What then are the product values of an HMO, and how well do they match the general need/demand for services? The following are four basic HMO product values.

1. *Comprehensive care:* Many customers of service and indemnity plans have been disappointed or upset when they find that their "comprehensive" insurance coverage only partially pays for services they have received. As part of the HMO promotional activity, comparisons of the level of comprehensiveness between the indemnities and the "Blues" and the HMO may assure the potential subscriber that HMO coverage is more comprehensive than that of existing plans. Additional services that emphasize prevention and ambulatory care also may be viewed by the customer as value added.

2. *Accessible care:* The consumer with a fee-for-service, private family physician too often finds that no service is available on weekends, one day a week when the physician has no office hours, and during evening and nighttime hours. The HMO attempts to provide 24-hour coverage and telephone consultation. Emergency care in HMOs, however, may be provided on a referral basis, through out-of-area coverage, or in a hospital's emergency room. Long waits and impersonal service may be the result for the HMO subscriber.

3. *Quality care:* Although this is a very difficult area to document, consumers value quality care very highly. They consider quality to be the ability to see a physician when one is needed, the degree of respect and sensitivity with which patients are handled, the impression provided by the facility, the degree of choice of physician, the use of the family or managing physician, and the closeness of the consumer's relationship to the personal physician. Consumers cannot easily judge the quality of the medical treatment they receive, but they can and do evaluate the quality of the personal treatment.

4. *Reasonable cost:* The price of the benefit package is truly important and can be used as a selling point if it is competitive with the current insurance program's premiums. In group selling, when an expensive indemnity benefit plan is offered at no cost to the group member, and the difference needed to pay for the enrollment is low (less than $10 to $15 per month), no premium problems should be encountered in enrollment. If the member must bear an increase in

excess of approximately $15 per month, the premium becomes extremely important, especially if it is deducted from the employee's salary. When skillfully explained, consumers will understand that, although the premium may be higher than their present coverage, they also may be receiving more services for their money in the HMO system.

The third market-mix element—place—also must be considered during data analyses. The geographic location of the plan's facility and service area is important because of consumer access; the more available the health care services, the greater the attraction of the prepaid plan. Generally, it is recognized that at least 65 percent of the projected service population must live within a 30-minute drive of the facility. For urban areas, it is suggested that the facility can adequately serve an area within a 10-mile radius. Together, travel time and distance is described as the "travel function"—an aggravation index that includes distance, travel time, congestion, normal travel patterns, and parking. In addition, the existence of an attractive facility that can be shown to prospective members is an important marketing device. Hours of operation and types of emergency coverage also will be important in continuing account maintenance. Larger HMOs have realized that the use of satellite facilities are important in providing accessible service. With these issues in mind, several management questions must be answered from the data collected:

1. If the HMO will be using existing facilities, are the locations appropriate and is the facility modern and aesthetically pleasing?
2. Are the population segments that were chosen to be target groups within a 30-minute travel time and/or within a 10-mile drive from the facility?
3. Are the hours of operation and the types of services offered appropriate for the service populations?

Promotion—Advertising and Public Image: The final element of the marketing mix is promotion—communicating the plan's services to the potential service population. If one realizes that all of the planning activities and the development of staff, equipment, and facilities are of no significance if the availability of the HMO's services cannot be communicated to the potential market, then one can understand that promotion does add value to the services offered. But, because of the somewhat archaic attitude concerning "marketing" and "selling" in medical-care delivery, it is essential to discuss their use. The health plan should choose its language carefully concerning the use of both "marketing" and "selling," and should have a clear and specific understanding about how promotional literature and "selling" activities are to be used. The principles of medical ethics state that a physician shall not solicit patients; in HMOs, the concern is not so much the advertising by physicians themselves, but advertising on behalf of physicians. There is a difference between advertising the availability of medical care under a specific system—such as an HMO or Blue Cross/Blue Shield—and advertising the individual physicians that work with the system. The American Medical Association's Ethical Relations Committee and Judicial Council are now debating these issues, and representatives have suggested that new guidelines be issued that will allow physicians more freedom to advertise their services and charges. This is evolving because HMOs have been advertising, and fee-for-service physicians are responding to this competitive pressure. In effect, what HMOs have been encouraging—free choice—is finally being achieved. An official of a major medical society recently stated, ". . . with the alternative systems (e.g., HMO) of medical care available, there has to be some information given to the public so it can make a choice."[18]

Promotion of HMO services varies. Most HMOs have taken a relatively "soft sell" approach because of the current AMA opposition to advertising. This approach has included public-service announcements on radio and television, mailings, and newspaper ads that inform the public about the availability of health care services. These ads are generally supportive of the entire medical community and suggest only that the HMO, another medical provider, is available. Somewhat stronger advertisements may describe the uniqueness of the HMO approach—its emphasis on ambulatory and preventive services, and its 24-hour accessibility; hard-sell or "Madison Avenue" type techniques in advertising have been used infrequently. Advertisements might, however, include a description of the programs offered and the major advantages of controlled cost and quality, comprehensive coverage, and high access when care is needed. The use of comparison charts pointing out the advantages of the HMO over its leading competitors is very effective and may be a part of the advertisement. But no matter which technique is used, it is imperative that the marketing director contact the local medical society and discuss the HMO's advertising plans prior to their use. Ugly confrontations that could adversely affect the entire medical community and tarnish the HMO image can

[18]Jack Martin. "New Dilemma for Doctors: HMO Advertising." *Medical Economics:* 71, August 19, 1974.

thus be avoided. In all situations, materials presented must be in good taste and factual—neither over- or understating the HMO's ability to provide services. Advertising should not only inform the public, it should educate it at the same time. After the health plan has obtained its initial enrollment, the most effective advertising is by word of mouth, and this depends on many factors—quality of care, access, friendliness of personnel, and so on.

Advertising is one of several activities in the promotion effort that builds the public image of the health plan. Other public relation activities that are continuous throughout the life of the HMO include the actual selling activities; improvement of sales literature and preparation of annual reports and periodic preventive health tips for distribution to the membership; training and utilization of the sales force to be effective yet courteous and helpful; and a courteous receptionist and telephone operator. As Gumbiner suggests in *HMO: Putting It All Together,* the HMO has a relationship with several publics, all of which react in various ways to the health plan and its activities. These publics include "the general public, the professional public (other doctors, pharmacists, dentists), its in-house public (its own staff, which should never be forgotten), and the consumer public that it serves. Then there are many subgroups: government agencies, industries, unions, insurance companies, and hospitals."[19]

Although the planning for selling activities is undertaken as a part of the analysis process, the topic of active marketing and selling is discussed in a later section of this chapter in the context of the four stages in the marketing process. Selling, like all other marketing activities, must be tailored to each population segment. Those selling strategies described on pages 230–232 complete the analysis of the service-area population. The HMO board of trustees, using the recommendations of the administrator, is now ready to decide whether to continue and to market its services or to radically change its objectives and thus its approach to the service-area population, or whether marketing the program cannot be successful. To continue commits the HMO to its plans, objectives, and hopes for success. The following is a recapitulation of some market factors identified during data analysis that may create marketing problems.

1. Lack of large firms, unions, or associations
2. Lack of a single large industry that is interested in the health plan program

[19]Robert Gumbiner. *HMO: Putting It All Together.* St. Louis, Mo., C. V. Mosby Co., 1975, p. 87.

3. Lack of several good-sized national firms or unions whose health benefit decisions are made locally

4. Lack of a single large industry interested in the health plan's program and willing to participate in the marketing/enrollment process

5. An attempt to enroll Medicaid, Medicare, or other welfare program recipients as the base group (nonbalanced enrollment)

6. Marketing to an area in which more than 90 percent of the population is currently covered by a health-insuring mechanism

7. Marketing in areas where there is major consumer or physician opposition to the HMO

8. Areas with unstable economies

9. Areas that are predominantly low income or high revenue (both extremes create marketing problems)

10. Federally qualified plans that must offer expensive programs in an area not capable of supporting such benefit packages

11. The use of "sweetheart" contracts to attract major groups of enrollees, which creates major financial hazards

12. Salesmen whose perception of the plan differs from that of other personnel, and who sell more than the plan can provide

13. The need for service being adequately met by fee-for-service physicians and local hospitals; a ratio lower than one physician to more than 700 people (e.g., 1:500) may indicate adequate access

MAKING CHOICE AVAILABLE

The second phase in the marketing activity is offering dual-choice plans to those firms, unions, associations, and government agencies that have been chosen as the target population segments. This has been the traditional HMO strategy for breaking into other insurers' markets, but it also facilitates the development of true consumer choice between programs. Most employees or unions customarily offer only one mandatory program. The decision of a group leader to offer the HMO option as a second choice will require a change in attitudes and in current methods of operation, which may not necessarily have been based on sound decisions (e.g., the organization's health insurance has always been provided that way). Negotiation using logical reasoning is needed to change current habits and opinions, and HMO representatives must fully understand the HMO approach, the possible benefit packages, and the range of premiums. Advantages to the employer or union should be well understood and communicated, and a thorough knowledge of potential disadvantages is helpful in presenting an acceptable argument for dual choice. Both positions are presented in the following listings.

Advantages of Dual Choice

1. Greater employee satisfaction with the fringe benefit package and, thus, with their jobs.

2. Potential over the long run for less employee sick time and, thus, higher productivity, as a result of preventive services and the use of the less time-consuming ambulatory mode of delivery.

3. HMOs as a cost-containment approach may save money for the employer who contributes to his employees' health insurance, since the cost of the employer's contribution may not increase as quickly as in other insurance programs.

4. The employees' share of the cost of the package also may be moderated—thus, providing greater employee satisfaction with the company.

5. A more comprehensive benefit package may entice desirable potential employees to join the firm and induce current employees to remain with the company.

6. The firm may feel a social responsibility to the community and its employees to make available a choice and, perhaps, more valuable health care programs.

7. The firm may wish to offer dual choice to enhance its public image.

8. According to law, a firm governed by the Fair Labor Standards Act must offer dual choice to its employees, if a federally qualified HMO is available.

9. Finally, the firm may offer dual choice to meet the competition for employees because other local firms are offering dual choice.

Disadvantages of Dual Choice

1. Costs of HMO benefit packages are customarily slightly higher than the plans in effect; therefore, the HMO option may be viewed as an increase in financial liability for the firm.

2. There are increased costs, both start-up and operational, to the employer in administering two plans rather than one (e.g., recordkeeping, collection of premiums).

3. By offering more benefits initially, the employer might envision a possibility of accelerating union/employee demands for more fringe benefits.

4. Employers are reluctant to interrupt production by allowing marketing representatives to solicit employees on the job, although firms

generally will arrange meetings with union stewards and second-level management.

5. The possibility of a substantial dollar increase in health insurance deductions from an employee's salary may contribute to loss of employees.

6. Employees and spouses are being asked to break established physician relationships.

Steps to Implementing Dual Choice: There can be wide variations in implementation methods for dual choice. Generally, however, the following steps can be considered basic:[20]

1. Employers, unions, associations, and others are approached by the HMO, and the group representative opts to allow dual choice.

2. The group decides on the level of benefits and the premium. The general approach is to continue with the current premium level initially, although the HMO benefit package might vary substantially from the incumbent plan.

3. The group representative will decide to allow the HMO to market directly to group members; will ask the HMO to coordinate its efforts through the incumbent plan and let the existing plan market, enroll, and complete all other marketing activities, including collection of premiums; or will allow the HMO to market and manage the accounts for itself and the incumbent plan. A contract is consummated describing the arrangement agreed upon.

4. Information describing the benefits of the two plans is made available to each of the beneficiaries.

5. The beneficiaries are permitted and encouraged to decide for themselves which plan they desire.

6. Each beneficiary is required to make an affirmative choice of plans.

7. Beneficiaries are then given an opportunity annually to transfer from one plan to the other. (Enrollment periods must be coordinated with labor agreements and other health plan anniversary dates.)

8. The insurance plans must agree in advance to accept the beneficiaries who select their plan, without percentage restrictions or other qualifications.

Further discussion concerning dual choice is provided in Chapter 6.

[20]Avram Yedida. "Dual Choice Programs." *American Journal of Public Health,* 49(11):1476, November 1959.

ACTIVE MARKETING

With the target groups selected by the dual-choice agreements, the third phase—active marketing—begins. Selling to the groups is the primary objective, with the largest groups first, smaller sized groups (50 to 500) second, welfare programs such as Medicaid next, and individual contracts last. Large-group marketing costs per enrollee are the lowest; the effort to sell to 5,000 employees is not much more expensive than selling to 3,000 employees. There is a somewhat higher per-enrollee cost when selling to smaller groups, and substantially higher per-enrollee costs for individuals. Selling to Medicaid recipients can be very time-consuming, and they may be the last group to be enrolled, although negotiation for a state contract begins very early in the marketing process. Another important reason for beginning the active marketing process with employee groups is that the companies, by preemployment screening, generally have already screened those individuals who were severe health risks as being unacceptable for employment. Because of this, a fairly good cross-section of healthy people is selected, which will help to keep health plan utilization expenses low. Full-coverage or better coverage plans like HMOs have a tendency to attract people requiring above-average medical services. This is natural because the paid-in-full, better coverage program means less money out-of-pocket for the subscriber.[21] Unions are large groups that may present some initial difficulties, because they operate with negotiated contracts; many employers will refuse to do anything that is not included in the contract and will defer any action until the contract is renegotiated. Even during the negotiation period, there may be little compromise, with the union expecting that their specific demands will be met. In general, the HMO manager must maintain the same control over the solicitation activities as over all other marketing and health plan activities; thus, it is imperative that solicitation strategies be carefully developed and strictly followed by the sales staff. Strategies, staff development, and enrollment of specific groups are discussed in the following sections.

Staff Versus Contract Marketing: Who should be involved in the marketing and selling activities? That depends very much on the program's design and sponsorship. If the sponsor is an insurance company, the parent company probably will manage the marketing activities. For

---

[21]American Group Practice Association. *Fee-for-Service Conversion to Prepayment: Proceedings of a Conference.* Alexandria, Va., 1973, p. 46.

plans that are independent organizations, there are essentially three broad marketing organizational approaches:

1. Develop a marketing staff as an integral part of the HMO organization.
2. Contract with an existing organization or with brokers, general insurance agents, and existing carriers to complete marketing activities.
3. Use a combination of HMO staff and some contract marketing.

Each approach has its own strengths and weaknesses.[22] The decision to choose one program over another is based on several factors. Foremost is the ability or inability to attract a competent and experienced marketing director and a marketing staff. Recently, many federal HMO grantees exhibited major deficiencies in their in-house marketing efforts primarily because they lacked competent marketing directors. Good directors command substantial salaries. For a newly developing HMO with financial problems, this added cost may be greater than it is willing to undertake; hence, it may be more attractive to contract with Blue Cross and Blue Shield, for example, to undertake the marketing activities. It is obvious, however, that if the HMO is unwilling to invest substantial funds in the marketing activity, it will not be successful; the marketing budget for a new HMO will be more liberal than one for a mature HMO that is relying on word-of-mouth advertising and account maintenance. Although it may appear that the use of an outside agency is the least expensive method of marketing, this may be misleading. These organizations, of necessity, must have a return on their investment, even if they are nonprofit, just to stay in business. Coupled with the possibility that service and indemnity plan sales personnel may be inexperienced in HMO solicitation, the ultimate cost to the HMO, in all likelihood, may be more than if it hired an in-house marketing staff. Questions of cost, ability to attract experienced staff, and *control* of the marketing activities must be weighed carefully before the decision is made to use either system.

Solicitation Strategy: The methods by which the HMO solicits enrollees are as varied as the groups that are approached; however, several general approaches are worth noting. The solicitation of groups of employees or union members begins with the development of dual-

[22]An excellent discussion of this issue is provided by John R. Kress and James Singer. *HMO Handbook.* Rockville, Md., Aspen Systems Corporation, 1975, pp. 146–148.

choice arrangements. If possible, HMOs sell to and enroll the key personnel in the organization first, thus assuring support through example. As an aside, the HMO will naturally want its own physicians and staff and their spouses to become members of the plan, to show confidence in the program. At this point, the solicitation strategies become individualized for each market segment—selling approaches are tailored to the very specific needs of the potential individual enrollee. Usually, the following concepts or ideas are presented in the promotional and selling activities.[23]

1. Subscribers need not be ill to benefit from the plan; preventive medicine and early disease detection keep the member healthy.

2. The individual selects a personal "family" physician.

3. The subscriber's health care is managed: HMOs provide comprehensive services at one location, and a "family" physician manages the total health care needs of the family.

4. The HMO offers broader coverage with fewer and smaller copayments. Outpatient care is a normally covered service; subscribers do not have to be hospitalized to receive covered services.

5. Quality of care is assured and enhanced through the use of group practice, high medical staff standards, peer review, and the ready availability of specialists and equipment.

6. Freedom of choice under dual choice enables an individual to best meet his family's requirements and to change his choice annually if he wishes.

7. HMOs are cost-efficient methods of delivery, and premiums will not increase as rapidly as those for Blue Cross/Blue Shield plans.

8. Unlike in Blue Shield, access to physicians is enhanced. The subscriber need only call or go to the HMO to find a physician, while Blue Shield members must find a physician from the community willing to accept them as patients.

9. Health education is a part of the entire program offered by the HMO—education concerning the use of the program and its services, habits to develop to live healthier lives, and the use of available preventive programs.

The array of solicitation methods from which a selling strategy may be developed might include some of the following:

[23]U.S. Department of Health, Education, and Welfare. *Marketing of Health Maintenance Organizations*, Vol. V, p. 11.

1. *Dual-choice arrangement*—the first approach to employee and union groups. It is used to inform union and management leaders and to open otherwise closed markets to the HMO.

2. *Enrollment of key group leaders*—support through example, which may influence other group members.

3. *Solicitation of other influential individuals*—face-to-face meetings with as many influential people in the group as possible, with enrollment lending credibility to the plan.

4. *Individual employee or union member solicitation*—the critical second stage of group solicitation. The strategy used will be tailored to the group. Normally, it is preferable to meet with employees or union members in small groups rather than one large group. Large gatherings are very impersonal, and one group member radically opposed to the program could affect many potential subscribers in a large meeting. These meetings are held during workshift changes and on weekends.

5. *Work with existing insurance companies.* Some companies rely completely on the advice of their existing carriers. If, in fact, the existing carrier markets the HMO program, payment for services may more successfully guarantee an acceptable selling job.

6. *Small- to medium-sized employers.* Consider premium contributions as the most important issue in offering the HMO option. Other subjects considered important are rates and copayments, employer administration of dual-choice benefit plans, the HMO's health services and benefits, and master contract provisions.

7. *Community education*—public service announcements, brochures, and other media advertisements designed to foster acceptance and public awareness of the HMO in the service area.

8. *Mail communications*—effective in group selling. Letters may be more carefully read than a brochure (see also 15).

9. *Wives play a crucial role.* Wives normally have a strong voice in the decision to give up an existing pattern of care and to enter into a new system. Information concerning the HMO choice and its services must, therefore, reach wives.

10. *Open house at the HMO* may provide the potential subscriber with an opportunity to see the facility and may lend credibility to the promises made in small group meetings, although open houses usually are not well attended.

11. *Door-to-door selling.* Generally, this approach is reserved as one of the last methods in dual-choice selling because, although effective, it is almost impossible to reach families under dual choice. It is one of the most important approaches in selling to individual subscribers *not*

under dual-choice arrangements and in enrolling subscribers of government-assisted programs such as Medicaid.

12. *Volunteer activities.* Enthusiastic and articulate enrollees may be willing to provide expert assistance in financing, underwriting, public relations, and so on.

13. *Endorsement of sponsors.* Rely on the reputation of the sponsoring organization by sending out letters of solicitation on its stationery and over the signature of one of its officers; including its name in the HMO's name may help. Use of a statement of "qualification" by the Federal Government may or may not be advisable.

14. *Watch the terminology.* Presentations should not use the word "clinic" or "internist" but should refer to the facility as "medical center" or "health center," and physician specialists should not be confused with students. A "physician specializing in internal medicine" is preferable to "internist."

15. *Flyers, payroll envelope stuffers, posters, and other take-home literature.* All three are useful in group selling, but remember that they may not make it home.

16. *Comparisons.* Comparing the HMO with other plans available is effective in identifying the HMO as a program providing more comprehensive services for a similar premium. If possible, all health care costs for a specific period (total expenditures for health) should be used, including premiums and out-of-pocket expenses.

17. *Word of mouth.* This is the best promotional mechanism over the long run, after the initial enrollment group has been secured, and is the major means of acquiring new enrollment.

Solicitation Strategy—Individuals: The primary emphasis in marketing is on group enrollment; however, plans may find it necessary to market to individuals who are not associated with a large employer, union, or association, among others and, thus, are not offered a choice. For example, an existing group practice may wish to offer a prepaid group practice program to its current patients. In effect, these individuals become another "group" that should be underwritten the same as other groups in the service area. Traditionally, because the "individual" group is normally more heterogeneous, it is a higher risk group than employee or union groups. The pricing of the benefit package may result in somewhat higher premiums using the experience-rating method. Again, the HMO will have established as a marketing objective the size limitation on this group in the underwriting process. Choice of a community-rating approach may help to reduce the cost of the program to the "individual" group by spreading some of their potential expenses to other subscribers. (See Chapter 10 for a discussion of these rating approaches.)

Selling strategies usually are built around a one-to-one selling activity. Physicians themselves, or the group practice staff, may solicit patients by mail, telephone, or in person when the patient visits the HMO center. Letters may be sent to all patients registered with the group practice requesting their enrollment. Enrollment also may be open to individuals who have entered the service area and are "shopping around" for a physician. These unattached subscribers are preferred, because they tend to be young and in relatively good health. The marketing to individuals, however, should be monitored closely because of the generally higher risk.

Enrollment and Closing the Sale: By requiring the potential subscriber under dual choice to make a decision, the act of completing the sale and of actually enrolling the individual is made easy for the HMO representative. For individuals not covered by dual choice, the process requires some effort on the part of the marketing representative. In either case, the subscriber's signature on the enrollment card provides for finalization of the marketing process. Enrollment cards or forms usually state the benefits in general terms and the amount of the premium. It is recommended that the subscriber be given a complete description of the benefit package (policy and certificates), including any copayments of deductibles and any limitations on service. This statement should be in layman's language—easy to read and understand—and the salesman should thoroughly explain the statements. Over the long run, such a practice will substantially reduce misunderstandings on the part of the subscriber and foster better subscriber relations.

Signature cards or enrollment forms provide data concerning the subscriber, including his/her name and the names of his/her spouse and dependents. The cards or forms also may include insurance classification, dates of birth, occupation, sex, annual earnings, and so on, as well as a statement signed by the employee authorizing payroll deductions for any portion of the cost that the employer has specified must be paid by the employee.

The employer or union is the policyholder and receives a master policy form, the legal instrument that describes the complete agreement between the HMO and the employer or union. Employees or union members who are then classified as beneficiaries will receive an insurance certificate. While these certificates do not legally constitute a contract, they are evidence of the benefit package in force and should reflect, as heretofore described, the benefits and other provisions of the master policy—the formal contract. Persons who have "individual" policies with the HMO are both the policyholder and beneficiary and also should receive a comprehensive statement of the benefits and premiums in force. Because these issues may be governed by law, state government representatives should be contacted concerning the specific requirements of the states.

ACCOUNT MAINTENANCE AND GROWTH

The final phase of the marketing activity concerns continuing subscriber relations and identification of new markets. Once the potential subscriber becomes a member of the HMO, part of the marketing effort should be directed toward keeping that member satisfied with the health care program. It has been suggested that, if possible, the marketing agent who sold the plan should be the contact point, if the subscriber has problems. This may not be possible; but there should be a person who acts as the consumer contact point in the HMO, whether it is a receptionist, a physician, or a consumer ombudsman. These issues are addressed in Chapter 6.

Experience has shown that the quality of subscriber relations has a direct bearing on future enrollment. Good relations foster perhaps the best form of marketing—word-of-mouth advertising. As a direct service plan, HMO programs are sold by satisfied people who refer their neighbors and friends. Indeed, significant increases in enrollment can be expected after the first or second year of operation, primarily as a result of satisfied customers. This also suggests that HMOs should develop "growth objectives." Orderly growth requires good management of present and future accounts and subscribers. It also requires the establishment of growth levels for groups of subscribers and control of the marketing activities to ensure that these levels are met, but also that they are not exceeded. The situation of overenrollment is, in many ways, just as bad as not meeting the minimum enrollment level.

Marketing to Low-Income and Underserved Populations

The experiences of HMOs during their initial marketing and enrollment efforts with low-income, medically underserved populations were analyzed in a study completed by Shouldice et al.[24] Ten plans were

[24]Robert G. Shouldice et al. "Marketing to Low Income/Underserved Populations." Washington, D.C., Health Resources Associates, Inc., 1973. Unpublished paper.

selected that had enrolled low-income persons for a period of time sufficient to allow evaluation and that reflected a variety of geographic locations, sponsorships, and organizational models. Most of the low-income, medically underserved persons described in the study were eligible for Medicaid and/or OEO benefits.

The findings suggest that each HMO uses a unique marketing and enrollment strategy for low-income populations. Each plan must confront a different set of circumstances at differing marketing and enrollment stages. There are some commonalities, however, that do exist among like plans (e.g., well-established plans, new plans, or urban plans, rural plans) and also among all plans generally. Of the seven factors common to all marketing and enrollment efforts, five are independent variables that must be carefully examined in the design techniques: contract negotiations, target population, product, price, and place. The last two factors, promotion and enrollment, are dependent variables and must be tailored to maximize the positive aspects of the independent variables. Several solicitation methods and strategies used by four of the plans are identified in Table 26.

Contract negotiations with government administering agencies that finance the medical care of low-income persons are critical in defining target population, product, price, and promotional and enrollment activities. In the 10 plans studied, informal agreements were frequently reached regarding government-agency assistance during marketing and enrollment efforts. This assistance included the provision of a list of Medicaid eligibles, agency mailing of information letters to members of the target population, and, in three instances, agency personnel carrying out the bulk of promotional and enrollment activities.

Evaluation of the impact of the target population on the success or failure of the marketing and enrollment strategy focused on two major factors: the definition of the target population and the assessment of that population. The target population is defined by contract provisions regarding eligibility requirements and service-area boundaries. Eligibility requirements and size of a target population influence the ease with which the population can be further identified and the manner in which it is approached. Assessing the target population will assist the marketing strategist in estimating the time necessary to enroll a certain number of persons as well as in identifying characteristics of the target population that influence the design of the strategy. The target population's familiarity with the plan and/or the concept of prepaid health care and the availability of and its satisfaction with existing medical-care services are primary determinants in the target population's receptivity to joining the plan.

TABLE 26 Summary of Marketing to Four Low-Income Underserved Populations

	Group Health Cooperative of Puget Sound, Seattle, Wash.	Group Health Association, Washington, D.C.	Penobscot Bay Medical Center, Rockport, Me.	Rural Health Association, Farmington, Me.
Government purchaser	Title XIX	Title XIX	OEO	OEO
Area	Urban	Urban	Rural	Rural
Enrollment limited to less than number eligible (first come/first served)	Yes	Yes	Yes	No
HMO benefits equal to or more comprehensive than other available options	Yes	Yes	Yes	Yes
Continued eligibility guaranteed	Unknown	Yes—3 years	Unknown	Yes—1 year
Government workers, etc., available to assist in marketing and enrollment	Yes	Yes	Yes	Yes
Necessary to hire additional HMO marketing staff	No	No	Yes (new plan)	Yes (new plan)
Training programs for all marketing workers provided by HMO	Yes	Yes	Unknown	Yes
Mail campaign	Yes	Yes	Yes	Yes
Foreign translations available	Unknown	Yes	Unknown	No
Mail campaign joint effort of government and HMO	Yes	Yes	Yes	Not applicable
Preaddressed, stamped, reply card	Yes	Yes	Yes	Not applicable
Mail follow-up	No	Unknown	Yes	Not applicable

Telephone follow-up	No	Yes	No	No
Personal home solicitation visits	Yes	No	Yes	Yes
Benefit comparison fact sheet	Yes	Yes	Yes	Yes
Other brochures, pamphlets, etc.	Yes	Yes	Yes	No
Attempt to reach other than "eligible" population	No	No	Yes	Yes
Television and radio public-service advertising	Yes	No	Yes	Yes
Press conferences and releases	Yes	No	Yes	Yes
Presentation to external groups (clubs, churches)	No	No	Yes	No
Health facility tours	No	Yes	Yes	No
Small-group meetings in health center	No	Yes	No	No
Formal and informal "poor-community" leaders and organizations asked to help	No	Yes	Unknown	No
Personal home follow-up visit	No	No	No	No
History and physical examination part of enrollment process	Yes	Yes	Yes	Yes
Government-funded research study included in contract	No	Yes	No	No
General marketing style	Low-key	Low-key	Low-key	Low-key

Source: Robert G. Shouldice et al. "Marketing to Low Income/Underserved Populations." Washington, D.C., Health Resources Associates, Inc., 1973. Unpublished paper.

Characteristics of the low-income population vary with each plan. Several general characteristics were identified. For all plans studied, recipients of Aid to Families with Dependent Children comprised the majority of the target population, and the heads of households were women. Accordingly, women were used almost exclusively to handle promotional and enrollment activities. Among the specific characteristics, it was important to several plans that their low-income target population was by and large homogeneous with the service-area community. As a consequence, promotional activities often were directed toward the population at large.

The plans studied can be categorized into two major groups with respect to the scope of benefits offered. The first group (four plans) offered a benefit package that included fewer services than were available to the target population under Medicaid regulations. The second group (six plans) offered more services than the Medicaid schedule. Enrollees in the first group were required, in effect, to participate in two health care systems to obtain all services provided under the Medicaid program. The results of such a dual system discouraged enrollment, created confusion on the part of the enrollee, and, in some cases, resulted in out-of-plan use. In the second group, the availability of all Medicaid services, plus additional services, had a positive effect on the decision of potential enrollees to join the HMO plans.

The location of the plan's facilities is a determinant in the plan's successful realization of its marketing goal. Accessibility, however, is a relative state, reflected in the fact that the study did not find any common definition or guidelines that, from an accessibility point of view, provide a basis for the distribution of facilities. Each plan did stress the accessibility of services in its promotional efforts.

Premium rates did not significantly affect the decision of potential enrollees to join the plan, except in the case of persons who were eligible for OEO benefits but not the Medicaid program. A competitive premium rate was of extreme importance, however, in negotiating a prepaid contract to serve the low-income population. Of greater importance to the Medicaid recipient was the lack of utilization control and restrictions that are applicable to regular Medicaid programs in many states. For all but one of the plans studied, these utilization controls were dropped.

The overall promotional effort had a primary goal of informing the target population of the availability of the plan as an option for Medicaid services and of providing information about the plan. Five general promotional techniques were identified in the plans studied, namely, general literature distribution, use of mass media, use of group

contacts, mass mailings, and one-to-one contact with potential enrollees.

The promotional technique used with the greatest frequency and
success by the plans studied was a mass mailing to members of the
target population. In general, the more established plans were able to
rely on this technique to generate a sufficient number of responses
from members of the target populations to reach their marketing goals.
Newer plans, however, had to use additional types of promotional
techniques to reach their goals. Mailings by all plans except one were
sent by the state or local agency administering the Medicaid program.

All new plans studied used one-to-one contact with potential en-
rolleeŝ—a very effective promotional technique. This is expensive
and, therefore, may not be appropriate to every plan's strategy. The
following factors should be considered in any decision to use this technique: The degree of familiarity of the target population with the plan
and the concept of prepaid health care; the necessity for the plan to
handle the actual enrollment; and the inability of the plan to specifically
identify the target population.

The enrollment activities of plans studied reveal several characteristics affecting both enrollment and the likelihood that new enrollees will
remain with the plan. The most convenient location for enrollment is
the potential enrollee's home. Those persons who do make a trip to the
plan facility are generally more committed to enroll, although there
may be some loss of potential enrollees who cannot come to the facility. Enrollment in the office of a caseworker is not as convenient as in
the home but perhaps more familiar to the enrollee than the plan facility. If outreach or similar activities are planned, implementation requires a more concerted effort when enrollment occurs in the caseworker's office or in the enrollee's home.

In all cases, enrollment involves one-to-one contact between an enrollment agent of the plan and the potential enrollee. The characteristics of the personnel are more critical when promotion is also a major
objective of the encounter. In these instances, personnel were predominantly women and either indigenous to the low-income community or
officials of an agency that worked with members of the target population.

The likelihood that Medicaid recipients would remain with the plan
after enrollment was influenced by their introduction to the plan.
Fewer problems resulted when Medicaid identification cards were re-
placed by plan membership cards. Moreover, outreach and similar
activities were most successful when new enrollees established themselves with the plan by selecting a physician and going to the plan

facility for an initial examination. For several plans, the opportunity to receive quality medical care without discrimination (i.e., identification as a Medicaid recipient) was, for many low-income persons, a major reason for joining and remaining with these plans.

Summary

Administrators of health care delivery programs, including HMO managers, have realized that marketing of their programs is a legitimate task of management. Forced by a free-market system where consumer attitudes and beliefs are important to program success, HMOs have developed their programs and marketed them to meet the needs of their subscribers. In HMOs, marketing is defined as the performance of a wide range of activities, including market surveys, benefit design, pricing, promotion, selling, and enrollment. The first task of marketing is the development of a marketing strategy—the selection of a target population and the development of a market mix, which is the choice of elements that the HMO intends to bring together in order to meet the needs of the target population. Four basic variables are identified in the market mix—product, place, promotion, and price.

Viewed as an HMO-wide set of activities, marketing is a four-step process: market analysis, making choice available, active marketing, and account maintenance. Market analysis is undertaken to determine what the consumer demand will be so that services can be adjusted to successfully serve the market and to determine whether a sufficient market exists to support the HMO. Data on the demographic, socioeconomic, epidemiological, and competitive situation are collected and analyzed to determine if the HMO is feasible. Analysis includes the tasks of population segmentation and estimates of penetration of each segment—tasks that allow the HMO manager to decide on target populations. The process then continues with estimates of demand of each population selected and a financial analysis or underwriting that allows the HMO to forecast the necessary capacity to provide services to meet the demand. The intermediate product of market analysis and underwriting is the development of the market mix.

The final products of the segmentation and penetration studies are a list of sources of membership and a projection of the level of subscribers from each source. In addition, each source is completely described, which information is essential to making the market feasibility decision and, later, in developing benefit packages and performing other underwriting and actuarial analyses.

One of the elements of the marketing mix—promotion—is a highly sensitive issue within the health-services industry. The HMO realizes that its activities are insignificant unless the availability of its services is communicated; hence, it chooses its promotional activities carefully, to stay within the guidelines of the American Medical Association. Although the AMA is reevaluating the issue of advertisement of medical services, the HMO manager should clear promotion activities with the local medical society prior to initiation of such activities.

The second phase of the marketing activity is the development of dual-choice arrangements in firms, unions, associations, and government agencies that have been chosen as target population segments. This is a traditional strategy of HMOs for breaking into other insurer's markets and for developing true consumer choice. Advantages to the employer offering dual choice include greater employee satisfaction, potentially higher productivity because of less sick time, cost containment, and becoming more competitive for desirable, potential employees. Disadvantages include the slightly higher costs of the HMO package, increased costs of offering two programs rather than one, and possible employee backlash because of increased salary deductions or loss of established physician relationships.

The third phase is the actual selling to groups and individuals identified as the target population. Selling to groups is the primary objective, with the largest groups first, smaller groups second, welfare programs next, and individual contracts last. This order, however, depends on the local situation and must be tailored to the characteristics of the target population; for instance, the patients of established doctors may be considered a "group" of individual contracts that may make up the target population. Solicitation strategies are as varied as the groups to be approached. Some of the methods used include dual-choice arrangements, enrollment of key group leaders, cooperation with existing insurance companies, community education, marketing to wives, open house of facility, door-to-door selling, comparison of plans, and word-of-mouth promotion.

The final phase concerns continuing subscriber relations and the identification of new markets. It is vital that an employee of the HMO act as the consumer contact point and that he be directed to keep the consumer satisfied with the health care program. Experience has shown that the quality of account maintenance has a direct relationship to future enrollment. HMO programs are sold by satisfied people who refer their neighbors and friends.

Marketing to special groups such as low-income and medically underserved populations requires special marketing strategies. Seven factors that are important to enrollment strategies for low-income populations include contract negotiations, target population definition, and the market-mix variables of product, price, place, promotion, and enrollment. Both promotion and enrollment, the last two factors, are dependent variables that must be closely tailored to each group to maximize success. In most instances, marketing to low-income populations includes one-to-one contact between an enrollment agent of the plan and the potential enrollee.

References

Bergwall, David F.; Reeves, Philip N.; and Woodside, Nina B. *Introduction to Health Planning*. Washington, D.C., Information Resources Press, 1974.

Burke, Richard T. *Guidelines for HMO Marketing*. Minneapolis, Minn., InterStudy, 1973.

Gumbiner, Robert. *HMO: Putting It All Together*. St. Louis, Mo., C. V. Mosby Co., 1975, pp. 68–90.

Kress, John R., and Singer, James. *HMO Handbook*. Rockville, Md., Aspen Systems Corporation, 1975, pp. 135–155.

LeCompte, Roger B. *Prepaid Group Practice: A Manual*. Chicago, Blue Cross Association, 1972, Chapter 4.

McCarthy, E. Jerome. *Basic Marketing*. 4th Edition. Homewood, Ill., Richard D. Irwin, Inc., 1971.

Schumer, Jeff M. "HMO Feasibility: The Marketing Decision." *Medical Group Management*, 24(2):37–40, March/April 1977.

U.S. Department of Health, Education, and Welfare, Health Maintenance Organization Service. *Marketing of Health Maintenance Organizations*. Volumes I–VI. Rockville, Md., 1972. DHEW Publ. Nos. (HSM) 72-100 and (HSM) 73-13006.

—————. *Marketing Pre-Paid Health Care Plans*. Rockville, Md., 1972. DHEW Publ. No. (HSM) 73-6207.

Arthur Young and Company. *HMO Feasibility Study Guide*. Rockville, Md., Bureau of Community Health Services, Health Services Administration, U.S. Department of Health, Education, and Welfare, 1974, pp. 32–58. DHEW Publ. No. (HSM) 74-13020.

9

Efficiency, Productivity, Utilization, and Economies of Scale

Many of the productivity elements in group practice health care services can and frequently do differ significantly from those in solo practice, fee-for-service delivery systems. In this chapter, an attempt will be made to isolate each of these elements and to describe their causes and effects from the viewpoint of economic theory.

Certain significant problems are inescapable in any attempt to make the productivity fit the traditional model of the practice. Defining a unit of output is the primary difficulty. In most studies on the subject (and throughout this chapter), the unit of output is defined as a physician visit. Many health professionals, however, argue that the physician visit is not an output, but only one input in the creation of the final product, which is good health or the cure of a specific illness. A more serious problem concerns the assumption that all physician visits are identical and therefore comparable between delivery systems; quality differences surely exist among physicians. There are the components of the visit itself: for example, history taking; measurement of pulse, blood pressure, and weight; general physical examination; diagnosis; and perhaps conversing with the patient to alleviate fears, nervousness, and so on. Not all visits contain every element or absorb the same amount of time.[1] Nevertheless, for purposes of economic analysis, it is necessary to assume that the visits are indeed identical with respect to

---

[1]The use of "encounters" rather than visits or services may help to reduce differences in data. Encounters are defined as any face-to-face contact with a provider of health care.

quality and mix of services. In a large-scale study on a nationwide level, the law of large numbers may cause this assumption to appear less than heroic.

A second problem concerns the patients or consumers: It must be assumed that the populations served are identical among delivery systems with respect to age, sex, race, income, education, habitat, and any other variables that may affect their demand (desire) for medical care and/or incidence of illness. Because many prepaid group practice plans serve only consumer groups whose actuarial predictions are within defined limits, they are not always comparable to randomly selected patients in the fee-for-service systems.

One of the major cost savings that has been consistently demonstrated by prepaid group practice plans is markedly lower hospital utilization rates for their subscribers, as compared with commercial carrier and Blue Cross/Blue Shield subscribers. A close look at Figure 33 will confirm this fact. There are two reasons why this occurs: the effect of insurance benefits on the patient's ability to pay for medical services, and the effect of the incentives (which do not exist in most prepaid group practice plans) generated by the fee-for-service financing mechanism. When it is recognized that hospital care is by far the largest and most expensive component of total national health expenditures (39.2 percent in 1974, as compared to 18.2 percent for physicians' services and 9.3 percent for drugs), and the one that is escalating most rapidly, the significance of any savings in this critical area will be obvious.

The Theory

All forms of insurance inevitably raise the demand for health services, which can be explained in an economic context by utility theory: Consumers will continue to purchase additional units of a commodity until the marginal utility of the last unit purchased is equal to its price. For services covered by insurance, the price is zero to consumers; therefore, they greatly increase their consumption of such services relative to the true social cost of the resources thus used, in comparison with the benefits derived. With the exception of direct-service plans, most health insurance contracts cover inpatient hospital care but do not cover outpatient care. Consequently, it is to the patient's financial advantage to be hospitalized for many tests, routine procedures, and minor surgery that could be performed on an outpatient basis at greatly reduced costs. This results in a misallocation of resources, in that services are shifted from outpatient to inpatient care so the burden of payment can be placed on the insurance company. In addition, physicians may tend to prescribe more services for patients who are covered by insurance than for those who are not, as a means of increasing their own income at no cost to the insured patient (who will therefore not be tempted to change doctors to avoid large bills).

In a prepaid group practice plan, the subscriber pays a fixed monthly premium that guarantees the provision of all covered medical services at no additional charge or at nominal charge; coverage is usually quite comprehensive. These premiums are the primary income of the health

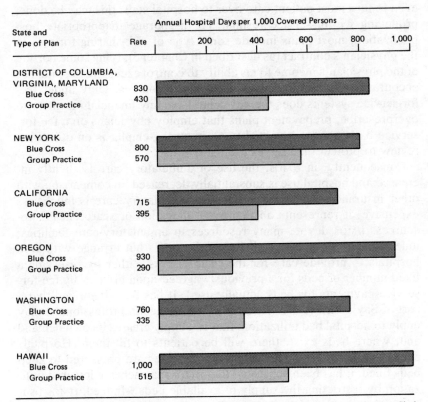

Source: Adapted from George S. Perrott and Jean C. Chase. "The Federal Employee Program. Sixth Term Coverage and Utilization." *Group Health and Welfare News, Special Supplement, October 1968.* Washington, D.C., Group Health Association of America, 1968, p. vii. The article does not specify the names of the group practice plans it reports on.

Figure 33   Federal Employees Health Benefits Program (January–December 1966)—comparing hospital utilization among several states for Blue Cross and Group Practice Plans (nonmaternity, in-hospital services, high-option plan).

plan; the more services it provides and the more costly these services are, the less its income will be. When the physicians constitute the health plan, as in a physician-provider model, the cost of care provided directly affects each doctor's personal income. The less costly the care provided, the greater the profits—in which each has a share—will be. If the physicians are compensated on a capitation or salary basis, again there will be no financial incentive to make unnecessary use of hospitalization or to overprescribe; no disincentive exists either, and, if it is indeed time-saving for physicians to visit hospitalized patients or even to turn most patient care over to hospital staff, this may be done, producing fee-for-service results. To discourage inappropriate hospitalization, most plans include some type of risk-sharing formula in the physician's contract (as described in Chapter 5); tying some portion of the physician's income to his ability to control excessive hospital use encourages efficient use of facilities and resources. Only under fee-for-service systems does the physician have any financial incentive to overprescribe; prepayment plans that employ physicians on a fee-for-service basis can be expected to place strong emphasis on utilization review to protect themselves against overuse.

Consequently, in HMOs, the use of ambulatory care is slightly increased and hospital use is substantially decreased, in comparison with other insurance mechanisms. Because ambulatory care is much less expensive, it represents an improved allocation of scarce health resources. HMOs devote many resources to ambulatory-care facilities; indeed, many do not own their own hospitals but arrange with area hospitals to provide care for their subscribers, either by reserving a fixed number of beds for a previously agreed-upon price or by fee-for-service payments for beds actually used. It has been theorized that a sort of Say's Law (called Roemer's Law by health professionals) may apply to hospital bed utilization; that is, supply creates its own demand and, where beds exist, there will be patients to fill them. Hospitals admit that physicians with admitting privileges are pressured to keep beds filled; it has been suggested that HMOs may achieve lowered utilization by restricting the supply of available beds.[2] Indeed, HMOs usually maintain a lower bed-to-population ratio than otherwise exists in the local community. Since most surveys indicate that HMO subscribers are at least as well cared for as members of other groups, it would appear that restricting bed supply would be advisable under other systems as well.

[2]Herbert E. Klarman. "Approaches to Moderating the Increases in Medical Care Costs." *Medical Care, VII*(3):177–179, May–June 1969.

There are two other reasons why hospital use rates are lower under prepayment plans. First, there is a much lower rate of elective surgery (e.g., tonsillectomies, hemorrhoidectomies, and sometimes hysterectomies); the difference in admission rates for elective surgery between prepaid subscribers and Blue Cross or commercial-carrier subscribers suggests that many surgeons may perform operations mainly for income, rather than because of medical necessity, since the prepaid plan population appears to suffer no ill effects from reduced surgical admissions.[3] Second, the prepayment philosophy places emphasis on preventive medicine, and patients are more likely to seek care at the onset of symptoms if no charge is incurred. Both factors result in early diagnosis; hence, many conditions can be treated successfully before they progress to the point where costly hospitalization becomes necessary.

In addition to lowered hospital use, two other strong economic advantages are frequently attributed to group practice of medicine: economies of scale and increased physician productivity. General discussions of the subject refer to the expected gains from both sources as increased productivity or efficiency, although economically they are separate effects and will be so treated here.

PRODUCTIVITY

Productivity is the output generated by only one input: for example, physician productivity, nurse productivity, capital equipment productivity. Specifically, the marginal physical product (MPP) of a factor of production is the increase in output that results from the addition of one unit of that factor of input, all other inputs being held constant. Under most circumstances, the greater the number of other inputs the factor in question is working with, the greater will be its MPP. The optimum condition for hiring inputs is to continue to employ additional units until the value of the marginal product (the price of the output times the number of units produced) is equal to its price, $MPP_1 = P_1$.

EFFICIENCY

Efficiency refers to the manner in which all inputs are combined to produce the final output, that is, the production function itself. The optimum or cost-minimizing condition for the employment of all fac-

[3] Avedis Donabedian. "An Evaluation of Prepaid Group Practice." *Inquiry*, VI(3):13–16, September 1969.

tors taken together is to continue to hire inputs until the ratio of the MPPs to their prices is equal for all inputs employed:

$$\frac{MPP_1}{P_1} = \frac{MPP_2}{P_2} = \frac{MPP_i}{P_i}$$

ECONOMIES OF SCALE

Economies of scale refer to the size of the final output. It is generally true that, as the amount of output increases, the per-unit cost of producing that output decreases. This is true because the production function may change as the size of the practice increases; factors may be used in different proportions—the purchase of new and better equipment that was too costly when spread over a small output may become feasible. This is illustrated in Figure 34, where AC is the long-run average cost curve for the production of good x. Firm A is able to produce 10 units of x when operating at its minimum cost level of output. From the graph, it is obvious that a firm between the sizes of A and B could produce those 10 units at a lower cost, as shown by the long-run AC curve (which assumes that all possible methods of production are available). The optimum size is C, producing 20 units at the least possible cost per unit, P_1. Firm C is more efficient than A (P_1 is less than P_2); therefore, if 20 units of x are desired, it would be better to have them produced by one firm of size C than by two firms of size A. Firms D and E are "too large" to be efficient; x is best produced by firms of size C.

Paul Feldstein states that economies of scale must be the result of either division of labor or the use of specialized machines:

Consequently, with an increase in volume, hence, greater specialization of labor and machines, there will be an increase in productivity and the per-unit cost of producing physician care will decrease; hence there may be said to be economies of scale.[4]

He outlines three ways to measure the extent of economies of scale:

1. To determine whether there is specialization, ratios of personnel may be compared between groups of varying sizes and also to solo practice ratios.
2. Cost per unit of output can be related to group size (one would expect to find an inverse relationship over some size range).

[4]Paul J. Feldstein. *Prepaid Group Practice: An Analysis and Review.* Ann Arbor, Mich., University Microfilms International, 1971, p. 26.

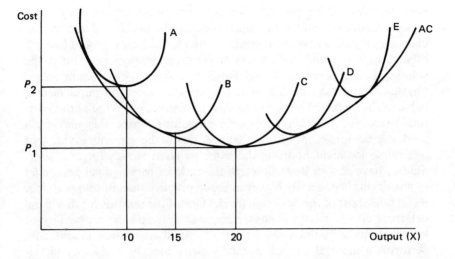

Figure 34   Long-run average cost curve.

3. Physician income may be compared by group size (those with the highest income should be the most productive).[5]

The last method is the least reliable, because it assumes no fee differentials among physicians and areas of the country and no quality differences in output.

There is no reason why scalar economies should not be operative in the delivery of medical care. Proceeding along the lines of the previous analysis, the average cost of a medical firm will decrease as the number of physicians, size of facility, value of equipment, and so on, increases. The administrative costs of coordination of activities should eventually place an upper limit on the optimum "plant" size. Unfortunately, there are as yet no definitive studies on the optimum size of a group practice; indeed, the optimum size will, in all likelihood, vary, depending on the composition of the group (e.g., single specialty or multispecialty) and, perhaps, on the characteristics of the subscriber/patient population.

The falling cost curve can be explained by changes in production made feasible by expansion, causing a shift in the least-cost expansion path and a downward shift in the corresponding total-cost curve. The increase in the overall number of patients seen by the group as a whole facilitates the employment of nurses, clerical staff, and paramedical personnel, because their salaries can be spread over a broader patient

[5]*Ibid.*

base than would be possible for solo practitioners and very small groups; laboratory and X-ray equipment can be purchased and technicians employed, whereas, in small practices, the high cost and low use of such inputs would make them prohibitively expensive. This is the solution to the problem of indivisibility; that is, the optimum nurse/physician ratio may be 2.5 to 1, but nurses cannot be purchased in halves. The standard response to this, of course, is "What about part-time employees?" There are some situations where this may be a workable compromise, but, in essence, this is the same as saying that one nurse for eight hours is the same as eight nurses for one hour. Studies have shown that, although the ratio of paramedical personnel to physicians is generally higher in group practice than in solo practice, it still falls short of the optimum level.[6] One of the reasons for this is the deterrent effect of both licensure requirements and the probability of legal responsibility if a malpractice suit should arise when a paramedic performs a medical service normally performed by a doctor. Physicians' attitudes toward the use of paramedics also may have a negative effect on their employment, although group practice physicians appear to be less resistant in this area than solo practitioners.

A similar argument concerns the advantage of maintaining specialized laboratory and X-ray facilities, that is, that solo physicians already have access to the most efficient laboratory and X-ray facilities. Why should they have to be under the same roof to be equally efficient? This view overlooks the time saved by obtaining immediate results and ignores the value of the patient's time and travel expenses when he has to be referred elsewhere for X-rays and tests.

Economies of space also are available to group practice plans. If one receptionist can serve several physicians, so can one waiting room, clerical office, and so on. Hence, the amount of floor space required per physician should decrease in group practice.

SUBSTITUTION OF INPUTS

In an HMO system, one would expect much greater reliance on paramedical personnel to perform those functions for which an M.D. degree is not necessary. The increased productivity of such paramedical personnel, when spread over a large number of patients, makes their employment relatively cheaper when compared to the use of

[6]See Uwe E. Reinhardt and Donald E. Yett. "Physician Production Functions Under Varying Practice Arrangements." Technical Paper No. 11. Los Angeles, Calif., Community Profile Data Center, Human Resources Research Center of the University of Southern California Research Institute for Business and Economics, 1971.

physicians to perform the same services. In Figure 35(a), the number of physicians needed to produce the output of isoquant 1 is reduced from X_0 to X_1, and the substitution of paramedical personnel is increased from Y_0 to Y_1, the least-cost expansion path shifts accordingly from $LCEP_0$ to $LCEP_1$; in Figure 35(b), total cost falls from TC_0 to TC_1.

Isoquants, or isoproduct curves, relate all of the possible combinations of two inputs that can produce the same quantity of output. For example, assume that the output of isoquant 1 in Figure 35(a) is 50 units; these may be produced by using X_0 of physicians and Y_0 of paramedics, or by using X_1 of physicians and Y_1 of paramedics, or by the X and Y values corresponding to any point along the curve. The optimal combination of the two factors is determined by their relative prices, depicted graphically by the straight-line tangents and the isoquants. These relative price lines represent the cost of production; as they move farther away from the origin, the total cost increases in the same way that successive isoquants represent higher levels of output. Consequently, the least-cost factor combination for a given level of output is at the point of tangency between an isoquant and the relative price line. Any other point on the relative price line (budget constraint) would intersect a smaller isoquant, that is, less output for the same cost.

The least-cost expansion path (LCEP) is the straight line from the origin that connects the tangency points for successive isoquants, given the relative prices of the two inputs. It reveals the optimal amounts of each factor that should be used as output increases. A change in the relative prices of the inputs will change the slope of the

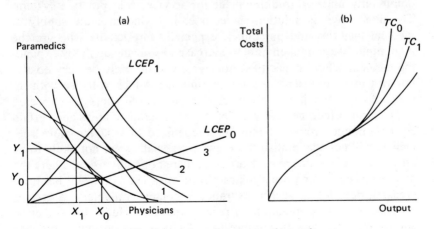

Figure 35 (a) Paramedics/physicians isoquants; (b) total cost curves.

budget constraint and thus change the optimal factor combination (by changing the point of tangency to each isoquant). This is represented as a shift in the least-cost expansion path.

The decreasing relative price of the paramedical input can be explained in terms of marginal productivity if the patient also is considered as an input. This again is the problem of indivisibility; that is, to employ an additional technician for a small number of patients would result in a very low marginal product for the last (which may be the first) input hired. Increasing the other input—patients—would raise the MPP of the paramedical input and make its employment financially feasible.

The increased use of paramedical personnel will, in turn, increase the productivity of the physician (usually defined as the number of patients seen in a given time period) by enabling him to devote his more valuable time to procedures that only he can perform. In effect, the supply curve for physician services shifts to the right, which means an effective increase in the supply of physicians. The analysis is symmetrical for the substitution of nurses for physicians to take histories, give injections, and so on, and for a clerical staff to handle billings, insurance forms, and other clerical tasks.

METHODS TO INCREASE PHYSICIAN OUTPUT

The possibility for increasing physician output may be one of the most significant advantages of group practice over solo practice. The United States has decided that it "needs" more medical services than can be produced with the existing supply of medical personnel, organized predominantly under a traditional fee-for-service, solo practice system. The most obvious solution, of course, is to increase the supply of medical facilities and personnel, especially physicians, who are the main input. Action taken now to increase physician supply by expanding medical school capacities, however, will not only be very costly, but will involve at least a six-year time lag, which will rise with increased specialization. Moreover, if the increased supply is expected to primarily affect medically underserved geographic areas and certain socioeconomic groups, it must be recognized that having more specialists will not accomplish these goals. Specialists are not likely to be attracted to a practice in such areas, and are not really useful where the greatest need is for primary-care physicians. The latter will be in increasing demand as health insurance becomes available to a greater proportion of the population. A recent American Medical Association survey reported that the proportion of physicians providing primary care (defined as general and family practice, internal medicine, pediatrics, and obstetrics/gynecology) has decreased from 49.4 percent in 1964 to 38.3 percent in 1974. Also, new additions to the physician supply would have to be incredibly large to add appreciably to the total supply; in 1967, Rashi Fein calculated that the number of medical school graduates would have to increase by 100 percent to raise the total supply by 5 percent.[7] Finally, there is no assurance that an increased supply of physicians will prevent further escalation in costs, let alone reduce them. The market for physician services is far from competitive, and, insofar as physicians are able to practice price discrimination and to create a demand for their services, it is extremely unlikely that their wages will ever be flexible in a downward direction.

With the aforementioned problems in mind, it would be wise to look for ways to increase the productivity (output) of the current supply of physicians, rather than to devote more resources to increasing the supply. Rashi Fein has estimated that even so modest an increase as 4 percent in physician productivity (and this is by far the lowest estimate of the HMO's gain) would add more physicians than the current graduating class to the effective supply.[8]

Physician productivity may be loosely defined as the output of medical services per a specific time period. The simplest methods used to measure physician productivity are number of patient visits per physician and annual gross billings per physician. The first has the drawback of assuming that all visits are standard. The second assumes that fee structures are identical among physicians and that there are no quality differentials (which may cause fee differentials). Other measures are being developed, including one by Joel Kovner of the University of California at Los Angeles, which breaks down visits into "identifiable medical procedures";[9] thus, the measure of output is weighted, which, while more definitive than simply counting number of visits, requires a greater complexity of data that may make its use less feasible in many instances.

Of course, the primary objective is to obtain increased medical services from each physician; one way to achieve such an increase would

[7]Rashi Fein. *The Doctor Shortage*. Washington, D.C., The Brookings Institution, 1967, p. 60.

[8]*Ibid.*, p. 138.

[9]Please see the studies completed by Joel W. Kovner, reviewed by Don Strope, Bonnie Cohen, and Ann Yonkers in *Increasing Productivity in the Delivery of Ambulatory Health Services: A Review of Literature and On-going Projects*. Rockville, Md., Office of the Secretary, U.S. Department of Health, Education, and Welfare, 1968.

be an incentive to work longer hours, the most probable inducement being greater financial compensation. This, however, is not a viable solution to cost containment. It would be preferable to increase the time available for purely medical tasks during normal working hours, thereby increasing productivity. Because group practice provides administrative and clerical services, the physician is free of practice management duties, problems related to billing and collections, physical plant responsibilities, and other duties that in no way require medical expertise but that do absorb a significant amount of the physician's working hours. This aspect of increasing physician output is attributable to the existence of scalar economies.

Other benefits derived from the economies inherent in group practice may more directly affect physician productivity per se. An increase in amounts and types of other inputs will inevitably raise the output of the first input, namely, physician labor. As the possibility for input substitution increases with group size (e.g., using paramedics to perform routine medical procedures), so does the possibility of introducing complementary inputs, that is, nurses, paramedics, and equipment. Perhaps there is equipment that can greatly enhance the speed with which a physician can perform certain tasks (e.g., autoanalyzers, multiphasic screening systems); in many instances, a solo practitioner either will be unable to afford such equipment and thus be forced to work less efficiently without it, or he will purchase it and allow it to stand idle much of the time, passing on the cost of under use to his patients via higher than necessary fees. Would it not be a better use of scarce resources to have one X-ray machine used full-time than two used only half-time? The purchase of many useful pieces of equipment is an all-or-nothing proposition to solo practitioners.

Technological improvement may be one of the most important methods of increasing physician productivity. But it will have no effect if its benefits are unaffordable to most doctors. A criticism of this argument for group practice (i.e., that group practice makes feasible the purchase of the "best" available machines) is that this equipment is available to solo practitioners through the use of such equipment in nearby hospitals. One rebuttal should be that this does not take into account the physician's travel time to the hospital. Second, he will charge his patients higher fees to cover his costs for using the hospital's facilities. Third, and most important, many tests and procedures will have to be performed in the hospital rather than in an ambulatory-care setting, thus increasing hospital utilization, the most costly form of delivery. Furthermore, in the long run, it will foster the expansion of hospital construction and divert scarce resources away from the construction of more efficient ambulatory-care facilities.

QUALITY

An argument frequently proffered against group practice is that, by substituting nurse and paramedic services for doctors' services, the quality of care will diminish. First, no data exist that support this reasoning. The physician is ultimately responsible for the total care of his patients in group practice and thus oversees the activities of the paramedics. A more important aspect of the quality problem has been pointed out by Rashi Fein; the question of whether other types of medical personnel perform less well than doctors should not be asked, for often the choice is not between best available care and poorer quality care, but between the latter and no care at all. "The comparison of 'some' care with much better, but unavailable, or insufficient, 'maximum quality' medical care is irrelevant."[10]

While on the subject of quality, that elusive and unmeasurable entity, it should be noted that there are reasons to expect that the quality of care may even be enhanced in multispecialty medical group practice and prepaid group practice plans. The following are some of the more important quality upgrading factors:

1. Because of the regular hours, financial advantages, and periodic sabbaticals available to many group physicians, there is both time for and encouragement of continuing education. The doctors in group practices may be expected to be "better" because they will be more aware of new discoveries.

2. Strict quality control is ensured through constant peer review and free exchange of patients among physicians within the group.

3. Patients with complications will be referred to a specialist immediately, as there is no threat to the primary-care physician of losing his fee or his patient.

4. Consultation with specialists in one's own group will be easier and faster than referral to an outside specialist.

5. The unit medical record facilitates good continuity of care; every test, X-ray, and diagnosis is recorded and available to each doctor the patient sees within the group. This also prevents costly duplication of tests, and ensures that treatments (especially prescriptions) for two different conditions by two different doctors will not conflict.

[10]Fein. *The Doctor Shortage,* p. 117.

6. Preventive medicine is an element of high-quality care, and this is emphasized by prepaid group practice.

This section of the chapter has covered the potential economic advantages of group practice over solo practice as an organizational form for the delivery of medical-care services and of prepayment over fee-for-service as a financing mechanism. In the next section, the extent of these potential gains will be demonstrated from existing studies. It must be recognized, however, that, if such gains are small or nonexistent, the fault may be outside the realm of economic relationships—for example, poor management in some plans, legal barriers that limit the use of ancillary personnel, behavioral motivations on the part of physicians and managers, that is, something that runs counter to purely economic logic. It may be that, in order to exploit the full economic advantages, some type of active promotion and encouragement of group practice will have to take place—perhaps something as simple as educating consumers and physicians about the nature of group practice.

Empirical Evidence: A Review of Selected Studies

A close look at the literature on the advantages of group practice reveals an unusual phenomenon—there are almost as many reviews of other researchers' studies as there are original studies. Relatively little usable data have been compiled to date, except in the area of hospital-use rates; therefore, it is difficult to get information on truly comparable user groups. Paul Feldstein's data (see pages 278–281) are as comprehensive as any.

Unfortunately, the information needed most for economic analyses—productivity and cost figures—is also the most difficult to obtain. Productivity is derived indirectly through gross income figures and, a little more directly, by physician-visit statistics. The income data have the overwhelming drawback of requiring an assumption of standardized fees among physicians, geographic areas, and practice modes (as well as assuming no quality differences in output), but such data are fairly easy to obtain. The productivity data are more rewarding, requiring the serious but less stringent assumption of comparable outputs vis-à-vis quality and components of physician visits, but such data are more difficult to obtain and have the added deficiency that all of the responding physicians may not follow the same guidelines on what to include. Cost data seem to be almost impossible to obtain.

Another major stumbling block to exacting research efforts is that almost no information is available on many topics from the solo practice, fee-for-service sector. In general, medical group practices generate much more data, which are compiled in formats comparable between groups, probably because such data are needed for internal controls. In fact, Paul Ellwood noted that HMOs have produced studies on quality of care far out of proportion to their share of services; he points out that the ease with which a research project can be performed is directly related to the ease of setting up an ongoing quality control system, and quality control is an area with which the Federal Government is becoming increasingly concerned.[11] The little information that is available on the solo practice system is usually highly aggregated and generally not comparable to that generated from group practices.

The studies reviewed in this section are included more as examples of the kinds of analyses being performed than for the actual content of the data. Most of the studies reached very similar conclusions; therefore, no attempt is made to demonstrate proof of these conclusions by the weight of the data presented here. The reader who is seriously interested in pursuing the available evidence should read the Roemer and Shonick article listed in the references to this chapter, as it is a comprehensive review of the literature on all aspects of HMOs.

REINHARDT AND YETT

Uwe Reinhardt and Donald Yett have produced the most rigorous and comprehensive study on physician productivity to date. Interested in methods of increasing physician productivity, they structured their study to provide answers to the following questions:

1. To what extent is it technically feasible to substitute paramedical effort for a physician's own time?

2. Given technical feasibility, to what extent is it profitable for a physician to substitute paramedical effort for his own?

[11]Paul M. Ellwood, Jr. "Restructuring the Health Delivery System—Will the Health Maintenance Strategy Work?" *In: Health Maintenance Organizations: A Reconfiguration of the Health Services System. Proceedings of the Thirteenth Annual Symposium on Hospital Affairs.* Graduate School of Business, Center for Health Administration Studies, Graduate Program in Hospital Administration, University of Chicago. Chicago, 1971, p. 7.

3. Does a physician function more efficiently in multiphysician practices (partnerships and/or medical groups) or in the traditional solo practice?[12]

Reinhardt and Yett obtained their data from 1965 and 1967 nationwide surveys of private medical practices by Medical Economics, Inc. of Oradell, New Jersey. Within certain limitations, which will be cited, these data appear to be the most comprehensive used in any studies on physician productivity, especially in terms of sample size.

Initially, Reinhardt and Yett specified a production function that would enable them to obtain values for differing input combinations in order to answer the three research questions and that would be compatible with statistical estimation. The equation used was

$$Q \text{ or } Y = A \cdot H^a \cdot K^b \cdot \left\{ e[cH + \sum_{i=1}^{i=3} (d_i L_i) + g \cdot (\sum_{i=1}^{i=1} L_i)]^2 \right\} \cdot \left\{ e \sum_{i=1}^{i=n} (h_i D_i) \cdot U \right\}$$

where

A = constant

Q = the physician's weekly rate of patient visits

Y = the physician's annual gross patient billings, in thousands of dollars (defined as annual gross income divided by the collection ratio)

H = the number of strictly practice-related hours worked by the physician per week

U = error term

L_1 = the number of R.N.s per physician

L_2 = the number of technicians per physician

L_3 = the number of office aides per physician

L_i = the number of paramedical aides per physician

K_t = an index of capital usage in hundreds of dollars

D_i = a set of variables further characterizing the physician vis-à-vis age, location, and so on

The constants a, b, e, d_i, g, and h_i are the parameters whose numerical values are to be estimated. Specific versions of the equation were determined for each medical specialty study, making comparisons more valid. Output was measured by patient visits and by annual gross billings, enabling them to verify the consistency of their findings.

When using patient visits as the measure of output, Reinhardt and

---

[12]Reinhardt and Yett. "Physician Production Functions," pp. iii–iv.

Yett assumed that there were no essential differences in the quality of services provided by the various physicians sampled (specifically, that an increase in a physician's hourly load of patients, if achieved through the employment of additional paramedical aides, will not cause a deterioration in the quality of his services) and that the mix of services provided does not vary subsequently over the physician population (i.e., that each visit for each physician consists of the same elements). Neither of these assumptions are that extreme, especially considering the breadth of the data.

Reinhardt and Yett are not happy with the use of gross billings as an output measure. It may be argued that the assumptions of both constant quality and constant mix of services are unnecessary if physician output is measured in terms of annual gross patient billings (defined as annual gross income divided by the collection ratio). This would be the case if differences in billings reflected differences in quality of service and/or in varying mixes of services. Unfortunately, this involves a set of assumptions even more stringent than those accompanying the use of patient visits. In particular, it must be assumed that relative, if not absolute, fees charged are identical for all physicians and are proportional to the costs of providing these services. It is most unlikely that this condition is met in practice.[13]

Because of the unusual depth and thoroughness of the Reinhardt and Yett study, it would be impossible to discuss all of their findings and conclusions; therefore, only those that bear on the scope of this chapter will be reported. First, it should be noted that the term "group" used hereafter will refer exclusively to *single-specialty* partnerships or groups, because the number of observations on multispecialty groups in the Reinhardt and Yett data was quite low. This is unfortunate, because multispecialty groups are the most interesting economically and as providers in HMOs.

Reinhardt and Yett found that the effect of multiphysician practice on output is much lower when estimated on the basis of a production function than when one merely compares the visit rate (which most studies have done). For example, a 1966 survey by Medical Economics, Inc. revealed a median weekly visit rate for solo practitioners of 118, while the median for groups or partnerships was 144; the corresponding averages were 183 and 213, respectively.[14] Reinhardt and Yett account for the difference in magnitude of their observations by the fact that the various practice modes differ systematically with respect to the relative amounts of inputs they use (e.g., solo practitioners

[13]*Ibid.*, p. 10.
[14]*Ibid.*, p. 31.

tend to work fewer hours and employ fewer aides per physician than do those in group practices). Hence, unless adjustment is made for input differences, the effect of increased inputs is loaded onto the practice mode. The production function approach serves to segregate the separate effects of input differentials from the practice mode per se. Even so, Reinhardt and Yett found a substantial difference in output between solo practices and groups, as shown in Tables 27, 28, and 29.

In Table 28, the smallest improvement in productivity was 4.0 percent for internists; in the billings approach depicted in Table 29, it was 3.7 percent, again for internists. In light of the infinitesimal number of physicians in group practices (as compared to the national population of physicians), even a 25 percent shift from solo to group practices would generate a significant increase in output. In addition, Reinhardt

TABLE 27   Estimated Optimal Aide Input at Various Assumed Weekly Salaries*—All Four Medical Specialties

Specialty and Mode of Practice	Weekly Salary of Aides (in dollars)								
	70	80	90	100	110	120	130	140	150
General Practitioners									
Solo	4.02	3.90	3.71	3.59	3.40	3.21	3.02	2.84	2.65
Group	4.12	4.00	3.81	3.70	3.53	3.37	3.19	3.00	2.81
Pediatricians									
Solo	4.04	3.95	3.82	3.72	3.64	3.51	3.39	3.26	3.14
Group	4.14	4.04	3.95	3.86	3.76	3.67	3.57	3.45	3.36
Obstetricians and *Gynecologists*									
Solo	3.70	3.64	3.54	3.48	3.39	3.32	3.23	3.14	3.04
Group	3.79	3.72	3.64	3.57	3.51	3.45	3.36	3.29	3.23
Internists									
Solo	3.83	3.74	3.64	3.55	3.49	3.36	3.30	3.17	3.08
Group	3.86	3.77	3.67	3.61	3.52	3.42	3.33	3.24	3.14

*The estimates are based on the assumption that the physician works 60 hours per week (approximately the sample average for 1965–1967), that he can sell additional services without having to lower his medical fees, and that he is a price maker in the paramedical aide market. Given these assumptions, the optimal level of aide input is defined as that level at which the incremental annual patient billings attributable to the marginal aide just cover the incremental wage and nonwage labor costs.

Source: Uwe E. Reinhardt and Donald E. Yett. "Physician Production Functions Under Varying Practice Arrangements." Technical Paper No. 11. Los Angeles, Calif., Community Profile Data Center, Human Resources Research Center of the University of Southern California Research Institute for Business and Economics, 1971, p. 75.

TABLE 28 Percentage by Which the Weekly Rate of Patient Visits of Members in Multiphysician Practices Exceeds that of Solo Practitioners at Given Levels of Inputs

Specialty	Additional Output (in percent)
General practitioners	4.5
Pediatricians	6.2
Obstetricians and Gynecologists	13.8
Internists	4.0

Source: Adapted from Reinhardt and Yett, "Physician Production Functions," p. 33 (derived from production function estimates based on Medical Economics, Inc. "Continuing Survey of Physicians' Income and Expenses." Oradell, N.J., 1965 and 1967).

and Yett advocate the formation of group practice because it increases the divisibility of inputs.

They also derive isoquants for physician hours per aide input and conclude that, although most of the physicians in the sample could increase their output by increasing their aide input, the maximum increase can be obtained by increasing inputs of physician time—which they do not view as a feasible means of generating increased productivity nationwide. They also analyze the profitability of increasing aide employment via a marginal cost/marginal revenue approach (using both

TABLE 29 Estimated Percentage by Which Annual Patient Billings of Members in Multiphysician Practice Exceeds that of Solo Practitioners at Given Levels of Inputs

Specialty	Additional Output (in percent)
General Practitioners	5.6
Pediatricians	10.5
Obstetricians and Gynecologists	12.2
Internists	3.7

Source: Adapted from Reinhardt and Yett. "Physician Production Functions," p. 59 (derived from production function estimates based on Medical Economics, Inc. "Continuing Survey of Physicians' Income and Expenses." Oradell, N.J., 1965 and 1967).

patient visits and gross billings data). Table 29 presents the results. Here again, Reinhardt and Yett observe that the overall optimal level of aide input is much higher (between 2.5 and 4.0 aides per physician) than the average input currently employed in practice (1.5 to 1.8 aides per physician).[15]

Why should physicians persist in producing below optimal factor allocations? Reinhardt and Yett assert that perhaps doctors are not wealth maximizers, as they assumed in their analysis, but are instead utility maximizers, that is, other goals may be more important than maximum earnings.[16] If there are subjective costs to the physician in employing aides, for example, administrative and supervisory duties that are distasteful, the price of an aide is higher than the market price by the amount of the marginal subjective cost. Since group practices almost invariably employ more aides per physician than do solo practices and since Reinhardt and Yett demonstrated that an increase in the aide input increases both productivity and profitability, can it not be hypothesized that there is something inherent in group practices that reduces the subjective cost of employing aides? The ability to overcome physician resistance to an increased dependence on aide input is certainly a strong argument for encouraging the formation of such practices. An interesting point, however, is that the optimal level of aide input is only slightly higher for groups than for solo practitioners, although groups currently are more likely to approach optimal levels in actual practice than are solo practitioners.

The conclusions of Reinhardt and Yett, from the production function approach, are essentially simple. Group practice as a mode of delivery does show increased physician productivity over the solo practice mode, although not to the extent that is usually predicted. This results from separating the effect of the practice mode per se from the effect of employing additional inputs per physician, which group practice consistently does. The major finding is that physician productivity may be significantly increased by the use of more aide inputs, in both solo and group practice.

BAILEY

Richard Bailey's "Economies of Scale in Medical Practice"[17] is one of the most frequently cited articles that criticize the advocacy of group

[15]*Ibid.*, p. 74.
[16]*Ibid.*, p. 89.
[17]Richard M. Bailey. "Economies of Scale in Medical Practice." Working Paper No. 4. Berkeley, Calif., Institute of Business and Economic Research, University of California, 1968.

practice on economic grounds. It is primarily a theoretical work that challenges the economic analyses of supporters of group practice; the empirical data are very limited.

Bailey's argument essentially is that the economies of scale attributed to group practice are derived solely from technological factors in laboratory, X-ray, and pharmacy areas; there is, he says, no evidence that justifies the belief in greater physician productivity as a result of scalar economies in group practice.

Economies of scale, Bailey claims, are primarily the result of technology and can be readily accessible to the solo practitioner through hospital and commercial laboratories and radiology facilities. They are not a part of the physician product, and it is wrong to lump all of these services together when citing the advantages of group practice. His line of reasoning is that group practices are really multiproduct firms; therefore, their output is not comparable to solo practice output. Rather, outputs of laboratories and radiology departments are "ancillary products," where the predominant input is physician time; each product can be said to have a separate and unique production function. Traditional analysis regards laboratory and X-ray products as inputs, not outputs. Moreover, they cannot be said to be "joint" products, in that the addition of a laboratory test to the product line in no way alters physician productivity relative to the output of patient examinations. The reason that physicians in group practice tend to have higher incomes than those in solo practice is not because they are more productive, but because their additional revenue is derived from the sale of ancillary products. Bailey also questions whether, given the opportunities for substitution of paramedical personnel for physicians inherent in group practice, such substitution actually takes place, or whether these personnel are simply used to provide new and additional services that previously were supplied elsewhere.

Bailey's data to support his arguments are shown in Tables 30, 31, and 32, reproduced from his article. His major conclusions are as follows:

In fact, an accurate measure of paramedical substitutability would consider only those personnel who assist in the production of physician products. Table [32] demonstrates that a considerable proportion of paramedical hours are [sic] devoted to ancillary products. At the same time the data confirm that as the size of the organization increases, more paramedical personnel are added. Theorists in the past have deduced that this latter phenomenon points to a substitutability that must directly increase physician productivity. The assumption is basically that certain physician functions lend themselves to a degree of paramedical assistance resulting in direct substitution for physician time. The average physician productivity data in Table [31] contradict this conclusion.

TABLE 30   Average Physician Production, 1966*

Production Measures	Firm Size†				
	Solo	2-man	3-man	4- to 5-man	Clinics
Physical Volume					
Office Visits	2,727	2,653	2,421	2,277	2,561
Dollar Volume					
Office Visits	$29,298	$29,385	$31,517	$25,064	$34,824
Physical Volume					
Hospital Visits	901	677	1,079	782	n.a.‡
Dollar Volume					
Hospital Visits	$10,225	$ 8,039	$13,884	$10,347	$ 9,040

*Based on data obtained from a selected sample of internists practicing in the San Francisco Bay Area.

†The number of practices represented in each category of firm size is: solo—12; 2-man—4; 3-man—6; 4- to 5-man—5; clinics—4.

‡Information not available.

Source: Richard M. Bailey. "Economies of Scale in Medical Practice." Working Paper No. 4. Berkeley, Calif., Institute of Business and Economic Research, University of California, 1968, p. 20.

Productivity in the large clinics (as measured by patient visits per hour) was found to be lower on average than in smaller scale practices. Total production, on the other hand, is about the same at the two extreme sizes. These data suggest that the addition of paramedical personnel does not directly affect physician production rates but may result in the substitution of paramedical time for physician time spent on certain tasks which are extraneous to patient-visit activities. In sum, our data suggest that adding paramedical personnel merely frees more of the physician's total monthly work hours for contact with patients.[18]

Bailey's last conclusion reduces his entire article to a mere exercise. As shown in Table 31, clinic physicians produce the same number of office visits as the solo practitioner, yet the productivity of clinic physicians, when weighted by time spent with patients, is less (2.9 patient visits as compared to 3.4). Can this not be taken as an implication that the quality of the visit therefore is higher for clinic physicians' output? The strong possibility of quality differences should not be ignored.

Bailey also fails to separate the effects of economies of scale from physician productivity. While the availability of such economies will affect physician productivity, this is not their primary effect. To lump

[18]*Ibid.*, pp. 23–24.

the two together and thus reject the theory of economies of scale in group practice because they fail to sufficiently increase physician productivity is absurd. From a standpoint of medical services actually rendered by solo versus group practice, the important thing is how many services (output) can be generated by each, and at what cost? For purposes of cost savings, who actually produces the services and how they are produced does not alter the argument, provided the services are comparable.

Related to this is the fact that economies of scale are a cost phenomenon, and physician productivity is a physical-rate phenomenon. If group practice fosters the employment of paramedical personnel (as Table 32 clearly shows) who are substituted for physicians in the production of medical services normally rendered by the physician in a solo practice, thus lowering the costs of the same output, it matters not whether they alter the production of purely "physician products." Bailey discusses a cost phenomenon, then produces only rate phenomenon data.

He espouses the use of hospital and commercial laboratories, rather than integrating them into the physician's own practice, on the grounds that the economies of size can be used by the physician regardless of who owns the facilities. This does not take into account the time absorbed by physicians or patients in making trips to outside facilities, nor does it recognize the impact of speedier test results on the quality of the purely physician products, diagnosis and treatment. Not only

TABLE 31   Average Physician Production and Productivity, April 1967*

Production Measures	Firm Size†				
	Solo	2-man	3-man	4- to 5-man	Clinics
Weighted Production: Office Visits per M.D.	286	278	291	243	286
Weighted Production of Office Visits per Physician Time with Patients	3.4	3.9	3.5	3.1	2.9

*Based on data obtained from a selected sample of internists practicing in the San Francisco Bay Area.
†The number of practices represented in each category of firm size is: solo—12; 2-man—4; 3-man—6; 4- to 5-man—5; clinics—4.

Source: Bailey. "Economies of Scale," p. 21.

TABLE 32   Physician-Paramedical Hours, April 1967*

Hours and Ratios	Firm Size†				
	Solo	2-man	3-man	4- to 5-man	Clinics
Average M.D. Hours	218	222	197	200	197
Average Paramedical Hours Worked per Physician	187	181	225	271	499
Average Technical Hours‡ Worked per Physician	7	11	9	44	122
Paramedical Hours per Physician Hours	.858	.817	1.142	1.353	2.531

*Based on data obtained from a selected sample of internists practicing in the San Francisco Bay Area.

†The number of practices represented in each category of firm size is: solo—12; 2-man—4; 3-man—6; 4- to 5-man—5; clinics—4.

‡Technical hours cover time spent by paramedical personnel using EKG machines and tapes, taking X-rays, and performing laboratory activities.

Source: Bailey. "Economies of Scale," p. 22.

does Bailey disregard the physician-time cost element, but he ignores the fact that the laboratory must make a profit as well. If the group practice-owned laboratories could be induced to pass this profit on to the consumer in the form of lowered costs, would not this reduce the escalation in the costs of medical care? Moreover, tests and X-rays may be final products to the laboratory, but they are also inputs in patient care.

A final criticism is that Bailey's data are sparse—12, 4, 6, 5, and 4 observations, respectively, for solo, 2-man, 3-man, 4- to 5-man, and clinic practices. Furthermore, all of the observations concern internists, who showed the least significant productivity increases in the Reinhardt and Yett study.

UTILIZATION

Because the cost of medical care is directly related to utilization of services, the ability to control such utilization is essential to the efficient operation of an HMO. A serious problem arises since there are no established norms for "proper" utilization, although the utilization experience of established HMOs provides the operating manager with examples of ranges of utilization. HMOs, through incentives and control mechanisms, can expect a greater control over utilization than is realized under a solo, fee-for-service system. Donabedian identifies several ways in which an HMO can alter utilization patterns:[19]

1. Utilization may be *increased appropriately* through educational programs that help subscribers identify their need for care; through deletion programs via regular physicals and more thorough clinical investigation at each visit; through removal of barriers to access to care.

2. Utilization may be *decreased appropriately* through early detection and prevention of illness; through effective management of illness vis-à-vis use of less expensive alternative treatment methods.

3. Utilization may be *increased inappropriately* by an absence of checks on excessive patient demand; by an absence of checks on over-treatment (utilization review); by the presence of incentives to over-treat, to hospitalize, to perform excessive surgery, and so on.

4. Utilization may be *decreased inappropriately* through neglect of patient education; through erection of financial and administrative barriers to care; by providing less care than is medically necessary.

For reasons that were discussed earlier, HMOs can be expected to decrease utilization of hospital services and to increase utilization of ambulatory services, thus lowering total cost of care by varying the mix of services provided and by substituting less expensive treatment methods when medically appropriate. The available evidence (which is considerable in the area of utilization) suggests that this actually does occur.

AMBULATORY USE

Studies concerning the use of health care services generally indicate that HMO subscribers use slightly more physician services than are apparent in any other payment or delivery form, although these studies also present a conflicting and confusing picture of the use of HMO ambulatory services.[20]

In his review of ambulatory services, Donabedian suggests that there

---

[19]Donabedian. "An Evaluation of Prepaid Group Practice," p. 10.

[20]Five authors have brought together the current studies on both ambulatory and hospital utilization in HMOs, group practice, and other delivery forms. Except for the Feldstein study, these studies will not be reviewed here but are recommended to the reader as general summations of the current work in the utilization area. In addition to the Feldstein (1971) publication, the other studies are Donabedian (1969), Klarman (1969 and 1971), and Roemer and Shonick (1973); all are cited in the references at the end of this chapter.

TABLE 33 Ambulatory Care Utilization by Persons in HMOs and Control Groups, by Type of Provider and Plan in 1975

| | | Annualized rate† | | |
| | | Physician contacts‡ | | Nonphysician contacts per 100 persons |
Plan	Total visits per 100 persons*	Number per 100 persons	Percent patient-initiated	
Prepaid Group Practice (Total)	396	348	56	48
Control (Total)	404	360	55	44
Central Los Angeles				
Health Project	§	384	§	§
Control	§	456	§	§
Consolidated Medical System	391	348	57	43
Control	386	348	51	38
Family Health Program	344	300	63	44
Control	364	324	56	40
Group Health Cooperative				
of Puget Sound	514	408	54	106
Control	606	480	44	126
Harbor Health Services	436	384	54	52
Control	292	288	66	4
Harvard Health Plan	274	252	58	22
Control	253	216	52	37
Health Insurance Plan				
of Greater New York	443	396	54	47
Control	461	420	59	41
Temple Health Plan	313	288	51	25
Control	395	372	56	23
Foundation and control:				
Redwood	517	408	53	109
Control	451	384	51	67
Sacramento	634	516‖	50	118
Control	469	396‖	53	73

*Tests of statistical significance not yet completed.
†Based on 1-month period.
‡Outpatient visits only.
§Data not available.
‖Differences statistically significant at the 95-percent confidence level.

Source: Adapted from Clifton R. Gaus, Barbara S. Cooper, and Constance G. Hirschman. "Contrasts in HMO and Fee-for-Service Performance." *Social Security Bulletin*, 39(5): 9–10, May 1976.

is "little" difference in ambulatory use between matched samples of fee-for-service and prepaid consumers, although he concludes that "there may be some small increase in utilization" under the broader prepaid group practice coverage.[21] Gaus, Cooper, and Hirschman also came to a similar conclusion in a more recent study of HMO performance in 10 plans in comparison with the fee-for-service system for a Medicaid population. As shown in Table 33, both groups had approximately the same number of total visits per person annually (total visits of 3.96 for prepaid plans and 4.04 for the controls) and practically the same number of physician contacts (3.48 for prepaid plans and 3.60 for the control group).[22]

Roemer et al.[23] provide the figures shown in Table 34, which clearly indicate that HMO organizations included in their sample of plans provided more physician visits (aggregate rate of approximately 3.4 doctor-patient ambulatory contacts/person/year) than the indemnity-commercial plans but less than the BC/BS plans. Roemer et al. suggest that the HMO plans are underreported, and that the true use figures should be close to those of the "Blues." They further suggest that commercial rates are lower because of favorable risk selection and cost-sharing deterrents. The latter are assumed to consist of the greater use of copayments and deductibles and the generally narrower coverage provided by the commercial carriers. Indeed, the analysis provided in Table 35, which brings together several of the studies on physician use, suggests that HMO and BC/BS plans show similar use rates, which are generally lower than physician-visit rates for the total United States. Klarman (1971) estimated that the rate of physician visits per capita was 4.50 per year for Kaiser-Permanente compared to 4.42 for the general California population, but these differences are not significant, especially when one considers the reporting difficulties, definitional problems, and numerous adjustments that were made.

Table 35 also provides the use rates for several HMOs (Western Clinic—1968 and 1969, Community Health Association—1969, and Marshfield Clinic—1972 and 1973) that provide services to both pre-

[21]Avedis Donabedian. *A Review of Some Experiences with Prepaid Group Practice:* Research Series No. 12. Ann Arbor, Mich., School of Public Health, Bureau of Public Health Economics, University of Michigan, 1965, p. 19.

[22]Clifton R. Gaus, Barbara S. Cooper, and Constance G. Hirschman. "Contrasts in HMO and Fee-for-Service Performance." *Social Security Bulletin,* 39(5): 9–10, May 1976.

[23]Milton Roemer et al. *Health Insurance Effects.* Research Series No. 16. Ann Arbor, Mich., School of Public Health, Bureau of Public Health Economics, University of Michigan, 1972, p. 27.

TABLE 34   Comparison of Physician to Population Visits in 1967–
1968

Plan Type	Doctor Visits per 100 Population per Quarter-year	Rates per Year
Indemnity/Commercial	77.7	310.8
BC/BS Provider Plans	99.6	398.4
HMO Group Practice Plans	83.1	332.4
All Plans (N = 2999 family units)	84.2	336.8

paid and fee-for-service patients in the same group practice facilities.
Use rates for these plans suggest that, for all except the Marshfield
Clinic, physician-visit rates for fee-for-service patients are similar to
those for prepaid subscribers. Comparable rates are expected; physician practice patterns in these plans should not change because of
payment mode. The Marshfield rates are suspect, because their HMO
program had only recently been instituted after a long history of fee-
for-service practice, and patterns of care may not have stabilized by
1973. It also has been suggested that the use of open enrollment and
community rating may have resulted in the enrollment of higher risk
subscribers in the Marshfield HMO plan, but socioeconomic data concerning the HMO and fee-for-service populations do not support this
conclusion.[24]
     Theoretically, the reasons suggested for potential increases in HMO
ambulatory use are based on the HMO philosophy, which emphasizes
that primary, ambulatory care and preventive services be provided on
an outpatient basis and deemphasizes the provision of these services in
hospital, the most costly delivery form. Naturally, there must be hospitalization when good medical practice demands it. But, good medical
practice also recognizes the value of ambulatory care as the primary
mode, because it is less traumatic to the patient and his family and less
costly to both the patient and society.
     Another method for evaluating the utilization of physician services
has been ratio analysis. The physician-to-population ratios are considered indicators of patient-doctor contact rates and physician productivity rates. The level of the ratio for HMOs has been approximately 1
physician to 1,000 population, although the actual ratios have been
somewhat larger (the range has been from 1:1,000 to 1:1,200). When

[24]Ingo Angermeier. "Impact of Community Rating and Open Enrollment on a Prepaid
Group Practice." *Inquiry, 13*:52–53, March 1976.

compared to the ratios for the entire United States (as noted in Table 36), the HMO ratios are substantially lower than those for the general population. Lower physician-to-population ratios may reflect either increasing productivity by physicians or decreasing use of physician services per person.[25] Because the rate of HMO annual services (both physician and paraprofessional) per person is the same as or even somewhat higher than that found in the general population, there does not appear to be a lower than normal use of physician and health plan services. Indeed, the use of ambulatory physician visits in HMOs may be higher than that experienced by other insurance programs. It is generally concluded, therefore, that lower HMO ratios are indicators of more efficient delivery mechanisms, although the current studies do not show consistent results, and much more evidence is needed to support this statement.

One final look at ambulatory care may help reconcile the theory that ambulatory rates should increase in an HMO and the empirical evidence that does not support such a theory. Milton Roemer and William Shonick suggest that the *relative* use of ambulatory services as compared to hospitalization rates under the HMO group practice model should be examined. Such an examination supports the statement that HMOs do place almost double the *relative* emphasis on ambulatory care, as can be seen in the Roemer-Shonick ratios between doctor visits and hospital days presented in Table 37.[26]

HOSPITALIZATION

In evaluating hospital utilization, standard indicators are used. Three of the best hospital utilization indicators are admissions per 1,000 persons per year; hospital days per 1,000 persons per year; and average length of stay per admission. In order to make comparative studies of hospital use between members of prepaid group practice plans and members of more conventional health insurance plans, matched populations should be used. Unfortunately, it is difficult to isolate homogeneous groups. Therefore, to assure more valid results in comparative studies, adjustments must be made for the age and sex compositions of the groups in question. Geographical differences in hospital utilization also must be considered. Even after these adjustments are made, differences in socioeconomic characteristics, which are very difficult to isolate, may affect the results of comparative studies.

---

[25] Klarman. "Approaches to Moderating the Increases in Medical Care Costs," p. 181.
[26] Milton Roemer and William Shonick. "HMO Performance: The Recent Evidence." *Milbank Memorial Fund Quarterly, Health and Society:*290–291, Summer 1973.

TABLE 35   Physician Visits per 100 Population per Year in Selected Health Care Programs.

HMO Programs				BC/BS and Indemnity Programs*			Total United States	
Year	Plan	No. of Visits	Average	Year	Plan	No. of Visits	Year	No. of Visits
1968	Kaiser (Oregon Region)	331		1968	BC/BS	398‡	1968	420§
1968	CHA†	268						
1968	CHA†	345	355					
1968	GHC†	390						
1968	GHP†	370						
1968	HIP†	358		1968	Western† (F-F-S)	384†		
1968	Western†	423						
1969	Kaiser (Oregon Region)	219					1969	430‖
1969	CHA†	234						
1969	GHA†	342	344					
1969	GHC†	373						
1969	GHP†	432		1969	Western† (F-F-S)	399†		
1969	HIP†	360						
1969	Western†	347						
1970	Kaiser (Oregon Region)	338					1970	460#
1970	Kaiser (So. Calif. Region)	357	391					
1970	HIP	539						
1970	GHC	470						
1970	Columbia	308						
1970	GHA	335						

1971	Kaiser** (Oregon Region)	348			490††
1972	Marshfield	369		1972 Marshfield	149‡‡	500††
1973	Marshfield	368		1973 Marshfield	173‡‡	500§§
1973	GHA	325 ‖‖			
1974	GHA	329 ‖‖		1974		490§§

Key:

BC/BS	=	Blue Cross and Blue Shield
CHA	=	Community Health Association, Detroit, Michigan (now Metro Health Plan)
Columbia	=	Columbia Medical Plan, Columbia, Maryland
F-F-S	=	Provision of physician care by the health plan on a fee-for-service basis

GHA	=	Group Health Association, Washington, D.C.
GHC	=	Group Health Cooperative of Puget Sound, Seattle, Washington
GHP	=	Group Health Plan, Inc., St. Paul, Minnesota
HIP	=	Health Insurance Plan of Greater New York, New York
Kaiser	=	Kaiser-Permanente Health Plan (region specified)
Marshfield	=	Marshfield Clinic, Marshfield, Wisconsin

Sources:

*BC/BS statistics for 1968 are from a special study of BC/BS subscribers. Because of limited BC/BS coverage for physician visits provided outside of hospital settings, there are no utilization figures for 1969 forward.

†Leon Gintzig and Robert G. Shouldice. "Prepaid Group Practice: An Analysis as a Delivery System." Washington, D.C.. The George Washington University. 1972, pp. 155, 169, 170. Mimeographed. (Face-to-face visit of patient with physician at the health plan clinic; excludes hospital visits.)

‡Milton Roemer et al. Health Insurance Effects. Research Series No. 16. Ann Arbor, Mich., Bureau of Public Health Economics, School of Public Health, University of Michigan, 1972, p. 27.

§U.S. Department of Health, Education, and Welfare, Health Resources Administration, National Center for Health Statistics. Current Estimates from the Health Interview Survey, United States—1968. Vital and Health Statistics, Series 10, No. 60. Rockville, Md., 1970, p. 22.

‖ U.S. Department of Health, Education, and Welfare, Health Resources Administration, National Center for Health Statistics. Current Estimates from the Health Interview Survey, United States—1969. Vital and Health Statistics, Series 10, No. 63. Rockville, Md., 1971, p. 23.

#Health Insurance Institute. Source Book of Health Insurance Data 1972–73. New York, 1973, p. 53.

**U.S. Department of Health, Education, and Welfare, Health Services and Mental Health Administration, Health Maintenance Organization Service. Some Information Descriptive of a Successfully Operating HMO. Rockville, Md., 1974, p. 13.

††U.S. Department of Health, Education, and Welfare, Health Resources Administration, National Center for Health Statistics. Current Estimates from the Health Interview Survey, United States—1972. Vital and Health Statistics, Series 10, No. 85. Rockville, Md., 1973, p. 26.

‡‡Joel Broida. "The Impact of Membership in an Enrolled Prepaid Population on the Utilization of Health Services in a Group Practice." Doctoral Dissertation. Baltimore, Md., The Johns Hopkins University, 1975.

§§Health Insurance Institute. Source Book of Health Insurance Data 1975–76. New York, 1976, p. 64.

‖‖ GHA News Annual Report Issue, 37(2):8, 1975.

TABLE 36   Physician-to-Population Ratios in 1971: Some Examples

		Ratio	
Year	Plan	HMO	U.S. (Regional)
1971	CHA, Detroit, Michigan	1:1,200	1:609
1971	GHA, Washington, D.C.	1:1,000	1:599
1971	GHC, Seattle, Washington	1:1,070	1:586

To illustrate the importance of making these adjustments in the measurement of hospital use in comparative studies, the following example is offered. In 1969, the Kaiser Foundation Health Plan (Northern California region) reported hospital utilization rates of 488 hospital days per 1,000 members. After adjustments were made to the California population distribution, however, this rate became 604 per 1,000; after adjustment to the U.S. population distribution, it became 613 per 1,000.[27]

HIP STUDIES

In 1955, the Health Insurance Plan of Greater New York (HIP) conducted systematic comparative studies of hospital use by members of HIP. The HIP data were first analyzed by Densen et al., but have become the basis of further studies by such prominent health care professionals as Dearing, Donabedian, and Klarman. A comparison was made of the hospitalization records of two groups, one consisting of HIP members and the other of a closely matched employee group with the same type of hospital-care insurance but with a different form of

TABLE 37   Ratios Between Doctor Visits and Hospital Days

Plan Type	Doctor Visits per 100 Population per Year (a)	Hospital Days per 100 Population per Year (b)	Ratio (a):(b)
Indemnity/Commercial	310.4	86.4	3.6
Blue Cross/Blue Shield	398.4	110.9	3.6
HMO-like Group Practice	332.4	52.6	6.3

[27]Anne R. Somers, ed. *The Kaiser-Permanente Medical Care Program.* New York, The Commonwealth Fund, 1971, p. 41.

medical-care insurance.[28] All persons in the HIP studies, including HIP enrollees, were insured for hospitalization through Blue Cross. The persons insured under both arrangements were members of the same unions in New York City. Although the groups being studied were rather homogeneous, some adjustments were made to account for minor variations in population composition.[29]

The 1955 HIP study (Table 38) compared the hospital use of HIP enrollees with that of Blue Shield members whose medical-care insurance was limited to the hospital. A 1957 HIP study compared HIP enrollees with members of GHI. GHI members have coverage for medical care both inside and outside the hospital; these services are provided by solo practitioners on a fee-for-service basis.[30] Also in 1957, a household survey conducted by the Health Information Foundation (HIF) and the National Opinion Research Center (NORC) compared the hospital use rates of members of three unions subscribing to HIP and GHI under conditions of dual choice.[31]

The findings of these studies (Table 38) show that HIP subscribers had the lowest hospital use rate, largely due to differences in admission rates. In both HIP-sponsored studies, the use rates of HIP subscribers were approximately 20 percent lower than those of the other matched populations. This is the figure that is widely published in the literature and strongly defended by Sam Shapiro, Director of the Health Services Research and Development Center at The Johns Hopkins University, among others.[32]

A comparative study in 1958 of GHA also supports the HIP findings. This study compared the hospital use of GHA subscribers to that of Washington, D.C. Blue Cross subscribers. It should be noted that GHA self-insures for hospitalization in local hospitals. The results of this study indicated lower hospitalization for GHA enrollees—76 admissions and 499 days per 1,000 persons, compared to Blue Cross enrollees—122 admissions and 762 days per 1,000 persons; the average length of stay was similar—6.6 and 6.2 days, respectively.[33]

[28]Herbert E. Klarman. "Effect of Prepaid Group Practice on Hospital Use." *Public Health Reports, LXXVIII:*957, November 1963.

[29]Walter P. Dearing. *Developments and Accomplishments of Comprehensive Group Practice Prepayment Programs.* Washington, D.C., Group Health Association of America, 1963, p. 18.

[30]Klarman. "Effect of Prepaid Group Practice on Hospital Use," p. 957.

[31]*Ibid.*

[32]Sam Shapiro. "Comments on Approaches to Moderating the Increases in Medical Costs." *Medical Care, VIII:*88–89, January–February 1970.

[33]Dearing. *Developments and Accomplishments,* pp. 18–19.

TABLE 38   Rates of Hospital Use in Matched Populations, Data for
1955–1957

Study Sponsor	Plan or Population Group	Admission Rate per 1,000	LOS* (days)	Patient Days per 1,000
HIP (BC) 1955	HIP-Blue Cross	77	7.6	588
	Blue Shield-Blue Cross	96	7.2	688
HIP (BC) 1957	HIP-Blue Cross	70	10.4	744
	GHI-Blue Cross	88	10.8	955
HIF-NORC 1957	HIP-Blue Cross	63	6.5	410
(household	GHI-Blue Cross	110	8.0	870
survey)				

*Length of stay.

Source: Herbert E. Klarman. "Effect of Prepaid Group Practice on Hospital Use." *Public Health
Reports, LXXVIII:*955, November 1963.

FEDERAL EMPLOYEE STUDIES

Information has been available since 1962 concerning the use of health
services by federal employees, their dependents, and annuitants. The
Federal Employees Health Benefits Program is the largest voluntary
health insurance program in the world. In 1971, federal employees had
a multiple choice in selecting health insurance carriers or plans, including Blue Cross/Blue Shield, indemnity plans, 15 employee organization
plans, and, in certain localities, some 20 comprehensive group practice
plans and comprehensive individual practice plans.[34]

The findings presented by Perrott, based on 1961–1968 federal employee health utilization data, indicate that members of prepaid group
practice plans have substantially lower hospital utilization rates than
members of alternate plans. Perrott found that lower hospital utilization was not dependent on age differences, since the inpatient days per
1,000 persons were lower for prepaid group practice members at each
age level that was studied. Perrott also found that geographical differences were not responsible for the lower rates (Table 39). In virtually every state with prepaid group subscribers, their hospital-use rates

[34]George S. Perrott. *The Federal Employees Health Benefits Program: Enrollment
and Utilization of Health Services, 1961–1968.* Washington, D.C., Health Services and
Mental Health Administration, U.S. Department of Health, Education, and Welfare,
1971, p. 1. See also Donald C. Riedel et al. *Federal Employees Health Benefits Program:
Utilization Study.* Rockville, Md., Health Resources Administration, U.S. Department
of Health, Education, and Welfare, 1975.

TABLE 39 Federal Employees Health Benefits Program, January–December, 1967–1968—Comparing Hospital Utilization Among Several States for Blue Cross and Group Practice Plans (Nonmaternity, In-hospital Services, High Option Plan)

State	Type of Plan	Admission Rate per 1,000	LOS* (days)	Patient Days per 1,000
District of	Blue Cross	83	10.1	838
Columbia,	Group Practice	40	9.4	379
Virginia				
Maryland				
New York	Blue Cross	64	11.2	725
	Group Practice	43	10.8	468
California	Blue Cross	97	8.5	825
	Group Practice	48	8.8	422
Oregon	Blue Cross	119	7.4	879
	Group Practice	46	5.9	272
Washington	Blue Cross	126	6.3	791
	Group Practice	55	5.2	241
Hawaii	Blue Cross	183	7.5	1,364
	Group Practice	49	8.2	404

*Length of stay.

Source: Adapted from George S. Perrott. *The Federal Employees Health Benefits Program: Enrollment and Utilization of Health Services, 1961–1968.* Washington, D.C., Health Services and Mental Health Administration, U.S. Department of Health, Education, and Welfare, 1971, p. 13.

were lower than for Blue Cross subscribers. The obvious factor responsible for lower hospital use was the difference in admission rates. Perrott found that the average length of stay was not a significant factor in the lower utilization of hospitals under prepaid group practice. He reported 924 hospital days per 1,000 persons under Blue Cross/Blue Shield, 987 hospital days per 1,000 persons for indemnity plans, and 471 hospital days per 1,000 persons with prepaid group practice.[35] Since federal employees represent a very large, diverse population, it is possible that further adjustments are needed to allow for socioeconomic differences in the population. Nevertheless, Perrott's study does qualitatively confirm the HIP findings. These statistics are also supported by the Gaus, Cooper, and Hirschman study reported earlier. Hospital use by 10 HMOs compared to fee-for-service providers

[35]Perrott. *The Federal Employees Health Benefits Program,* pp. 11–15.

for Medicaid populations was significantly lower (two and one-half times) in group practice plans than in the fee-for-service system. Admissions per 1,000 persons were 46/1,000 for HMOs and 114/1,000 for the fee-for-service system. Average length of stay was 7.4 for HMOs and 7.7 for the fee-for-service system. Days of care per 1,000 persons were 340/1,000 for HMOs and 888/1,000 for the fee-for-service system.[36]

DONABEDIAN

By examining hospitalization according to diagnosis, it should be possible to determine the kinds of admissions prepaid group plans are able to reduce. The use of various diagnostic labels, however, does differ among physicians and institutions, and such data are somewhat difficult to interpret. Donabedian, in summarizing the work of Densen et al., compared HIP and Blue Cross/Blue Shield (New York City) for hospital admission rates involving conditions that often require surgery. Without exception, HIP rates were lower for elective surgical procedures, including tonsillectomies, appendectomies, and removal of hemorrhoids and varicose veins.[37]

FELDSTEIN

Paul J. Feldstein summarizes all the relevant data on hospital utilization, physician utilization, nursing home services, and additional patient outlays for noncovered services for various plans as shown in Table 40. He is careful to caution the reader about drawing certain conclusions on the basis of this data:

It is really impossible to prove why there are cost savings and from what they result, whether from a limitation of beds within the plan, the methods used to reimburse physicians, etc. There are just not sufficient data to prove any of the above hypotheses. The idea that the mere institution of a prepaid group practice will automatically save money must be disclaimed. This conclusion should not be drawn based upon any of the data in this report nor upon that which have been published to date.[38]

His point is that, although most of the studies conducted thus far do

[36]Gaus, Cooper, and Hirschman. "Contrasts in HMO and Fee-for-Service Performance," p. 8.

[37]Donabedian. *A Review of Some Experiences with Prepaid Group Practice*, pp. 23–25.

[38]Feldstein. *Prepaid Group Practice: An Analysis and Review*, p. 45.

point to substantial savings in certain aspects of medical services delivery under prepaid group practice plans, it has not been determined with any degree of rigorousness to which HMO elements these gains can be attributed.

Feldstein concludes that the gains of prepaid group practice plans are felt in three different areas. The first, and most recognized, is a lower hospitalization rate; the average hospital utilization of prepaid group practice plans appears to be only 40 percent of that of fee-for-service group practice plans. Second, subscribers to prepaid plans average a lower out-of-pocket expense for services that are not covered by the premium (prepaid group practice plans normally charge a higher premium than the "Blues" or commercial indemnity plans, but the coverage offered is more comprehensive). Third, the percentage increase in medical-care costs has risen less rapidly for persons in prepaid group practice plans than for those in nongroup plans.

The use rates for physician services are generally slightly higher for prepaid groups, which supports statements made heretofore, although there is a wide range of visit rates under both types (388 to 519 visits per 100 population for prepaid group, 410 to 550 for nongroup). Theoretically, physician visits should be higher under prepaid group practice plans, because outpatient care is being substituted for hospital care. The age composition of the population served, however, can be an important factor in the difference in visit rates; for example, from Health Insurance Plan of Greater New York (HIP) observations, the physician visit rate per 100 persons per year is 428 for those under 65 and 791 for those over 65 (obviously, the inclusion of a majority of plans whose subscriber group is biased in either direction will seriously alter the results). The internal structure of the plan itself also can be the cause for widely varying rates, again suggesting that comparable data are not available.

The comparison between prepaid group practice plans and fee-for-service plans is more definitive for hospital use; prepaid plans undoubtedly have a lower rate, that is, the mean days shown in Table 40 are 552, as opposed to 1,155 days per 1,000 population for nonprepaid plans.

The data on per capita expenditures are not as reliable, because the prepaid data are mainly from the Kaiser plan. Kaiser charges a higher premium than Blue Cross/Blue Shield, but Kaiser subscribers have lower out-of-pocket expenditures for noncovered care. Also, the percentage increase in per capita medical expenses under Kaiser is approximately one-half that of BC/BS. Thus, the Kaiser data should not be extrapolated to include all prepaid plans, as there may be some factor peculiar to Kaiser that accounts for the very significant differences.

TABLE 40   Summary Table Showing Utilization Rates and Expenses for Group and Nongroup Plans

	Group (Prepaid Group Practice)		Nongroup (Nonprepaid Group Practice)	Percentage, Group to Nongroup
Physician visits per 1,000 population	mean = 4,920* range = 5,190 3,880		4,733† 5,500 4,100	1.04
Hospital patient days per 1,000 population	mean = 552‡ range = 696 400		1,155§ 1,444 954	.48
Premium paid by enrollee per year ‖	$284		$ 256	1.11
Out-of-pocket expenses per enrollee per year ‖	$ 89		$ 194	.45
Total annual costs to enrollee (premium plus out-of-pocket) ‖	$373		$ 450	.83
Percentage increase in medical expenses (1960–1965)#	19.1		43.5	.44

*This figure is the average range of three group plans:

   Kaiser (1958) = 5,900 visits per 1,000 population
   GHA   (1967) = 3,880 visits per 1,000 population
   HIP   (1968) = 4,980 visits per 1,000 population

†This figure is the average of the following group plans:

   GHI (1958)   = 5,500 visits per 1,000 population
   Major Medical (1958) = 4,600 visits per 1,000 population
   BC/BS (1958)   = 4,100 visits per 1,000 population

‡This figure is the average of the hospital utilization data from seven group plans presented in the tables on hospitalization rates. The plans and the data are:

   Kaiser = 534   GHC = 572   GPP = 523   HIP = 549
   GHA   = 587   CHA = 698   CHA = 400

§This figure is the average of the hospital utilization data for four nongroup studies as described in the tables on hospital utilization:

   BC (U.S. Blue Cross) (1965)   = 1,209
   BC (Michigan Blue Cross) (1965)   = 1,444
   FEBC (Blue Cross, High Option) (1963–1964) =   954
   FE Indemnity (1963–1964)   = 1,020

‖ These figures came from D. Dozier et al. "Report to the Medical and Hospital Advisory Council to the Board of Administration of the California State Employees Retirement System." Sacramento, Calif., 1964, as follows:

TABLE 40   (continued)

| | Group | Nongroup | |
	Kaiser	CWO	BC/BS
Premiums	$284	$227	$285
Total cost (all services)	373	416	485
Out-of-pocket expenditures	89	189	200

#Group data represent all Kaiser California plans while the comparable nongroup data represent all U.S. per capita medical-care expenditures.

Source: Paul J. Feldstein. *Prepaid Group Practice: An Analysis and Review*. Ann Arbor, Mich., University Microfilms International, 1971, pp. 50, 51.

Feldstein's conclusion that the average hospitalization rate (patient days per 1,000 population) for HMOs is lower than for non-HMOs also is supported by Gintzig and Shouldice, in a review of three plans that provide health services to both prepaid subscribers and fee-for-service patients in the same facilities. Table 41 shows that hospital days for subscribers of prepaid group practice plans are approximately one-half the number of those for fee-for-service patients seen in the same medical offices. This apparently results from a conscious effort by the physicians to lower admission rates for prepaid subscribers. It also suggests that the physicians involved are not lowering their professional standards of care and are maintaining quality but through less hospitalization and ostensibly more ambulatory services.

MEDICAID RECIPIENTS

Because HMOs may offer potential savings to Medicaid recipients, a study by Gaus, Fuller, and Bohannon on utilization rates of a selected Medicaid population before and after enrollment in an HMO will be reviewed.[39] The data are for 776 persons who were in the Aid to Families with Dependent Children category of Title XIX from October 1970 to March 1971 and were subsequently enrolled in Group Health Association, Washington, D.C. from October 1971 to March 1972. Tables 42, 43, and 44 present the study results in the areas of ambulatory physician encounters, hospital admissions, and patient days for the population before and after enrollment in an HMO. Total ambulatory use was slightly higher for the group as a whole after enrollment in

[39]Clifton R. Gaus, Norman A. Fuller, and Carol Bohannon. "HMO Evaluation: Utilization Before and After Enrollment." Paper presented at the Annual Meeting of the American Public Health Association, Atlantic City, N.J., November 15, 1972.

TABLE 41   Prepaid Group Practice Subscribers and Fee-for-Service Patients in Three Prepaid Group Practice Plans—Hospitalization

Plan	Year	Hospital Days per 1,000 Population			Admissions per 1,000 Population		
		Subscribers (A)	Fee-for-Service Patients (B)	A/B %	Subscribers (C)	Fee-for-Service Patients (D)	C/D %
Community Health Association, Detroit, Michigan	1968	465	980	47	61.8	113.3	55
	1969	468	938	50	71.0	117.6	60
Kaiser-Permanente, Hawaii	1968	492	903	54	86.5	122.9	70
	1969	492	781	62	85.7	135.6	63
Kaiser-Permanente, Northern California Region	1968	397	1,108	36	77.0	128.5	60
	1969	488	1,011	48	78.5	145.6	54

Source: Leon Gintzig and Robert G. Shouldice. "Prepaid Group Practice: An Analysis as a Delivery System." Washington, D.C., The George Washington University, 1972, pp. 160, 163. Mimeographed.

TABLE 42 Ambulatory Physician Encounters (Office, Outpatient Department, and Emergency Room) and Annualized Rates per Enrollee by Age Group for the 6-Month Period Before and After HMO Enrollment

Age Group	Population at Risk	BEFORE HMO ENROLLMENT October '70–March '71		AFTER HMO ENROLLMENT October '71–March '72		p-value of difference
		Number of Encounters	Visits Enrollee/yr.	Number of Encounters	Visits Enrollee/yr.	
1–4	125	147	2.34	243	3.89	.001
5–9	142	110	1.54	107	1.51	*
10–14	158	136	1.71	165	2.10	*
15–19	141	200	2.82	250	3.55	*
20–24	53	197	7.40	111	4.19	.04
25–34	65	273	8.37	207	6.40	*
35–44	47	220	9.32	199	8.47	*
45–54	33	180	6.48	162	9.82	*
55–64	12	28	4.67	36	6.00	*
All Ages (1–64)	776	1491	3.64	1480	3.85	*

* = p-value > .10

Source: Clifton R. Gaus, Norman A. Fuller, and Carol Bohannon. "HMO Evaluation: Utilization Before and After Enrollment." Paper presented at the Annual Meeting of the American Public Health Association, Atlantic City, N. J., November 15, 1972, p. 7.

TABLE 43   Hospital Admissions and Annual Rates per 1,000 Enrollees by Age Group for the 6-Month Period Before and After HMO Enrollment

Age Group	Population at Risk	BEFORE HMO ENROLLMENT October '70–March '71		AFTER HMO ENROLLMENT October '71–March '72		p-value of x^2
		Number of Admissions	Admiss./1000 Enrollees/yr.	Number of Admissions	Admiss./1000 Enrollees/yr.	
1–4	125	12	192	1	16	.001
5–9	142	4	56	1	14	*
10–14	158	2	25	4	50	*
15–19	141	13	184	14	199	*
20–24	53	13	490	3	113	.005
25–34	65	10	308	4	123	.035
35–44	47	5	213	8	340	*
45–54	33	6	364	1	61	*
55–64	12	2	333	1	167	*
All Ages (1–64)	776	67	172	37	95	.005

* = p-value > .10

Source: Gaus, Fuller, and Bohannon. "HMO Evaluation," p. 8.

GHA, primarily because of the increased use by children ages 1–14; however, the rate was less for the 20–44 age group. This suggests that the HMO system may help allocate resources (services) more appropriately to those subscribers who have greatest need. Total hospital admission rates per 1,000 enrollees are significantly lower after enrollment in GHA—45 percent less for all groups combined. Annual inpatient days per 1,000 enrollees also were much lower in the after-enrollment group—31 percent lower for all age groups combined. These findings indicate a potential for substantial cost savings if Medicaid recipients are enrolled in HMOs; Gintzig and Shouldice conclude that savings of as much as 20 percent, primarily the result of decreased hospital utilization, might be achieved.[40]

A more detailed study of before- and after-enrollment utilization rates for Medicaid recipients was done by the Department of Health, Education, and Welfare in 1976 to evaluate whether or not Medicaid patients enrolled in an HMO could receive care of comparable quality

[40]*Ibid.,* p. 13.

TABLE 44   Hospital Patient Days and Annual Rates per 1,000 Enrollees by Age Group for the 6-Month Period Before and After HMO Enrollment

Age Group	Population at Risk	BEFORE HMO ENROLLMENT October '70–March '71		AFTER HMO ENROLLMENT October '71–March '72	
		Number of Patient days	Pt. Days/1000 Enrollees/yr.	Number of Patient days	Pt. days/1000 Enrollees/yr.
1–4	125	52	832	1	16
5–9	142	9	127	1	14
10–14	158	29	367	23	291
15–19	141	50	709	83	1177
20–24	53	66	2490	15	566
25–34	65	36	1108	15	462
35–44	47	41	1744	92	3914
45–54	33	29	1757	1	61
55–64	12	29	4833	5	833
All Ages (1–64)	776	341	879	236	608

Source: Gaus, Fuller, and Bohannon, "HMO Evaluation," p. 10.

but at less cost than under the existing fee-for-service program.[41] Medical services utilization was compared for 12, 18, and 22 months before and after enrollment:

Significant and consistent *decreases* in all four categories of utilization (physician encounters, drug prescriptions, hospital admissions, and hospital days) were reported. Overall ambulatory physician encounter rates decreased 15 percent, drug utilization was down 18 percent, hospital admissions decreased 30 percent, and hospital days declined 32 percent after enrollment in the prepaid group practice. . . ."[42]

Annual per capita costs for the same benefit package for Medicaid enrollees were 37 percent lower after enrollment in a prepaid group practice plan over the three-year period 1972–1974; even with a more comprehensive benefit package than that provided by the Washington,

[41]U.S. Department of Health, Education, and Welfare, Bureau of Medical Services. *Report on a Study of Medicaid Utilization of Services in a Prepaid Group Practice Health Plan.* Rockville, Md., 1976.
[42]*Ibid.,* p. 96.

D.C. Medicaid Plan, the study of prepaid group practice enrollees showed an average saving of 21 percent over the same period.[43] Again, the savings are attributed primarily to decreased hospital use.

The two aforementioned studies are especially significant because the population groups were comparable, whereas in many of the other studies reviewed in this chapter, the uncertainty of comparability between groups caused the findings to be suspect. These findings are, however, consistent with earlier studies completed by Kaiser (Oregon Region), HIP (New York), and Group Health Cooperative (Seattle, Washington).[44]

PROPOSED EXPLANATIONS FOR UTILIZATION

There are several explanations for the unique utilization patterns of HMOs, although considerable research is needed to fully understand them.

1. The emphasis on health insurance for ambulatory care and on preventive medicine and health maintenance may result in a slight increase in physician and out-of-hospital plan services.

2. The emphasis on use of X-ray, laboratory, and other diagnostic services and the use of health plan center facilities to perform minor surgical procedures that do not require postoperative hospitalization may tend to reduce hospital admissions and hospital days.

3. Access to beds or low bed-to-population ratios may limit hospitalization.

4. Low hospital use might indicate a failure to diagnose and treat medical conditions or might force subscribers to seek hospitalization outside the HMO system. The former has not been supported by studies on the appropriateness of care rendered by HMOs.

5. From the fee-for-service viewpoint, hospital use may be high because health insurance benefits are limited to inpatient care.

6. The capitation mechanism offers physicians no financial incentive to hospitalize patients unnecessarily.

7. The use of group practice provides the plan with a mechanism for peer and utilization reviews that undoubtedly influence hospital admission. Controls over admission, whether formally structured or merely the result of peer review and pressure to maintain professional standards, appear to be a key factor in the low hospital use by prepaid group practice plans. In fact, some authors attributed the utilization and prac-

---

[43]*Ibid.*, p. 98.
[44]Chapter 6, pp. 149–155.

tice patterns of prepaid group practice physicians to the influence of the medical group practice mode rather than exclusively to a physician capitation payment.

8. Education of subscribers in use of the health plan may affect the use rates of both in- and outpatients.

The implications for cost savings due to reduced hospitalization under prepaid group practice plans are difficult to consider in quantitative terms. The HIP studies indicate that a 20 percent reduction in hospital use can be realized; the Perrott studies suggest greater reductions. Klarman, however, believes that the 20 percent figure should be reduced to approximately 10 percent after adjustments are made to compensate for differences in access to hospital beds, age differences in subscribers, and other differences in population characteristics.[45] Inasmuch as certain adjustments were made in the original HIP studies, perhaps Klarman may adjust downward too heavily. In any event, even 10 to 20 percent reductions could result in savings of billions of dollars per year on a national scale.

Costs

THE MEDICAL GROUP MANAGEMENT ASSOCIATION COST SURVEY

The Medical Group Management Association's (MGMA) 1975 cost survey is included here because of its data on multispecialty groups, which are scarce. This is confidential information obtained from MGMA member clinics via a questionnaire, to which 34 percent of the members responded. Unfortunately, it is necessary to use gross receipts as a proxy for output, with the attendant deficiencies in the method mentioned previously. It also must be noted that the responses are primarily from fee-for-service groups.

The information in Table 45 indicates that the 6- to 10-man group is the most productive in terms of output as measured by gross receipts (the proportionately large number of respondents in this category tends to strengthen the accuracy of the data). Note that this category employs an average of 3.37 ancillary personnel per physician, whereas the largest group, more than 30 physicians, employs 3.85. (Unfortunately, there is no information on the types of ancillary personnel included in the category.) In terms of cost, however, the 11- to 15-man and the 16- to 20-man groups are most efficient (least cost). These two size group-

[45] Klarman. "Approaches to Moderating the Increases in Medical Care Costs," p. 183.

TABLE 45 Average Income and Expense per Physician in Percentage of Total Multispecialty Groups—1974

	Number of Physicians in Clinic						
	All Groups	3–5	6–10	11–15	16–20	21–30	More than 30
GROSS ANNUAL RECEIPTS	$117,134	$122,867	$127,765	$111,077	$114,835	$109,078	$114,172
Nonphysician Salaries							
Administrative	6.4%	7.4%	6.6%	6.1%	6.4%	6.4%	5.3%
Physician support personnel	7.5	6.5	6.8	7.7	8.3	8.1	8.4
Technician	3.2	3.1	3.1	3.1	2.8	3.3	3.9
Other support personnel	3.2	3.1	3.3	3.4	2.4	3.0	4.0
TOTAL	20.3	20.1	19.8	20.3	19.9	20.8	21.6
Nonphysician Employee Benefit Cost							
TOTAL	3.6	5.2	3.9	3.2	3.3	3.2	3.2
Computer Cost							
TOTAL	1.2	1.0	1.0	1.2	1.4	1.8	1.3
Laboratory Expenses							
TOTAL	2.8	2.9	2.8	3.0	3.0	3.1	2.4
X-ray Expenses							
TOTAL	1.5	1.2	1.6	1.6	1.6	1.3	1.7
Medical and Surgical Supplies							
TOTAL	2.9	3.0	3.1	2.7	2.8	2.8	3.0
Building and Occupancy Expense							
TOTAL	6.9	5.9	6.4	7.3	7.2	7.1	7.2
Furniture and Equipment Expense							
TOTAL	1.3	1.6	1.1	1.0	1.1	1.2	1.9

Office Supplies and Services TOTAL	1.5	1.4	1.5	1.7	1.8	1.8	1.7
Legal and Accounting TOTAL	0.3	0.3	0.4	0.4	0.5	0.6	0.4
Telephone and Telegraph TOTAL	1.2	1.2	1.2	1.2	1.2	1.2	1.2
Insurance TOTAL	1.5	1.4	1.2	1.4	1.8	2.2	1.6
Consultant Fees TOTAL	0.1	0.1	0.1	0.3	0.2	0.2	0.2
Other Nonphysician Expenses TOTAL	1.1	1.1	1.8	0.8	1.8	1.3	1.3
TOTAL OPERATING EXPENSES	48.2	47.7	46.5	46.4	46.6	48.2	46.8
NET INCOME BEFORE DISTRIBUTION	51.8	53.2	53.4	53.6	53.4	51.6	53.0
GROSS ANNUAL RECEIPTS (%)	100.0*	100.0	99.9	100.0	100.0	99.8	99.8
Physician Benefit Expenditure TOTAL	5.4	5.0	3.8	5.3	6.0	3.9	5.2
NET INCOME	46.4	48.2	49.5	48.3	47.4	47.6	47.8
Collection Percentage	93.03	93.51	93.43	94.83	93.38	94.23	93.83
Accounts Receivable Ratio	3.93	4.00	3.98	3.89	3.46	3.44	3.73
Number of Full-time Equivalent Employees	3.85	3.38	3.16	3.12	3.37	3.26	3.33
Number of Respondents	42	42	40	75	91	39	329

*May not equal 100% because of rounding.

Source: Adapted from Medical Group Management Association. *1975 Cost Survey.* Denver, Colo., 1975, pp. 3–4.

TABLE 46 Average Income and Expense per Physician (Census Division: All Single-Specialty Groups — 1974)

	Number of Employees per Physician		
	All Groups	Nonlabor Intensive Groups*	Labor Intensive Groups†
1. Gross Annual Receipts	100%	100%	100%
2. Nonphysician Salaries			
Administrative	5.4	5.7	4.5
Physician support personnel	4.5	4.2	5.7
Technician	5.1	3.5	9.9
Other support personnel	2.8	2.5	4.0
TOTAL	17.8	15.9	24.1
3. Nonphysician Employee Benefit Cost			
TOTAL	3.5	3.7	2.9
4. Computer Cost			
TOTAL	1.4	1.1	2.4
5. Laboratory Expenses			
TOTAL	2.0	0.9	5.7
6. X-ray Expenses			
TOTAL	1.9	2.1	1.2
7. Medical and Surgical Supplies			
TOTAL	2.5	2.5	2.5
8. Building and Occupancy Expense			
TOTAL	5.5	5.7	4.9
9. Furniture and Equipment Expense			
TOTAL	2.3	1.9	3.7
10. Office Supplies and Services			
TOTAL	2.0	2.0	2.1
11. Legal and Accounting			
TOTAL	1.1	1.1	1.0
12. Telephone and Telegraph			
TOTAL	1.1	1.1	1.2
13. Insurance			
TOTAL	1.3	1.5	0.5
14. Consultant Fees			
TOTAL	0.1	0.1	0.0
15. Other Nonphysician Expenses			
TOTAL	2.5	0.9	7.6
TOTAL OPERATING EXPENSES	45.0	40.5	60.0

TABLE 46   (continued)

| | Number of Employees per Physician | | |
	All Groups	Nonlabor Intensive Groups*	Labor Intensive Groups†
NET INCOME BEFORE DISTRIBUTION	55.0	59.5	40.0
Physician Benefit Expenditure TOTAL	7.8	8.9	3.9
NET INCOME	47.2	50.6	36.1
Collection Percentage	94.73	94.43	95.72
Accounts Receivable Ratio	2.63	2.74	2.23
Number of Respondents	22	17	5

*Less than four employees per physician
†Four or more employees per physician

Source: Medical Group Management Association. *1975 Cost Survey*, pp. 27–28.

ings also employ the lowest number of ancillary personnel, 3.12 and 3.16 per physician.

The tentative conclusion, therefore, is that the 11- to 20-man range appears to be the optimum size for multispecialty group practice and that probably 3.1 to 3.4 is the range for the optimal number of ancillary personnel per physician if both physician productivity and cost-efficiency are examined. To be really accurate, however, one would have to determine the per-unit cost of output, which cannot be done with the data currently available. Moreover, using gross receipts as a proxy for output assumes not only that the products themselves are identical over the group-size ranges, but that the price of the output is an accurate reflection of the value of the inputs used in its production.

Table 46 is included here only because it reinforces the above conclusion concerning ancillary personnel ratios, that is, that the greater use of ancillary personnel, while it undoubtedly increases productivity, may well be inefficient. According to Table 46, the labor-intensive groups devote 60 percent of gross receipts to costs, whereas the non-labor intensive groups devote only 40.5 percent; that is, they are able to generate 76 percent of the income at only 49.7 percent of the cost. Given only five respondents in the labor-intensive category, however, the results are entirely suspect. These five may be very poorly managed (not only is the nonphysician salary component much greater for labor-intensive groups, but the laboratory expenses, excluding personnel, are much greater in the labor-intensive groups, that is, 5.7 percent as compared to 0.9 percent, for a relatively small difference in total output) or the difference may be the result of the cost of productivity factors peculiar to the particular specialty groups reporting.

Summary

The group practice organization of delivery and the prepayment method of financing may offer partial solutions to the problems facing the health industry. This chapter has presented the economic rationale for the belief that the HMO has the potential for greater efficiency and productivity than can be achieved under a solo practice, fee-for-service organizational mode. A few of the reasons for these differences follow:

1. Economies of scale in the use of equipment, facilities, and personnel are available to group physicians, which should result in lower per-unit costs of output. Not only will physicians have immediate access to specialized equipment otherwise obtainable only from hospitals and commercial laboratories, but the grouping of physicians also can eliminate costly duplication of equipment and its attendant underutilization.

2. Physician productivity can be increased substantially through the greater use of paramedical and other ancillary personnel. This has been shown to occur more frequently under group than solo practice arrangements, although whether it is a result of the greater patient base and/or administrative skill available in group practice, or of the more favorable attitudes toward paramedics by physicians who tend to join group practices, has not been proved conclusively.

3. Prepayment for services rendered makes the cost of providing medical services to a given population predictable. Moreover, it increases incentives to substitute ambulatory care for hospital care and deters unnecessary use of *all* components of care.

4. Formulas for physician compensation, based in part on productivity/capitation and not straight fee-for-service, predominate in group practice organizations. These may provide incentives to physicians to perform in a more economically rewarding manner, that is, less "overdoctoring" may occur, lower cost alternative methods of treatment may be sought, and so on.

5. Professional management expertise can be used by groups, which should facilitate improvements in billing, collection, recordkeeping, and personnel recruitment and management.

Theory is one thing; proof is another. A review of studies clearly reveals the paucity and poor quality of data available from the health-services industry. The solo practice, fee-for-service sector generates almost no useful data, which makes comparisons among systems difficult at best; group practice and the prepaid group practice plans unquestionably produce more useful data, but, here too, much information is sorely needed that can be derived only indirectly from that which is already produced.

In many instances, it can be shown that, generally, there are certain results under prepaid group practice plans, but the particular factor that causes these results cannot be isolated. For example, hospital utilization in general, especially admission for elective surgery, is always substantially lower for prepaid group practice subscribers than for comparable groups with other types of insurance. There is still some question, however, whether this results from the method used to reimburse the physician, the extent of the insurance coverage for the patient, effective management control over utilization through the use of the group practice mode, or an arbitrary limitation of hospital bed supply on the part of many HMOs. If a federally financed demonstration project hopes to effect cost savings by reducing hospital utilization, which of these factors should be emphasized in order to produce the desired result? It may even be that all of these factors must be present in some degree for the result to obtain.

In other instances, virtually nothing of what has been postulated has been proved, especially in the area of economies of scale. Per-unit costs have not been compared, because usable output data are scarce. Little is known about the optimum size of groups, which should probably differ between single-specialty and multispecialty groups. If the recommendation is government-sponsored encouragement of group practice, optimum size should be determined. Also, more work is needed on the effects of subscriber composition (characteristics) on use and costs. The production function approach as used by Reinhardt and Yett appears to offer the best methodology for isolating factor contributions and separating the effects of each element in the production function.

Within the foregoing limitations, however, a substantial body of information has been collected on the economic consequences of HMOs. The weight of the existing evidence is by far in favor of HMOs for economic reasons, although whether it is sufficient to state conclusively that HMOs will consistently produce superior results in every given situation remains doubtful; however, the hypotheses have still to be disproved conclusively.

The reader should be aware that there are many noneconomic arguments for and against medical group practice and HMOs that were not discussed in this chapter. They, too, must be evaluated and weighted before a position of advocacy can be taken. Consumer and physician attitudes toward group practice can be very important to its implementation. It does appear, however, that the attitudes of both groups become much more favorable as they learn more about the concept and its benefits. Quality of care and health outcomes under both systems should be evaluated. If a dependence on paramedical personnel should be a major element, then the feasibility of their recruitment and training also must be investigated.

The alternatives to changing the composition of the present delivery system from predominantly solo practice, fee-for-service organizations to include increased reliance on HMO models are relatively few. Substantially increased government control over quality and utilization is a probable means; methods to significantly increase the supply of physicians is another. Both imply enormous costs, which must be weighed against the costs and benefits of fostering the development of HMOs. In addition, it must be determined who is to receive the benefit of these additional medical services, especially those sponsored and paid for with public funds. If the primary recipients are to be the current medically underserved segments of the population, for whom both accessibility and affordability of care are problems, providing more funds and increasing the supply of physicians may not be a solution. There is no guarantee that an increased supply of doctors would flock to slum and rural areas, or even that the skills they choose to acquire in medical schools would be the ones most needed in these areas. It may be necessary to actively provide the needed care itself, and not merely the money to pay for it, even if the money can somehow be obtained by the patient. The HMO concept does seem to offer a better solution in such situations.

Although much of the evidence is still rather inconclusive, there are strong theoretical arguments that prepaid group practice can provide significant economic improvement over the way in which most medical service delivery firms are now organized. It is vital that our knowledge be expanded with respect to the nature and extent of the potential gains available from this source.

References

Bailey, Richard M. "Economies of Scale in Medical Practice." Working Paper No. 4. Berkeley, Calif., Institute of Business and Economic Research, University of California, 1968.

Donabedian, Avedis. "An Evaluation of Prepaid Group Practice." *Inquiry, VI*(3):6–27, September 1969.

Fein, Rashi. *The Doctor Shortage.* Washington, D.C., The Brookings Institution, 1967.

Feldstein, Paul J. *Prepaid Group Practice: An Analysis and Review.* Ann Arbor, Mich., University Microfilms International, 1971.

Gaus, Clifton R.; Cooper, Barbara S.; Hirschman, Constance G. "Contrasts in HMO and Fee-for-Service Performance." *Social Security Bulletin, 39*(5):3–14, May 1976.

Klarman, Herbert E. "Analysis of the HMO Proposal—Its Assumptions, Implications, and Prospects." *In: Health Maintenance Organizations: A Reconfiguration of the Health Services System. Proceedings of the Thirteenth Annual Symposium on Hospital Affairs.* Chicago, Graduate School of Business, Center for Health Administration, Graduate Program in Hospital Administration, University of Chicago, 1971, pp. 24–38.

_____ . "Approaches to Moderating the Increases in Medical Care Costs." *Medical Care, VII*(3):175–190, May–June 1969.

Mechanic, David. "The Organization of Medical Practice and Practice Orientations Among Physicians in Prepaid and Nonprepaid Primary Care Settings." *Medical Care, XIII*(3):189–204, March 1975.

Reinhardt, Uwe E., and Yett, Donald E. "Physician Production Functions Under Varying Practice Arrangements." Technical Paper No. 11. Los Angeles, Calif., Community Profile Data Center, Human Resources Research Center of the University of Southern California Research Institute for Business and Economics, 1971.

Riedel, Donald C. et al. *Federal Employees Health Benefits Program: Utilization Study.* Rockville, Md., Health Resources Administration, U.S. Department of Health, Education, and Welfare, 1975. DHEW Publ. No. (HRA) 75-3125.

Roemer, Milton, and Shonick, William. "HMO Performance: The Recent Evidence." *Milbank Memorial Fund Quarterly, Health and Society:*271–317, Summer 1973.

Strope, Don; Cohen, Bonnie; and Yonkers, Ann. *Increasing Productivity in the Delivery of Ambulatory Health Service: A Review of Literature and On-going Projects.* Rockville, Md., Office of the Secretary, U.S. Department of Health, Education, and Welfare, 1968.

Ward, Richard A. *The Economics of Health Resources.* Menlo Park, Calif., Addison-Wesley Publishing Co., 1975.

10

Financial Management

One of the yardsticks for evaluating the success of a business is its return on investment—its ability to bring into the organization more money than it disperses. In the health-services industry, success is measured by an organization's ability to provide high-quality medical services and still remain solvent. The HMO planning activities described in the first nine chapters are drawn together here through a discussion of several financial planning models and completion of the financial planning activities. The financial planning models are discussed first; some are theoretical in nature and, thus, have not been applied to practice. Risk management and the use of underwriting techniques are then described, as well as the actuarial aspects of capitation and premium development. Note that both risk management and underwriting and actuarial techniques are an integral part of the financial planning activities and models. The chapter concludes with a discussion of some sources of capital financing and some financial management activities that provide the HMO manager with tools required for successful delivery of services.

Financial Planning

The marketing strategy was described in Chapter 8 as a two-step process—the selection of target populations and the development of a marketing mix (those elements that the HMO brings together to meet the target population's needs); also covered were the demographic, socioeconomic, and epidemiological data that are collected and analyzed to allow the manager to fully define market segments of the population and the strategy to be used for each. Decisions concerning target markets and marketing strategies are a part of the broader issues in the financial planning process; for example, estimates of the level of utilization to be anticipated from a population segment reflect what it will cost the HMO to provide needed services and, thus, help to determine a premium that will cover these costs. In essence, a part of the marketing and underwriting process is an actuarial analysis to determine the extent of risk involved in enrolling targeted populations. The following discussion addresses the marketing and financial planning issues—specifically, capacity and funds flow analysis—that were discussed in Chapter 8; these issues were outlined in Figure 30 and are reproduced in Figure 36. Throughout this section, several broad issues are discussed that the HMO manager must address regarding financial planning; special attention should be paid to these areas, which include the level of anticipated enrollees, the benefit package composition, staffing levels, size and operation of the facility, out-of-plan utilization, and debt service. Good financial management in these areas will help assure success of the health plan.

The HMO, whether it is a newly developed or long-established organization, periodically evaluates its reason for being, that is, its goals and objectives as a health care provider. Objectives are established that reflect the desires of the board of trustees or directors and the medical group, and the needs of the consuming public. Boards are usually interested in service to particular segments of the community (nonprofit) and return on investment (proprietary). Physicians desire convenience in practice, the ability to continue their education, research and teaching opportunities, and acceptable incomes. The needs and desires of the public are reflected in the construction of benefit packages, location of facilities, staffing patterns, and types of physicians employed. Thus, the major objectives of the HMO may reflect the following:

1. The location and the service area
2. The population's segments to be marketed
3. The target population size and composition
4. An acceptable return on investment (profit or surplus)
5. The demand and capacity of the organization
6. Physician-related goals

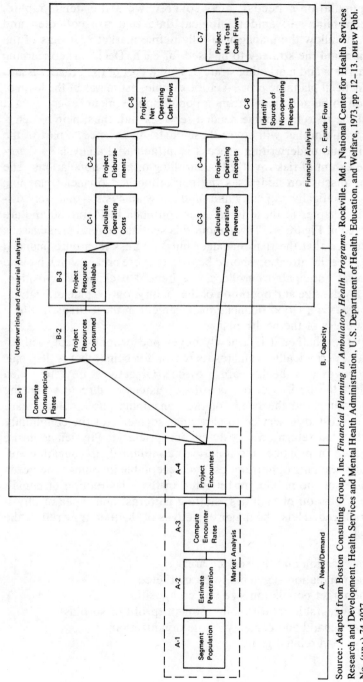
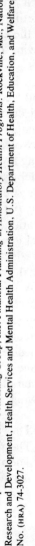

Source: Adapted from Boston Consulting Group, Inc. *Financial Planning in Ambulatory Health Programs.* Rockville, Md., National Center for Health Services Research and Development, Health Services and Mental Health Administration, U.S. Department of Health, Education, and Welfare, 1973, pp. 12–13. DHEW Publ. No. (HRA) 74-3027.

Figure 36   The marketing/financial planning process.

These objectives help to guide the manager in daily operational decision making.

In financial planning, the manager will have available the data described in the planning and marketing chapters (7 and 8). He also will be required, especially for a new HMO, to make some planning assumptions to help complete financial planning activities. In establishing programs, operational data may be available that will substantially reduce the guesswork normally found when using assumptions. Good estimates are available in the prepaid system, but such guidelines should be used with caution. The areas in which new HMOs must make some assumptions before their financial plans can be carried out are discussed in the following section.

FINANCIAL PLANNING ASSUMPTIONS

Staffing Ratios: Physician staffing ranges from 1:950 subscribers to as low as 1:1,100. The staffing ratios for physicians should be specified by specialty; in addition, paraprofessional staffing ratios must be determined (examples of these ratios are provided in Chapter 5). The issue of whether to use physician assistants must be addressed, and physician ratios adjusted accordingly.

Risk Assumption: HMOs, like other health insurers, seek to arrange the distribution of risk among the various HMO components and to exert control over the type of risk they are willing to assume. The various incentive and risk-sharing systems that HMOs use to spread the risk — to the physician groups, hospitals, indemnity insurers — were reviewed in Chapter 5. Decisions concerning the control and type of risk are classified as *underwriting* — the evaluation of categories of potential subscriber groups to determine the basis on which they will be acceptable to the HMO, taking into consideration legal requirements and other external factors and the HMO's underwriting rules and general philosophy (and objectives).[1] External factors are relatively simple to define: The HMO does or does not fall within the control of the state attorney general or the state insurance commissioner; state laws may regulate the organization and operation of the HMO; federally qualified HMOs must meet the federal regulations. These factors have been fully de-

[1] Health Insurance Association of America. *Principles of Group Health Insurance I.* Chicago, 1972, p. 93.

scribed in several publications that are available from the DHEW/HMO office in Rockville, Maryland. The HMO underwriting rules deal with more elusive issues, especially for the new HMO that has no underwriting experience. These rules must consider several selection factors: type of group; size of group; industry or type of company; composition of group; location of risk; plan of insurance, including eligibility and benefit package; cost sharing; and previous coverage and experience of the group.[2] Assumptions concerning these selection criteria, plus sound data, permit the HMO to predict, within reasonable limits, the probable utilization by and, thus, the cost of each group of enrollees. If, based on common sense and past experience, a decision on the level of a particular group cannot be reached, that group should not be enrolled. Underwriting allows for control of the risk by good selection of groups to be enrolled, defining differential rates for "classes" of risks, and providing different levels of benefits for the "classes" of risks.[3] These issues are fully discussed in the section of this chapter entitled "Risk Management and Underwriting."

Another risk category for which planning assumptions must be considered is the possibility of underenrollment. Substantial losses caused by initial enrollment being lower than projected levels used in the planning process create financial risks that may be totally unacceptable to the new program. Avoidance or minimization of such risks must be a management goal throughout the planning process. Premium rates also may include up to 5 percent additional to help reduce initial losses from underenrollment and start-up costs.

Utilization Rates: Depending on the level of sophistication of the financial planning model used, a variety of utilization rates must be assumed. These include encounter and consumption rates for hospital care, health plan care (doctor and paramedical personnel visits and health plan), ancillary services (laboratory tests, radiology, prescriptions), emergency services, and out-of-area services. Hospital rates may be in the form of hospital days per 1,000 members per year, admissions per 1,000 members per year, and average length of stay per admission for each group of enrollees, or they may be presented as rates for major specialty areas such as internal medicine, surgery by procedure, obstetrics, pediatrics, and so on. A highly sophisticated system of use projection may require hospitalization rates by disease categories, using the *International Classification of Diseases* specifi-

[2]*Ibid.*

[3]Roger B. LeCompte. *Prepaid Group Practice: A Manual.* Chicago, Blue Cross Association, 1972, Chapter 2.

cally "adapted" for use in hospitals (H-ICDA) or some other classification system. Services of the health plan (ambulatory services) include utilization rates for doctor office visits per enrollee per year for each of the physical specialty areas and/or H-ICDA categories. In addition, laboratory and X-ray service rates, prescription levels per member per year, and out-of-area and emergency service rates also must be estimated. A determination of encounter rates for physician assistants and other personnel also may be necessary.

Local utilization rates for HMOs are seldom available unless a functioning prepaid group practice plan already exists in the same area. If this is not the case, or if sharing of use data is impossible, where would one find such information? Several of the larger, long-established prepaid group practice plans have consistently collected and analyzed their utilization rates—especially the Kaiser Foundation Health Plans and the Health Insurance Plan of Greater New York—which data have been reported in the literature over the years and are available to the trained researcher.[4] Some of these data are presented in Chapter 9; other data are provided by the National Ambulatory Medical Care Survey, which is available from the Scientific and Technical Information Branch of the National Center for Health Statistics in Rockville, Maryland, and the National HMO Census of 1977 completed by the Group Health Association of America, Washington, D.C. Caution is advised in the use of such data; because they relate either to specific plans or include national averages, the data must be "localized" prior to being used in financial planning. "Tabular" rates of morbidity used by the commercial insurance industry also might be used. These rates, however, are *not* adjusted for the special underwriting characteristics of particular target groups, nor are they adjusted to match the unique operating objectives of the HMO—emphasis on outpatient care, economies resulting from the use of group practice, incentive systems that are opposite those in fee-for-service, and so on.

---

[4]Please refer to the sources listed in the References to Chapter 9. In addition, some data are provided in Boston Consulting Group, Inc. *Financial Planning in Ambulatory Health Programs.* Appendix 3. Rockville, Md., National Center for Health Services Research and Development, Health Services and Mental Health Administration, U.S. Department of Health, Education, and Welfare, 1973; Anne Somers, ed. *The Kaiser-Permanente Medical Care Program.* New York, The Commonwealth Fund, 1971; and E. Saward, Janet Blank, and Henry Lamb. *Some Information Descriptive of a Successfully Operating HMO.* Rockville, Md., Health Maintenance Organization Service, Health Services and Mental Health Administration, U.S. Department of Health, Education, and Welfare, 1974.

Morbidity, Mortality, and Disability Rates: Underwriting also will require some assumptions concerning the local levels of morbidity, mortality, and disability, which will allow the actuary to perform the following:

1. Analysis of mortality data
2. Analysis of morbidity data
3. Analysis of disease-specific data
4. Estimation of the coverage of the target population by health and related services
5. Estimation of the role of extrasectoral factors in the demand on the HMO sector

Sources of these epidemiological data are provided in Chapter 8, pages 209–210.

Models for Financial Planning

All models for financial planning require the establishment of the organization's objectives, the collection of data concerning the community, and the statement of assumptions in the four areas discussed above. Some models are simplistic and provide only indications of what might be expected. Others are highly sophisticated, providing more detailed projections, and require extensive data. In the following discussion, several models are presented that may be used to project and analyze the HMO's financial position. The utility of each approach must be weighed carefully in terms of the time, data required, cost, output of the model, and the manager's requirements, and should be cost effective for the circumstances. Models that provide an analysis of utilization and, thus, cost per member per year, may be very time-consuming and costly to prepare and may not be useful in a capitated system. On the other hand, such a system may provide the managerial control needed in a new HMO that is heavily in debt and anxious to make the most of every premium dollar.

AMBULATORY FACILITY- AND PHYSICIAN-FOCUSED MODELS

Among elementary ambulatory health-services models that have been used throughout the health care field are the "facility-focused" and "physician-focused" approaches. In each instance, a ratio is used to project the required facility size or number of physicians. The facility-focused model uses a standard facility-to-population ratio. This model enables the planner to determine the number of facilities or treatment rooms needed or demanded, either by comparing facility-to-population ratios or by translating projected facility visits into the number of treatment rooms and facilities demanded. Similarly, the physician-focused approach provides a statement of the number of physicians needed by comparing existing physician-to-population ratios to standard ratios. The physician-focused approach provides only indirect indications of facility needs. Because of problems with unsubstantiated ratios and lack of consideration of a host of intervening factors, neither of these approaches are recommended. The physician-focused approach may be used to provide a crude estimate of need/demand for general ambulatory health care and need/demand in rural areas or in areas without major outpatient facilities.[5]

AMBULATORY VISIT-FOCUSED MODELS

The approach that provides the basis for the highly rigorous approaches described later in this chapter is the ambulatory visit-focused model. This model is valuable in that it produces information on the total number of ambulatory visits needed/demanded by comparing existing visits to visits required to meet standard visit-to-population ratios. These data can be used to develop facility need/demand. Moreover, the model uses the basic activity unit of a "visit" or "encounter" and considers relationships between outpatient facilities and other sources of care and, thus, can be substantially refined.[6] For the HMO, this is the basic approach to general as well as financial planning and the determination of need/demand as discussed in Chapter 7.

COMPREHENSIVE COST-INCOME MODEL

The Health Maintenance Organization Service of the Department of Health, Education, and Welfare and Michael Herbert of InterStudy developed comprehensive financial planning models that combine the ambulatory visit-focused, the facility-focused, and the physician-focused approaches and also include an estimate for hospitalization.[7] Costs are developed for several expense areas based on generally rec-

[5]Marsha Gold et al. *Final Report, A Study for Evaluation of Methods for Determining Outpatient Facility Needs.* Cambridge, Mass., Abt Associates, Inc., 1974, pp. 31–34.
[6]*Ibid.*, p. x.
[7]U.S. Department of Health, Education, and Welfare, Health Services and Mental Health Administration, Health Maintenance Organization Service. *Financial Planning Manual.* Rockville, Md., 1972; and Michael E. Herbert. *A Financial Guide for HMO Planners.* Minneapolis, Minn., InterStudy, 1974.

ognized rule-of-thumb ratios; these should be adjusted for the specific area and for inflation. Sources of premium revenue, together with revenue for copayments, Medicare reimbursement, fees for service, and the like, are then developed, and a budget and funds flow analysis are prepared. The following provide the cost areas of this model and the basic computations:[8]

A. Physician Salaries and Fringe Benefits:

　1. Projected number of enrollees *divided* by the physician-to-population ratio *equals* the number of physicians required.
　2. Number of physicians required *times* the prevailing income for a particular specialty *equals* the total physician-income costs for that specialty.
　3. Compute physician-income costs for each specialty, then total all costs.
　4. Total physician-income costs, plus 20 percent of physician income costs for fringe benefits, *equals* the total cost of physician incomes and fringe benefits (note that 20 percent is a rule of thumb).

B. Nonphysician Salaries and Fringe Benefits:

　Total nonphysician-salary costs, plus 15 percent of nonphysician-salary costs *equals* the total cost of nonphysician salaries and fringe benefits (note that 15 percent is a rule of thumb).

C. Supplies, both Business and Medical:

　Four ambulatory physician services per year *times* the projected number of enrollees *times* $2.50 per ambulatory service *equals* the total cost of supplies (again, the figures are rules of thumb).

D. Out-of-Area Benefits:

　Three dollars *times* the projected number of enrollees *equals* the total cost of out-of-area benefits per year.

E. Drugs and Appliances (if included as a benefit):

　Sixteen dollars *times* the projected number of enrollees *equals* the total cost of drugs and appliances per year.

F. Building and Occupancy:

　The projected square footage required *times* the anticipated square-foot rental rates *plus* $0.75 (cost of utilities) *equals* the building and occupancy costs. (It is estimated that 2 square feet per

---

[8]This listing draws on Herbert's *A Financial Guide for HMO Planners* (based on 1972 data).

enrollee are required at the 10,000 enrollment population, 1.5 feet at 20,000, and 1.0 foot at 30,000 or more.)

G. Depreciation of Furniture and Equipment:

The number of physicians *times* the cost per physician *equals* the annual total depreciation of furniture and equipment. Approximate cost per physician by group size is:

Group Size	Cost per Physician
0– 4	$1,950
5– 9	1,291
10–14	1,274
15–19	1,279
20–29	1,244
30+	1,867

H. Hospitalization:

The projected number of enrollees *times* 600 hospital days per 1,000 enrollees *times* the average daily hospital expense *equals* the total hospitalization costs.

I. Amortization of Start-up Costs:

Costs can be amortized using a variety of methods, but the cost of amortization per subscriber should be less than 5 percent of the total premium per subscriber.

J. Other:

It is estimated that a $4.50 per-enrollee-per-year miscellaneous expense should be included in cost estimates; $4.50 *times* the projected number of enrollees *equals* the total other expenditures.

K. Administrative Reserve:

The total annual plan revenues *times* 2.5 percent *equals* the total administrative reserve for debt service.

The total of A through K provides the annual cost of the HMO. Monthly per capita costs are obtained by dividing total costs by total enrollment and then by 12 months. Premium rates are built around the product of this computation, with adjustments for differences in the characteristics of the groups enrolled. A pro forma operating statement and cash flow analyses can then be completed. Usually costs and income will not be equal, and adjustments must be made to the costs—

especially staffing levels—and premiums. For a more detailed discussion concerning this model and many rules of thumb, see DHEW's *Financial Planning Manual* and Michael Herbert's *A Financial Guide for HMO Planners.*

COMPREHENSIVE UNITS-OF-PRODUCTION MODEL

Another, quite unique, financial planning model, including both ambulatory care and hospitalization, was developed by Larry Butler while he was employed by the Boston Consulting Group, Inc.,[9] on a contract for the National Center for Health Services Research and Development, DHEW. The first objective of the model is to determine demand in terms of encounters with (or visits to) health care delivery personnel both on an outpatient and inpatient basis. The second step in the model is to match the required plant capacity (staff, equipment, facilities) to the demand statement, so that resources will be available to provide adequate services; this step uses "consumption rates" for each resource required to provide services to subscribers. Multiplying the total number of encounters by the consumption rate for each resource consumed provides the total amount of resources needed to meet the projected demand. Because resources are limited, a comparison of total available resources with those resources that are needed, identifies possible deficiencies/surpluses in staffing or in other resources. The HMO also may elect not to make available certain resources, thus consciously deciding not to provide selected services (e.g., identifying a need for mental health services but realizing that obtaining the services of a psychiatrist is not feasible). The third step in this approach allows the planners to apply a "cost per unit" of resource (disbursements) and a "revenue per encounter" (receipts); cash budgeting can then be completed. Depending on the results of the cash-flow projections, adjustments to reduce possible operating deficits may be necessary.

The steps necessary to complete this model are presented graphically in Figure 36 and are superficially reviewed in the outline that follows. Detailed steps and worksheets for the process are provided in DHEW's *Financial Planning in Ambulatory Health Programs.*

A. Develop a statement of demand by

[9]Boston Consulting Group, Inc. *Financial Planning in Ambulatory Health Programs.* Rockville, Md., National Center for Health Services Research and Development, Health Services and Mental Health Administration, U.S. Department of Health, Education, and Welfare, 1973.

1. Segmenting the target population.

2. Estimating penetration of each segment chosen, following the method provided in Chapter 8.

3. Computing encounter rates; total encounters are found by multiplying the projected number of enrollees by the encounter (or visit) rate per person. Encounters by type of service also should be determined by multiplying the encounter rate per service per person by the number of enrollees.

4. Projecting encounters over a period of time by estimating the number of times per month enrollees will use services.

B. Determine capacity and resources by

1. Defining the universe of resources necessary to provide the types of services (medical, surgical, obstetric, pediatric) for which there will be encounters (demand). These resources should be compared with benefits listed in subscribers' benefit packages to ensure that the HMO will have the specific resources necessary to provide each benefit. Some broad resource categories, in addition to medical specialists, may be other personnel; outside services, including a detailed description of types of inpatient services; space and rentals; consumable supplies; equipment; and employee benefits.

2. Computing consumption rates by determining the average number of units of a resource consumed by *one* encounter. Personnel resource units may be defined in terms of time, facilities in square footage, supplies in numbers of items, and other resources in terms of a proportionate share of their total consumption. To determine the number of units to be consumed for each type of encounter, multiply the total number of each type by the consumption rate for each resource consumed. (Completing for only the variable direct resources simplifies the process; cost of indirect [fixed] resources can then be added to the total costs in step C5.)

3. Projecting resources available by identifying the types of resources that are available and describing each in terms of the numbers of units of service that can be provided by the resource. For instance, a laboratory technician might provide one service every 6 minutes—10 per hour, or 2,000 per month (200 hours per month times 10 per hour). Multiply the encounters by service projected per month by the resources' consumption rate. Compare the product of this multiplication with the available resources to determine over- or underutilization of that resource and, thus, whether more or less increments are needed. (This may be completed for only variable direct resources.)

C. The funds flow analysis reduces the resources to a common denominator—dollars—so that disbursements and receipts can be compared; a positive cumulative cash flow over a 2- to 3-year period must be the outcome. The steps in this process are to

1. Determine the cost per unit of resource, and multiply the unit costs by the units of resource available.

2. Determine total monthly disbursements according to established personnel policies or contractual agreements.

3. Compare the costs of resources to the disbursement.

4. Determine the charge or revenue per encounter, and multiply by the number of each type of encounter per month. Reduce the total revenue by the percentage that will not be collected. (Uncollectables may amount to 5 percent of total premium revenue.) At this point, capitation and premium rates can be proposed.

5. Add indirect costs to disbursements if not included in steps B2 and B3. Then compare operating receipts with disbursements. Differences between the two represent the net operating cash flow. Cumulative cash flows can then be presented.

D. Adjustments will likely have to be performed to bring receipts and disbursements into close alignment.

The units-of-production model requires a high level of sophistication and an understanding by the HMO manager of the industrial production function. To use the model successfully, the HMO manager must have available the data to estimate encounters per type of service and consumption rates for resources. Aggregate rates of encounters and consumption are available from several sources, including Appendix 3 of DHEW's *Financial Planning in Ambulatory Health Programs,* but rates per medical service are much more difficult to obtain. If this major data requirement can be met, the units-of-production model has the capability of providing very useful estimates of demand capacity and funds flow analysis, because it builds upon the most elementary units—encounters per service, consumption of resources per encounter, and costs per unit of service. Decisions concerning projected utilization are made at the most basic levels and concern small segments of the total demand; thus projections of aggregates, such as total visits per 1,000 enrollees, are avoided, which, if erroneous, could create fallacious cost projections of major negative impact.

The model requires that the HMO manager think in terms of units of service and project costs and revenues on a basis similar to that of the manager in the fee-for-service sector. This is a reversal of the established, yet naive, method of relying on aggregates of services and using them as the basis for capitation arrangements with physician groups and in the development of premium rates for groups of subscribers. But, because of its sophistication and complexity, the cost of the units-of-production model may outweigh the benefits derived. Thus, the manager should evaluate the time, energy, and expense necessary to use the model and determine whether this level of detailed financial planning is necessary for his HMO.

Because the model requires that units of production be identified with the several medical-care services of the health plan, the HMO manager may decide to use these projections as the basis for an accountability mechanism as well as a budgeting device. Indeed, since physicians control the provision of services, they can be held accountable for their activities. Accountability can occur only if the physicians are involved in the planning process for establishing production levels and rates, and this model allows for such activity on a monthly basis.

COMPREHENSIVE INSURANCE UNDERWRITING MODEL

A potential financial planning model may be built around the activities associated with the insurance functions of underwriting—risk taking, actuarial analyses, incentive/risk-sharing formulas, and establishing rates. One such model, similar to that used by the Blue Cross/Blue Shield-sponsored HMOs, segments a service-area population and tentatively chooses groups of potential subscribers, much the same as the units-of-production model. A penetration-rate study is completed, and demographic, epidemiological, and socioeconomic data are collected concerning the target populations. Underwriters are then asked to analyze these populations to determine the types and levels of services required (i.e., the risk that the plan is to underwrite). From these studies, the HMO manager can develop lists of services that the target population will require, as well as estimates of the utilization rate for each service. Two categorization approaches from which the lists of services can be developed are the H-ICDA system previously discussed and the California Relative Value Study (CRVS); the latter has the capability of quantifying, in terms of "relative value," the degree of effort and other issues involved in each type of service. At this point, the HMO manager may decide to base the remainder of the financial analysis on one of the comprehensive models previously described or by the following method.

A. Determine, based on knowledge of available health resources, which services will be provided (i.e., describe the benefit packages to be offered).

B. Develop a protocol for each service to be provided (classified by the H-ICDA or the CRVS). Protocols basically are decision-logic trees that chart a course of treatment: they allow the physicians to establish practice patterns that ensure quality of care; permit the development of standard courses of treatment that become the basis for outcome studies; and enable the professional staff to determine the level of functioning of various paraprofessional personnel such as physician assistants. The administrator establishes a detailed description of the resources needed to provide care based on the protocols.

C. Determine the cost of the protocols for each service to be provided and multiply this cost by the number of each service category. Normally, only direct costs will be involved in this process; therefore, indirect costs such as heat, light, and amortization of debt should then be added to arrive at total costs or disbursements.

D. Per capita costs can be computed by dividing the total costs by the estimated number of enrollees. Loading and discounting the quotient, if experience rating is chosen, permits the manager to develop premiums.

E. Revenue, including premium income, sales of prescriptions, fees for service, copayments, and so on, are compared to total costs and adjustments are made.

In general, the insurance underwriting model permits the HMO manager to take advantage of the expertise of the underwriters and actuaries whose profession it is to determine the risks involved in insuring populations. Their recommendations normally are conservative but accurate. This model also requires involvement of the physicians in establishing protocols that can be used in financial analysis and physician capitation negotiations and that also can be used in professional review activities. Protocols that precisely describe the activities required of the physicians should also allow for the collection of productivity data to be used in the physician incentive system. Generally, this model does not require the sophisticated encounter and consumption rates of the units-of-production model, but the development of protocols is difficult and time-consuming. There are, however, examples of ambulatory and inpatient protocols currently available; these would provide a place to start the development of a protocol system.

EXPENSES AND INCOME

Following is a summary of the income and expense items mentioned in each of the models heretofore described. Expenses fall into three primary categories:[10]

1. *Medical care costs:* These costs include all medical service and supply expenditures for both inpatient and outpatient care.
2. *Hospitalization costs:* Included in this category are all hospital-related charges incurred during the delivery of inpatient care.
3. *Administrative costs:* All expenditures incurred by the health plan that are related to the administration and support of either the medical and/or hospital services.

Income items include:

1. *Premiums:* Revenue from membership dues directly related to the level of enrollment.
2. *Fees for service:* Income from services provided on a per-unit-of-service basis to non-HMO subscribers—patients of HMO physicians who, prior to joining the health plan, were in private practice; emergency services to local residents; services provided as a courtesy to residents in close proximity to the health plan; or income derived from planned fee-for-service activity.
3. *Copayments:* Revenues from charges of $1 or $2 levied at the time selected services are provided—for office visits, laboratory tests, radiology, injections, and so on.
4. Sale of drugs, supplies, and prosthetic devices.
5. *Federal, state, and local welfare program payments:* Includes revenue from the provision of services to recipients of programs such as Medicare, Medicaid, workmen's compensation, and local welfare programs.
6. *Loans, grants, and gifts:* Income from federal programs, such as the HMO Act, and philanthropy.
7. Investments and interest income.

[10]U.S. Department of Health, Education, and Welfare, *Financial Planning Manual,* p. 7.

Risk Management and Underwriting

Health maintenance organizations are health-delivery mechanisms, but they also have the role of insurer for those who seek their services. Many argue that HMOs do not insure but that they provide "assurances" of services, thus attempting to avoid regulation by the state insurance commissioners; this issue concerns every HMO manager who has offered a benefit package to subscribers. Of concern here are the insurance functions of risk management that must be performed by the HMO to assure financial stability of the organization. The HMO seeks to distribute the risk of providing care to a selected population within a financial budget and, therefore, attempts to control the type of risk that it is willing to assume. The process by which the risk of accepting populations as enrollees is evaluated and determined is called *underwriting*. Associated with the underwriting process are the *actuarial analyses*—the calculation of premium rates for each unit of service (unit of exposure or benefit unit) that is included in the benefit package. Thus, underwriting and its associated actuarial analyses provide a method of *rate making* for the HMO—a method for determining the types of services to be provided, the level of utilization of services, the risk involved in the provision of such services, and the rates that must be charged to subscribers to cover the cost *and* the risk involved in the provision of such services.

UNDERWRITING GROUPS

Figure 36 outlines the several activities that may be included in underwriting; note that this activity is a part of both the marketing process and the financial planning process, and it includes analyses of need/demand, capacity, and funds flow. There is no step-by-step process to be followed by HMO underwriters, but each group of potential subscribers is evaluated according to several underwriting assumptions, or rules, that are agreed upon by the board of the HMO and that describe the general acceptability of the risks involved. A description of these rules follows.[11]

1. *Types of groups:* The most common type of group is *individual employers*, who insure their employees for health insurance benefits. Consideration should be given to the character of the employer company or firm and its reputation as an employer in the community. A

[11]This discussion draws upon the Health Insurance Association of America's *Principles of Group Health Insurance,* Chapter IV.

second type is the *union group*. Of major concern in underwriting unions is the source of funds to pay the premiums, since the Taft-Hartley Law prohibits employer contributions to be transferred to a union. Thus, the entire premium payment for a union member's coverage must come entirely from union members, whether it is from dues, a separate collection, or from general union funds. *Multiple employers* (i.e., a number of employers in the same industry) sometimes band together to purchase health insurance as a single group, which can be considered a third type of group. Such an arrangement may be made by using a negotiated trusteeship, as required by the Taft-Hartley Law, for employees covered under a bargaining agreement. Eligibility requirements for benefits should be flexible enough to allow a substantial number of employees to join but still exclude transient employees. Voluntary trade associations also may establish a fund for their members and employees. Other important groups which may not be included in these three categories are jointly administered programs and federal, state, and local government groups. Again, the major concern in underwriting such groups is the capability of receiving and maintaining a high level of participation from each employer group.

2. *Size of the group:* Generally, the larger the group enrolled, the greater the degree of accuracy in mathematically predicting the probability of loss. Thus, HMOs attempt to attract large groups in which the expense ratio (ratio of expenses to earned premiums) is relatively low and in which there is a consistency of losses over time. Small groups have higher expense ratios because of the inability to spread the risk and the possibility that there will be wide fluctuations in use and, thus, cost. More rigorous underwriting rules may be applied to smaller groups.

3. *Industry or type of company:* Disability and morbidity rates for certain industries are high because of physical conditions in which employees must work. If a disability is job-related, it is covered by the workmen's compensation law, but secondary effects on an individual employee's health are not covered. Long-term effects must be carefully evaluated prior to underwriting more hazardous occupations and industries.

4. *Composition of a group:* The risk of underwriting varies with the makeup of a group. Factors such as age, sex, and dependents affect the use patterns. Generally, groups of extremely young or old persons tend to have high use patterns. Female employees, according to surveys conducted by the Department of Health, Education, and Welfare, have 25 percent more disabilities than male employees and have more short-duration disabilities during their younger years. Dependent

coverage presents another set of problems: In organizations with a high percentage of married women, the percentage participation of these employees may be very low, because many of their husbands will have coverage for themselves and their dependents through their own employers. Generally, the objective of the HMO in underwriting groups is to provide a benefit package broad enough to cover all activity at work, full-time employees, union, or association members. Thus, the benefit package should not be directed at any one class of employee or earnings level.

5. *Location of risk:* The ability to adequately provide service and to attend to administrative activities is an important factor in the HMO's selection of a group of potential enrollees. Long travel times or distances will compound the problems of service delivery.

6. *Plan of insurance, including eligibility and benefit package:* Eligibility determines who will be included as a potential subscriber. Normally, employee- and union-member eligibility is based on conditions that pertain to employment; thus, eligibility cannot be determined by age, sex, or race because, by law, these cannot be conditions of employment. Moreover, the coverage provided generally is extended to dependents; size of family and ages of dependents are, therefore, important data in assessing the risks of underwriting the group.

HMOs are recognized for their willingness to develop tailor-made packages for particular groups of employees. Special note should be made of extremely minimal or rich benefit packages; these situations may create underenrollment through lack of employee interest or adverse selection.

7. *Cost sharing:* There are two basic methods for payment of premiums—noncontributory, in which the policyholder (employer, union, association) pays the entire premium, or contributory, in which the enrollee may pay a portion or all (fully contributory) of the cost. Underwriters prefer noncontributory programs because they assure full employee participation, which simplifies marketing and administration. Fully contributory plans have many drawbacks (lack of employer interest, marketing problems, possible loss or lack of participation) and should be used only under special circumstances, such as supplemental packages to other health insurance programs and programs limited to higher salaried employees who generally do not have personal financial difficulties.

8. *Previous coverage and experience of the group:* The cost of prior coverage appears to be the main reason that groups shop for new health insurance coverage. Underwriting such groups is based on a review of previous coverage *and* experience. Information about the group's

coverage and use patterns for the three previous years at least is mandatory and may be evaluated as described in the following example:[12]

a. Review rate and loss experience:

Current Benefit Packages	Number of Insured	Monthly Premium
Employee	115	$24 per employee
Dependents	75	$34 per dependent unit

Year	Premiums	Utilization Experience
1st policy year	$ 65,600	$ 64,000
2nd policy year	67,000	62,000
3rd policy year	66,400	65,000
	$199,000	$191,000

b. Determine the present insurer's expected annual premium:

Employees   115 × $24 × 12 months = $33,120
Dependents   75 × $34 × 12 months = 30,600

Total premium, 12 months $63,720

c. Develop ratio of actual premium to premium calculated in step b:

$$\frac{\text{Actual premium 1st year} \quad \$65,600}{\text{Calculated premium} \quad \$63,720} = 103\%$$

$$\frac{\text{Actual premium 2nd year} \quad \$67,000}{\text{Calculated premium} \quad \$63,720} = 105\%$$

$$\frac{\text{Actual premium 3rd year} \quad \$66,400}{\text{Calculated premium} \quad \$63,720} = 104\%$$

d. Determine through actuarial analyses the new rates the HMO must charge:

Employees   115 × $26 × 12 months = $35,880
Dependents   75 × $37 × 12 months = 33,300
Total premium, 12 months $69,180

[12]Health Insurance Association of America. *Principles of Group Health Insurance*, pp. 103–105.

e. Adjust total premiums developed in step d by factors from step c:

1st policy year	$69,180 × 103% = $71,255
2nd policy year	$69,180 × 105% = 72,639
3rd policy year	$69,180 × 104% = 71,947
	$215,841

f. Determine the loss ratio of the HMO:

$$\frac{\text{Total three-year actual incurred expenses} \quad \$191,000}{\text{Total three-year premium of new HMO rate} \quad \$215,841} = 88\% \text{ loss ratio}$$

g. A management decision must be made to determine how high a loss ratio will allow for a surplus when other expenses are added. Assuming a loss ratio of 80 percent in this example, the HMO's premium rates must be increased to an amount equal to 110 percent (88% ÷ 80% = 110%) of the HMO's average rates for an equal benefit package (or, if using commercial insurance manuals, 110 percent of manual rates).[13] If the acceptable loss ratio was 90 percent rather than 80 percent, adjustments to manual rates would be a reduction of approximately 2 percent (88% ÷ 90% = 98%) to determine the premiums to be charged.

To summarize, certain factors are considered in underwriting and enrolling groups of subscribers, including difficulties in administration (especially with small groups), negotiated trusteeships, and groups that are partially or fully contributory. In addition, the law requires that employer groups provide a conversion privilege for employees leaving an employment group. Conversion may not always be to an individual membership in the HMO; or the HMO may offer individual enrollment but with highly restricted benefits. Dual choice may offer potential underwriting problems if, in fact, it creates an adverse selection mechanism; high users from the group might select the HMO option because of its broader coverage. (It has been shown, however, that there is *no* adverse selection in dual choice HMO programs; high risk individuals do not appear to concentrate in either the HMO program or in alterna-

---

[13]Manual rates are a commercial insurer's standard rate tables, included in its rate manual or underwriters' manual, that are used to develop premium rates. Because they have been developed on the basis of experience in the fee-for-service system, they should be used with caution. It is more appropriate to develop rate manuals for HMOs based on HMO experience, as discussed on pages 324–328.

tive health insurance packages.) Overall utilization does not appear to be affected.[14] For those groups that appear to be high risk/high utilizers, rate adjustments with loading factors may be used as described under rate making.

UNDERWRITING INDIVIDUALS

There are circumstances under which the HMO may wish to offer individual subscriptions outside of the usual group arrangement. This may be provided not only because of the HMO's sense of social responsibility to the community, but also as a marketing technique to attract the patients of physicians who join with the HMO, and others who are moving into the community, are self-employed, or are otherwise not associated with a group. Because the chances for adverse selection and billing difficulties are higher among such potential subscribers, underwriting rules for these individuals may be highly restrictive. In addition to a statement of health, their contracts may include preexisting condition limitations or exclusions. Higher premiums because of the greater risk are inevitable for individual subscribers.

HANDLING RISK

The discussion concerning underwriting of groups and individuals has provided some guidance on how to determine and cope with the risks involved in HMOs. Some other options for protection against these risks are described as follows:

1. *Out-of-area use:* Out-of-area occurrences may be controlled by limiting coverages and costs in the subscriber contract. Out-of-area use also may be reinsured or covered by a carrier participating with the plan.
2. *Catastrophic illness:* Rare, unusual, and expensive services that normally are outside the capability of the HMO providers, or illnesses that are very expensive to treat, may be included in the benefit package or limited by placing a ceiling on the amount or costs of such services. Another method may be the use of reinsurance for expenses over a selected level, say, $5,000 per enrollee per year for smaller HMOs.
3. *Epidemic or disaster:* These occurrences could be excluded or reinsured through commercial carriers.

---

[14]LeCompte. *Prepaid Group Practice,* Chapter 2; see also pp. 145–147 for more information concerning the consumer selection process.

4. *Adverse selection and excess utilization:* The risk of loss because enrollees exceed projected levels of utilization could be reduced by using the aforementioned underwriting rules, including accurate actuarial predictions of utilization of services, or by buying insurance to protect against loss from this exposure; reinsurance at $5,000 per person per year is recommended for smaller HMOs.

5. *Low enrollment levels:* Probable causes of low enrollment are lack of market analysis and an appropriate marketing strategy, lack of underwriting expertise, and setting of unrealistic enrollment goals. All three issues—goals, marketing, and underwriting—must be properly managed to protect against loss from this critical failure.

6. *Hospitalization:* The plan is the risk taker for excess hospitalization. Protection to a certain degree may be provided in contracts with hospitals by including a capitation arrangement or a ceiling on per diem and other charges. These risks also may be passed on to the physician group and other components of the HMO system (the hospital, commercial carriers) according to contractual arrangements. Methods of risk sharing are described in Chapter 5. These systems may also contain retrospective adjustments, on a periodic basis, according to utilization levels.

7. *The subscriber's contract:* The contract, or policy, between the HMO and the policyholder is useful in controlling and reducing risk, because it describes the rights and responsibilities of each party; it may be written to exclude or limit services, to specify conditions under which services will be provided, and even to specify the benefit package. Copayments and deductibles provided for in the contract may be used to help limit the use of services and/or to defray the cost of those services. It is important, however, to note that most HMOs attempt to provide full coverage and "first dollar/first day coverage" similar to or more comprehensive than competing Blue Cross/Blue Shield plans. Limitations, specific conditions, exclusions, copayments, and the like, should be used only in conjunction with other underwriting techniques in the reduction of risk.

BENEFIT PACKAGES: INCLUSIONS

The benefit packages offered by the HMO are its "products and services"; as such, they are at the heart of the organization and serve several important functional objectives—to meet the need/demand of the subscribers, to reduce financial deterrents to early care, and to develop a wide range of treatment alternatives that are available to the

HMO's providers.[15] There are several models that the HMO can use to help develop benefit packages, for example, traditional Blue Cross/ Blue Shield and indemnity programs, as well as existing HMOs. Because the HMO's packages will be competing with the existing programs, the structure of the packages must be similar to the BC/BS plans—comprehensive and offering first dollar/first day coverage, with few copayments and deductibles. In addition, the Health Maintenance Organization Act provides a list of required "basic health services" and a list of supplemental health services that may be provided at the option of the HMO; these two lists are provided in Chapter 3, pages 52 and 53. *Basic benefits* are those services that are considered essential to the provision of health care and that are included as benefits in most health care plans. *Optional benefits* are those additional services that are normally selected to meet a unique need of the target population or to increase the market acceptance of the plan.[16] Unlike the BC/BS and indemnity packages, the list of services offered by HMOs is somewhat more comprehensive and places equal emphasis on outpatient as well as inpatient services, including some preventive health services as regular "basic" benefits. Basic health-service packages also are defined by both the Medicare and Medicaid programs and may include additional services and more detailed requirements in the contract between the HMO and the responsible government agency. HMOs, however, are most concerned with meeting the level of competition and minimums established by law and, more importantly, with meeting the *special* needs of target populations. These objectives form the bases for benefit-package development, constrained by cost.

The basic and optional benefits that are commonly included in HMO benefit packages are listed in Table 47. It is important to note that most of the services are provided through both an ambulatory and an inpatient delivery mode (where applicable).

According to DHEW's *Financial Planning Manual*, the services listed in Table 47 can be categorized as follows:[17]

1. *Outpatient care:* Diagnostic services, office visits, physical examinations, medical consultations, and laboratory tests
2. *Inpatient care:* Services provided in hospitals and extended-care facilities, and the ancillary services provided to inpatients

---

[15]Roger W. Birnbaum. *Prepayment and Neighborhood Health Centers.* Washington, D.C., Office of Health Affairs, Office of Economic Opportunity, 1972.

[16]U.S. Department of Health, Education, and Welfare. *Financial Planning Manual,* p. 7.

[17]*Ibid.,* p. 8.

TABLE 47 Basic and Optional Services Commonly Included in HMO Benefit Packages

Basic Benefits	Optional Benefits
Physician services	Psychiatric treatment
Hospital services	Treatment of alcoholism and drug
Emergency health services	addiction
Home calls	Eye examinations and prescriptions
Diagnostic laboratory services	Ambulance service
Diagnostic and therapeutic radiologic	Visiting nurse service
services	Artificial limbs, eyes, and orthopedic
Specialist care and consultation	braces
Maternity care	Dental services
Well-baby care	Provision of allergens
Treatment of allergies	Prescription drugs
Physical examinations	Loan of crutches, wheelchairs, and so on
Immunizations	Treatment of conditions requiring care in
Anesthesia	other than general hospitals
Educational activities	Home health care
	Extended-care facility services

Source: Adapted from U.S. Department of Health, Education, and Welfare, Health Services and Mental Health Administration, Health Maintenance Organization Service. *Financial Planning Manual*. Rockville, Md., 1972, p. 7.

3. *Out-of-area and emergency care:* Services required in emergency situations within the HMO's service area and services provided for emergencies that occur outside the service area
   4. *Catastrophic illnesses:* Services to meet unique health needs
   5. *Drugs and appliances:* Prescription drugs, eye glasses, and other prosthetic and corrective devices
   6. *Other special care:* Services that might include home health care, therapeutic and rehabilitative care, and health education

BENEFIT PACKAGE: EXCLUSIONS, LIMITATIONS,
AND COPAYMENTS

Exclusions to the benefit package and limitations on services that are included in the package may be used for various reasons—to limit or control risk and thus maintain financial solvency, or to prevent inappropriate use of services. Most often such limitations and exclusions include war clauses, coordination of benefits with other insurers, serv-

ices covered under workmen's compensation or other public programs, physical examinations for employment or required by insurance
companies, preexisting conditions beyond a dollar limit of care, inten-
tionally self-inflicted injuries, personal comfort items while hospitalized, and private hospital rooms unless medically ordered. In
many of these circumstances, the liability for the service logically resides with other groups, such as an employer, a life insurance company, and local or federal governments. Antiduplication or coordination of benefits (COB) clauses are included so other carriers will bear
their fair share; for example, working wives may be covered first by the
plan where they work, with the HMO assuming the difference in cost for
care.

Copayments require the subscriber to pay a nominal "out-of-
pocket" amount each time selected services are used. The rationale for
such a system is that the total premium cost can be reduced somewhat
by the inclusion of copayments and that copayment charges will erect a
low economic barrier between the patient and the plan. Copayments
provide a mechanism for rationing among subscribers' health care
services—an outcome of the pricing system; since consumers will pay
something out-of-pocket ($1 or $2 fee) every time they receive a certain
service, they will not indulge unnecessarily.[18] Also, subscribers with
possible hypochondria may limit their use of health services. Copayments appear to work, more or less, according to this rationale. They
do increase revenues so that premium levels can be reduced and appear
to decrease utilization of physician services,[19] and they bring the
hypochondriac patient to the attention of his physician so that more
appropriate care can be provided.

Reservations still exist concerning copayments: They may not be the
most efficient or equitable way to control utilization and thus cost. This
is especially true in an HMO, where prevention and early detection is
such a large part of the philosophy of medical care. Copayments also
discriminate against the poor; this should be considered and the use of
copayments weighed against the objectives of the health plan.

BENEFIT PACKAGE: DESIGN AND FORMATION

The question of what should or should not be included in a package has
not been fully answered. As stated previously, the HMO must meet the

[18]"Coinsurance and Deductible Effect." *Medical Care Review, 30*(10):1096,
November 1973.
[19]*Ibid.*

competition; it also must meet the requirements of any government programs whose recipients will receive its services. It also was suggested previously that the HMO should have enough flexibility to allow the physician to choose from a range of treatment alternatives; the range of benefit categories should be broad enough to provide this flexibility. The major constraint in the benefit package will be the physicians themselves; can they and will they be willing to offer certain services? Will additional physician specialists be available to call upon if the health plan cannot perform the services? Physicians *must* be involved in the benefit package formulation to ensure that it is comprehensive and appropriate and to ensure their commitment to provide the services offered.

The formulation of the benefit package is an integral part of the marketing and financial planning process. Benefits should be *directly* related to the need/demand statements developed for the target populations, limited of course by costs and the availability of medical personnel. Moreover, benefits can be packaged in several ways. Programs offered to group subscribers may include the individual (self only) or the employee and family (self and family). Some plans provide additional programs for family membership based on the number of dependents (self and one dependent, self and two dependents, self and three dependents, and so on). Another common offering is a choice between low- and high-option programs, which differ in comprehensiveness, copayments, and deductibles. Such programs are developed with relative ease, using the basic unit of pricing—the "per capita" cost, which is the quotient of total costs divided by the total number of subscribers. By offering optional programs, the health plan may more effectively meet the needs and expectations of its subscribers. Generally, three methods of package design are followed, two of which provide programs tailored to specific groups of enrollees.

1. Standard and supplementary sets of benefits that roughly match the requirements of the population and providers are developed from the lists in Table 47. The health plan will then make available to groups the standard package *and* the option of adding benefits from the supplementary set to develop benefit levels that meet the group's particular needs.

2. Totally custom-made packages for all groups may be developed. Thus, there may be as many benefit packages as there are groups of subscribers.

3. The health plan may offer a standard plan only, with no custom

programs or supplementary sets of benefits. A similar method is followed by the Health Insurance Plan of Greater New York.

There are advantages and drawbacks in all three methods. Freedom of choice and flexibility in meeting special needs are the most important advantages of the custom package, but they are difficult for the HMO to manage. The standard plan offers great administrative ease, but lacks the custom approach peculiar to HMOs. Both the standard plus supplemental packages and custom packages require that each benefit be "costed" to determine its financial effect on the cost of the benefit package. Although the practice of identifying benefit costs is required for custom packages and is accepted practice, the identification of unit benefit costs is not mandatory for the development of the standard plan and may not be easy for a new plan to develop. Finally, costing benefits is a process of balancing the comprehensiveness of benefits against the use of deductibles and copayments and meeting the competition. Thus, initial packages will likely go through a metamorphosis as cost estimates are more fully developed and cost flow analyses are completed.

Actuarial Aspects

CAPITATION DEVELOPMENT AND PREMIUMS

A part of each of the financial planning models consists of *rate making*, the process of pricing the services that are to be sold. In the case of health plans, the price is called a *premium*—a fixed fee, paid in advance, that provides a plan member with all specified medical care and services. Before premiums can be calculated, rates (or charges) for each benefit unit (service) or unit of exposure must be developed. In the commercial insurance industry, the process of developing rates is the responsibility of an actuary. In HMOs, however, this process normally is the responsibility of the manager, but it may be delegated to the financial officer. Only advanced capitation models require the development of rates by benefit unit. Benefit units are described in the preliminary benefit package and include services listed in Table 47. Once rates have been established for each benefit unit, the calculation of the capitation rate can be completed by one of several methods. The *capitation rate* should be sufficient to cover all costs incurred by the plan when assigned equally to each member enrolled in the plan, and includes costs before adjustments are made. *Premium rates* are developed by adjusting the capitation rate for the unique characteristics of the plan and subscribers. Descriptions of methods for capitation rate calculation follow.

Rate Making: The rate-making process follows generally accepted procedures to assure that rates will be adequate to cover the total costs of providing the benefits, will allow for a surplus to cover any accumulated operating deficit, and will provide funds for utilization fluctuations and improvement of the health plan and its programs.[20] Rates developed must be evaluated in terms of their ability to compete with other programs in the community. The rate for each benefit unit must be equitable for all classes of policyholders so that each will be charged a rate reflecting the risk associated with his group or with all the groups of enrollees. In this regard, two rating systems are available, although one—community rating—has been described as embodying the philosophy of HMOs to provide for the social welfare of all enrollees on an equal basis without exclusive regard to demographic, socioeconomic, and morbidity differences.

Community rating, thus, is a rating system that embodies the total experience (or projected use level) of the enrollees and uses this data to determine a capitation rate that is common for all groups, regardless of the utilization experience of an individual or of any one group. This rating system spreads utilization and expense costs over the total membership of the health plan. Distinctions may be made among the major risk classes (i.e., over age 65 versus under age 65, individual versus group enrollees, indigency versus solvency), but premiums are not adjusted or loaded according to the loss experience of any one enrollee or group. Thus, each person or family who enrolls under a specific benefit package should pay exactly the same premium as every other enrollee in the same package. Given the attitude that no windfall from lowered utilization or loss from above-average use should accrue to any group or individual, but that the surplus or deficit should be spread over the entire enrollee population, there is no advantage to the HMO manager to incur the expense of projecting use data by particular classes or groups of enrollees. By carrying this operating philosophy one step farther, the reader should understand the rationale behind capitation, that is, equal assignment of costs to each plan member. Under a purely community-rated system, no adjustments to this capitation rate would be permitted, thus, the capitation rate and

[20]Health Insurance Association of America. *Principles of Group Health Insurance,* pp. 131–132.

premium rate would be the same. Some social welfare advocates suggest that this is desirable, because it is a good way to insure the high-risk segments of our population by averaging the costs across the entire membership. With the passage of federal welfare programs designed to cover some costs of high-risk groups (i.e., Medicare and Medicaid), however, community rating becomes less important for cost redistribution.

The second rating system used by HMOs and health care insurers is *experience rating*. This system allows for a variation in the rates for benefit units, computed on the basis of the experience (or projected use) of the group or individual. Information on past use and expenses incurred by the HMO for each group of enrollees is used to adjust rates for benefit units that have been developed in the actuary process or those rates that are found in rate manuals maintained by commercial health insurance carriers. It is a method by which premiums paid by a group policyholder are directly related to the actual utilization and expense experience of the group. Consequently, the experience-rating system modifies manual rates or rates developed in the underwriting process for broad classes of risk, usually based on a group of employees, union, or association.[21]

Although Blue Cross/Blue Shield plans and HMOs were historically established on a community-rating basis, both programs now increasingly lean toward the experience-rating system used by commercial carriers. This is accomplished through "discounts" or "loading" factors that provide adjustments to rates for major classes of risks. The basis for defending this system of rate making is that there is greater equity among policyholders: those with greater risks pay higher premiums. Moreover, competition among the many insurers has forced health plans to more systematically evaluate policyholders and to attempt, with reasonable premium rates, to retain groups with favorable experience. This widespread policy of experience rating places HMOs that qualify under the HMO Act at a disadvantage for adverse selection; qualified HMOs must use open enrollment and community rating (except for some distinction for major risk classes). Hence, groups with poor experience and high premiums may look toward the more liberal, qualified HMO for coverage. A second disadvantage concerning experience rating is that the process requires the fee-for-service approach of pricing out every unit of service and attributing such prices or rates to specific providers before a capitation for both providers and enrollees can be determined. For HMOs that serve a small number of groups

[21]*Ibid.*, p. 142.

or classes of risk, this task is manageable, but when many groups or risk classes are enrolled, the rate-making process becomes overwhelming. A combination of averaging all costs over the enrollee group and identifying and allocating each unit-of-service cost to categories of risk may be followed. Certain fixed costs may be averaged over the total population while the most variable costs, such as physician specialists and some supplies, may be apportioned on a piecemeal basis. The latter approach probably will result in the most cost-effective system of financial planning and rate making. Several approaches to capitation development, using both experience and community rating, are discussed in the following sections.

UNIT-OF-EXPOSURE APPROACH

In the commercial insurance field, it is customary to develop a manual of rates containing schedules of premiums (charges for each benefit unit) for broad classes of risks that reflect the most important factors affecting morbidity and expenses. Adjustments are then made using the experience-rating method previously discussed. Manuals are developed from the common experience of the insurance industry by the Society of Actuaries and individual insurance companies. These data are periodically published in the *Transactions of the Society of Actuaries* and should be valuable to the HMO in establishing its own utilization/cost rates. One approach to HMO rate making for physicians' services and other ambulatory care could be the use of manual rates and the basic tables from commercial insurance, adjusting the rates to HMO operations and experience. This adjustment (yearly) may be performed following this formula:

$$\frac{\text{Local total fee-for-service charges per specialty}}{\text{Local total number of office visits per specialty}} \times \frac{\text{HMO prototype office visit incidence per specialty}}{\text{Office visit incidence per specialty for prototype locality}} \times \frac{\text{Office visit incidence per specialty in HMO's area}}{12} = \frac{\text{Rate per specialty}}{}$$

A second adjustment could then be made to load or discount, based on the experience or projected use of broad classes of enrollees. Factors that will affect the manual rates, for which adjustments must be made, include age, sex, income, occupational hazards, locality, the secular trend of general increases in costs, size of group, and dependent coverage. The HMO should anticipate increases in medical-care costs and should increase premium rates by an inflationary factor.

It is likely that some larger, well-established HMOs have developed rate manuals that are used in the establishment of premium rates. The basis for the development of such manuals for the Oregon region of the Kaiser Foundation Health Plan were reported by Greenlick et al. as "a method of studying the factors which determine medical-care utilization for various types of morbidity."[22] The well-structured study used both the California Relative Value Study and the *International Classification of Diseases, Adapted for Indexing of Hospital Records* as coding systems for time, place, type of service, type of provider, symptoms, episodes, content of visit, and diagnosis of the presenting morbidity and all associated diseases. The tables generated from the study sample of enrollees provide the frequency and percentage distribution of 33 classifications of diseases in physician clinic visits and cross tabulations between health care services for these disease categories and age, sex, occupation, and religious preference. By adding cost factors to these data, a manual of rates can be developed.[23]

THE PRAGMATIC APPROACH

Kress and Singer report a simple approach to the development of the capitation rate. Assuming a breakeven population of 20,000 to 25,000 enrollees, a ratio of one physician for each 1,100 enrollees becomes the proxy indicator for the capitation rate. At this staffing level, physician income and fringe benefits "will equal the sum of all other operating expenses of its medical group."[24] The capitation rate is computed by the following formula:

$$\frac{\text{Average physician income}}{1,100} \times 2 = \text{Capitation rate}$$

To this rate should be added a hospitalization cost and an administra-

[22]Merwyn R. Greenlick et al. "Determinants of Medical Care Utilization." *Health Services Research*:296–315, Winter 1968.

[23]Please see the studies completed by Joel W. Kovner, reviewed by Don Strope, Bonnie Cohen, and Ann Yonkers in *Increasing Productivity in the Delivery of Ambulatory Health Services: A Review of Literature and On-Going Projects*. Rockville, Md., Office of the Secretary, U.S. Department of Health, Education, and Welfare, 1968, pp. 40–49.

[24]John R. Kress and James Singer. *HMO Handbook*. Rockville, Md., Aspen Systems Corporation, 1975, pp. 121–122.

tive cost to produce the total capitation rate. Hospitalization costs can be based on estimated days per 1,000 enrollees multiplied by a per diem cost. Administrative costs usually range from 5 to 10 percent of hospital and physician service costs. Naturally, the capitation rate developed by using this method should be adjusted to reflect major differences in the characteristics of groups of subscribers. A premium rate is thus developed by making such adjustments to the capitation rate. In general, this method is useful to new HMOs with little or no experience concerning how services are used by their subscribing groups, and it requires no actuarial estimates. But, because of its simplicity, it may provide a false sense of appropriateness when, in fact, rates developed by the method may not reflect actual variations in costs and revenues that might be identified by other methods.

TRADITIONAL, STANDARD, OR BUDGETARY APPROACH

The budgetary approach is used when the medical group is engaged completely in prepaid operations. The major source of revenues is the annual or monthly collection of premiums. Any income from fee-for-service operations is either totally absent or is inconsequential. The following steps illustrate this method:[25]

1. Determine the level of membership to be served—a membership level that will permit the HMO to break even. This level is equivalent to that for which the facility and program were designed so that the greatest contribution to fixed costs can be made.

    a. Determine the size of the potential market and the expected penetration levels of each component of that market

    b. Determine the availability of resources: manpower, equipment, and capital

    c. Determine the optimal size of the facility

2. Develop a set of planning assumptions.

    a. Utilization rates: physician services, laboratory tests, X-ray examinations per enrollee per year

    b. Staffing ratios: physicians, nurses, and other health personnel per fixed number of enrollees

3. Convert planning assumptions into an expense budget by developing cost estimates for five broad categories of health-center opera-

---

[25]Birnbaum. *Prepayment and Neighborhood Health Centers*, pp. 29–36.

tions at a breakeven level of membership (i.e., at the membership level where capitation income will equal costs).

    a. Salaries and wages
    b. Supplies
    c. Outside services
    d. Overhead (including depreciation, expansion, and capital acquisition costs)
    e. Administration

    4. Convert the expense budget into a capitation rate by determining how much money is required per enrollee to support the facility. Essentially, this is accomplished by dividing the expense budget by the number of enrollees. The capitation rate usually is divided by 12 to reflect a monthly breakdown. A more refined approach would be to divide the budgeted costs at the breakeven month by the breakeven membership level.

    5. The capitation rate is adjusted or "loaded" to reflect a variety of factors, including:

    a. Start-up costs
    b. Reinsurance arrangements for initial operating losses incurred before the breakeven membership is reached
    c. Relationship of the capitation to competitive packages in the market
    d. Reinsurance arrangements for special services
    e. Expected revenues from optional benefit charges and copayments
    f. Specific age, health status, social, and mobility characteristics of the enrolled population
    g. Family-loading factor reflecting the difference between those enrollees who are covered and those who actually pay

    The final capitation includes only the cost items calculated before adjusting or loading is done (i.e., before step 5). The premium, thus, would be the rate established by loading or discounting, as described in step 5, and with a cost factor added for hospitalization.

FEE-FOR-SERVICE APPROXIMATION APPROACH[26]

This capitation technique is used when HMO enrollees are incorporated into an existing fee-for-service medical group. The usual breakeven

---

[26]LeCompte. *Prepaid Group Practice*, pp. 2.29–2.34.

enrollment of 20,000 to 30,000 members in a predominantly prepaid situation is missing. Therefore, the provider must absorb prepaid enrollees in a system that has an opposite financial basis, which is accomplished by prorating the operating costs of the fee-for-service system for each prepaid enrollee. The methodology for this approach follows:

1. Determine the utilization rates of the enrolled population. Usually, the utilization characteristics of a newly enrolled prepaid group are unknown, and utilization rates for other prepaid group practices are adopted and adjusted.
2. Determine costs for various services, based on the fee-for-service charge structure of the existing medical group.
3. Develop a capitation per enrollee, based on the above cost and utilization factors.
4. Make final adjustments in accordance with loading factors previously described in step 5 of the budgetary approach, and add a cost factor for hospital use.

ADJUSTMENTS TO THE CAPITATION RATE

Hospital portions of the premium rates for HMOs that use nonplan hospitals may be calculated by using methods developed by the commercial carriers and Blue Cross; these adjustment mechanisms for the "hospitalization" portion of the premium would be useful in the final step of the budgetary and fee-for-service approximation approaches just described. The following example provides another method of projecting inpatient capitation rates.[27]

1. Data from community:
   a. 1,600 days per 1,000 non-HMO (i.e., BC) subscribers = A
   b. 950 days per 1,000 non-HMO (i.e., BC) subscribers' dependents = B
   c. Family size of 2.8 members = C
   d. 600,000 subscriber contract months of exposure to risk = D
   e. 400,000 dependent contract months of exposure to risk = E

2. Assumption:
   HMO will realize 700 inpatient days per 1,000 enrollees = F

[27]Ronald Becker. Appendix II to *Prepaid Group Practice,* by Roger B. LeCompte, pp. 2.55–2.66.

3. Solve for R = reduction factor because of HMO delivery system:

$$\frac{(D \times A \times R) + (E \times C \times B \times R)}{D + (E \times C)} = F$$

$$\frac{(600{,}000 \times 1{,}600 \times R) + (400{,}000 \times 2.8 \times 950 \times R)}{600{,}000 + (400{,}000 \times 2.8)} = 700$$

R = .8405

4. Rates for inpatient care can then be calculated:

		Subscriber		Dependent
Incidence		.15		.30
Length of stay	×	9.60	×	8.30
Reduction factor	×	.8405	×	.8405
Days per contract		1.21032		2.10
Per diem cost	×	$153.00	×	$140.00
Cost per contract		185.18		293.00
	÷	12	÷	12
Net monthly cost		15.44		24.42
Administrative loading	÷	.90	÷	.92
Gross monthly costs		$17.15		$26.54

5. Assumptions:

   a. Rate of incidence of inpatient care for the subscriber is .15 per year and .30 for his dependents per year.

   b. Length of stay for subscriber is 9.60 days per incident and 8.30 days per incident for dependents.

   c. Per diem cost of inpatient care is $153 for the subscriber and $140 for dependents.

The rates developed in the example would then be included in the capitation rates for the other medical-care services. Note that other in-hospital medical-care services (i.e., maternity, surgery, obstetric care) also might be logically adjusted by using the same method.

In the section of this chapter on benefit package design, several packaging systems (individual; individual plus spouse; individual, spouse, and one child; and so on) were described. Premiums are adjusted for each of these packages, using one of several available mechanisms. The simplest approach to adjusting the crude capitation rate to reflect composition of the population and risks is described as a "straight-rate system." No loading or discounting is used in the straight-rate system; thus, the base capitation rate is multiplied by the

TABLE 48   Simple Adjustment Methods

	Class of Enrollment			
	Individual	Individual + 1	Individual + 2	Family (Multiple Child)
Straight rate	1 X	2 X	3 X	N X
Two-step	1 X	2 X	2 X	2 X
Three-step	1 X	2 X	3 X	3 X
Three-step discounted	1 X	2 X	2.75 X	2.75 X
Three-step loaded	1 X	2 X	3.5 X	3.5 X

number of individuals to be covered by the contract. An individual's premium would be multiplied by 1, individual and spouse by 2, family with one child by 3, and so on, in a step-wise expansion of the base rate. A two-step system would assign the base rate to an individual and 2 times the base rate to an individual plus family. Another method used is described as a three-step system (times 1 for individual, times 2 for two-person families, and times 3 for families with more than two persons). Discounting, then, is accomplished by multiplying the base rate by less than 1 for each additional family member included in the family policy (i.e., the multiplier for a family with one child might be 2.75 rather than 3). Likewise, loading is accomplished by increasing the base rate by more than 1 times the base for each additional family member, as illustrated in Table 48.

Capital

Capital financing has generally been recognized as one of the critical considerations in HMO development. The private financial community, whose job essentially is to carefully evaluate risk and then to make an investment decision, has not especially welcomed potential HMO sponsors with open arms. As cold as this seems, it serves a very useful purpose. Not only does it protect the limited assets and profits of the financial organization, it protects the consumer—under a free-enterprise system—from the penalties of extremely high business bankruptcy and oversaturation and helps promote those ventures that can clearly demonstrate potential viability. Therefore, would-be HMO sponsors must learn about the needs and attitudes of the financial community and then present a well-prepared proposal that can compete with numerous other contenders for the same funds.

NEED FOR CAPITAL

Establishing an HMO requires a significant amount of capital. Gintzig and Shouldice,[28] through a financial analysis of three prepaid group practice plans established between 1964 and 1971, found that the overall costs ranged from a minimum of $4 million to a maximum of nearly $6 million. These total costs were allocated among the following:

1. Capital for construction or acquisition of facilities
2. Capital for research and development of the formal structure of the plan—$95,000 to $250,000
3. Capital for start-up operating costs—$75,000 to $100,000
4. Capital to underwrite possible operating and/or insurance losses

The Nixon Administration, in developing their original HMO appropriation proposals, reportedly used the following estimates:

For group practices serving a general population, planning costs are estimated between $100,000 and $300,000 with initial operating costs (deficit) estimated at approximately $2 million; for group practices serving poorer areas, planning costs are estimated between $300,000 and $500,000 and initial operating costs (deficit) between $2 million and $3 million. Capital funds (not including facilities) are estimated at approximately $1.5 million for both categories. For medical care foundations, the pre-operational planning costs are estimated between $50,000 and $150,000. These allocations combine to a range of $3.6 to $5.0 million.[29]

SOURCES OF CAPITAL

When considering and evaluating private sources of capital for HMOs, sponsors must remember that, with the exception of philanthropic foundations, nearly all potential financiers are motivated primarily by one thing—profit. Therefore, to appeal to them only on the basis of social need or participation in a national priority program is naive. In

[28]Leon Gintzig and Robert G. Shouldice. "Prepaid Group Practice: An Analysis as a Delivery System" Washington, D.C., The George Washington University, 1972, pp. 8–10. Mimeographed.
[29]Faith B. Rafkind. *Health Maintenance Organizations: Some Perspectives.* Chicago, Blue Cross Association, 1972, p. 128.

addition, sponsors will most likely find it impossible to obtain a commitment from an investor without a specific "deal" in mind—a detailed business plan with pro forma cash flow and profit-loss projections showing specifically how the funds will be used and when and how they will be repaid.[30]

HMO Act: A limited number of grants and loans are available through P.L. 93-222. These are described in Chapter 3.

Commercial Banks:[31] Bank loans frequently are one of the lower cost and more flexible methods of funding capital requirements. New HMO loans, however, generally will be too risky to make without some form of guarantee, such as provided in the HMO law. Some banks may experiment with a short- or medium-term loan to provide community support for the venture, or to gain experience themselves, but this should not be assumed.

The kinds of loans commonly made by banks for similar commercial ventures include short-term lines of credit on a yearly basis, term loans for periods of one to five or seven years, and interim financing during facility construction (after construction, the long-term loan normally would be assumed by a savings and loan association, savings bank, or insurance company).

An HMO loan most likely would be handled by bank officers who are familiar with hospital loans. Historically, hospital loans have been a problem for banks, especially in urban areas where hospitals provide a large volume of welfare care. The poor perception of hospital loans is often magnified, because banks must expend considerable effort to learn the peculiarities of hospital financial management.

If the bank approves an HMO loan without a federal loan guarantee, it probably will require a considerable list of covenants. These might include a limitation on additional debt, maintenance of certain working capital and other balance sheet ratios, a pledge of assets (accounts receivable, facilities, inventory), personal loan guarantees of the sponsors, maintenance of compensating demand deposits, and submission

---

[30]Kappa Systems, Inc. "An Evaluation of Private Sector Interests in the Development of HMOs." Arlington, Va., 1973, pp. 7–11. Unpublished contract study prepared for the U.S. Department of Health, Education, and Welfare.

[31]In part from A. T. Kearney and Co., Inc. "Private Sector Financing and Development of Health Maintenance Organizations." New York, 1973, pp. V-1, V-4–V-15. Unpublished paper prepared for the U.S. Department of Health, Education, and Welfare.

of annual and interim financial statements. Should the borrower violate any of the covenants without the prior knowledge or approval of the bank, the borrower technically is in default.

Banks are more receptive to HMO loans if they are backed by some form of guarantee, but express mixed feelings about many of the existing government loan guarantee programs. They often find the reduced risk an inducement to experiment with new types of loans, but they dislike the delay, red tape, and noncompetitive interest-rate ceilings commonly associated with such programs. They also point out that a guarantee does not automatically make an unsound loan acceptable. What frequently occurs is that banks make loans under federal guarantee programs when the money supply is expanding and loan demand is low, but curtail such loans when demand is high and money is in short supply.

The HMO sponsor should approach the bank loan officer as he would other potential sources of capital, with a well-prepared plan. The plan should include a feasibility study; information on the local market and competition; specific cash flow and loan pay-back projections; background data on the management team; a complete capital structure, including long-, medium-, and short-term needs and anticipated sources; and any other information that might help the bank better understand the proposed project.

Other nonlending aspects of large commercial banks can represent resources for the HMO. These include checking services, computerized payrolls, accounting, billing, or other data-processing services. The bank also may have a trust department or subsidiary venture-capital group willing to make risky investments at high potential rates of return, or a municipal bond department that might underwrite bonds if local or state tax-exempt bonds are approved for HMO financing. New Federal Reserve Board regulations permit bank holding companies to diversify into debt and equity investments in ventures that would aid community or area development. An urban HMO would probably fit that definition, and some big city banks have indicated an interest in the potential of such investments. Finally, banks have been historically generous donors of charitable gifts to qualified community projects, and bank officers might represent a valuable source of board members.

Savings Institutions: Savings banks, savings and loan associations, and other savings institutions have traditionally provided long-term mortgage financing for land and facilities. Some are now expanding the scope of their loans, at least to include interim construction financing, and should be included in the list of potential HMO capital sources.

Investment Bankers: The principal function of investment bankers is to manage issues of equity or long-term debt financing. Most firms work with ongoing businesses, but a few specialize in new ventures. One researcher has concluded that HMOs presently are not suitable for equity financing.[32] Obviously, most are not for profit, and those that are designed for profit are viewed as high-risk but low-return ventures. Debt financing through bond issues therefore appears to be a more promising avenue, but only a limited market at best exists for high-risk bonds.[33] Bond investors generally want safety of principal and a moderate interest return, while stock investors more often will risk depreciation of principal for a probability of appreciation of principal.

Insurance Companies: Major insurance companies that sell health insurance, including Blue Cross, are already highly knowledgeable about HMOs. The smaller companies generally have not experimented with HMOs and are adopting a wait-and-see attitude, which probably will not change until profit potential is clarified after several years of experience by the larger firms. At present, major insurance companies are the best-qualified financing sources to assess the feasibility of an HMO venture—they know hospitals, physicians, health insurance customers, and the legislative and regulatory climate. They have experienced actuaries to examine risks, pricing, and benefit packages.

There are several reasons why major insurance companies are actively interested in HMOs:[34]

1. Health insurance has been declining in profitability recently.

2. Health insurance generates a large premium volume; major health insurers, especially Blue Cross, have a lot to lose if the nature of the business changes dramatically. Basically, many of them want to maintain participation in a development that may have a profound impact on their own future.

3. Some insurance companies foresee a potential for substantial profits from services related to HMOs—the sale of marketing services, management services, actuarial services, and claims processing. HMOs will require insurance for excess risk protection and out-of-area benefit coverage.

[32]*Ibid.,* p. V-2.
[33]*Ibid.,* p. V-18.
[34]*Ibid.,* pp. V-2, V-21–V-25.

Insurance company financing may be available in several forms, including initial working capital, mortgage money for construction, and guarantees to cover operating losses for a specified number of years. When approaching insurance companies for capital financing, the HMO sponsor should remember several points. Insurance companies must be able to earn a profit on their investment; they probably have a stake in the health insurance business; and retail insurance companies are sometimes prone to invest in deals that are philanthropic and that might improve their public image in the community.

Pension and Welfare Trust Funds: A limited amount of such funds has been invested in HMO development by union-sponsored plans. Normally, however, HMO loans are too high a risk to place them in a significant position in the portfolios of these trusts.

Major Corporations: Several corporations have examined the HMO business, and some for-profit HMO companies have been founded. Generally, the major national corporations feel that, presently, HMOs do not offer a significant profit potential but they may be useful in containing the company's costs for health insurance benefits for its employees. From this viewpoint, some companies have reportedly assisted fledgling HMOs in small towns where they have plants, to help provide adequate employee medical care and to contain the company's costs on this fringe benefit.

Charitable Foundations:[35] Several large foundations have made demonstration grants to help develop HMOs and, perhaps, now are waiting to evaluate the success of these ventures. Foundations are interested in demonstration projects only as a means to test new concepts and are not interested in supplying funds for ongoing needs. Foundations also have limited resources and typically make demonstration grants in amounts significantly lower than those required by an HMO for start-up capital. Nationwide, the majority of grants are for under $100,000.

If a foundation makes an award to an HMO with the normal I.R.C. 501(c)(4) nonprofit status, the foundation is required to assure a prescribed form of supervision over and responsibility for the way in which grant funds are spent. As a result, most foundations have been hesitant to grant funds to HMOs unless a hospital or other charitable organization with the 501(c)(3) exemption can be the direct recipient of the grant.

[35]*Ibid.*, pp. V-2, V-28–V-31, VI-2–VI-3.

Financial Management

Financial management is a logical place to close a book on the planning, development, and operation of medical group practice and health maintenance organizations. Financial tools allow the manager to evaluate the organization's progress and to recognize its level of success in meeting its objectives. This is especially true in an HMO where—more than in any other health-delivery system—close fiscal management is the key to growth. Three financial tools are essential—the pro forma operating statements and cash flow analyses, the budget, and ratio analysis. All of these can be used to evaluate the potential level of operation during the development activities as well as after operations have begun. Cash flow and cumulative cash flows are most important indicators of current operations and should be positive after the first year or so. Budgets must be used to help set operating levels and then to periodically evaluate the actual levels obtained. Financial ratios and their use in analysis enables rapid and comprehensive digestion of routine financial statements in a minimum amount of time, with a maximum acquisition of useful information. Financial ratios help signal the need for new decisions about significant operational and financial issues and for reevaluation of certain areas of operation.

For HMOs in the early stages of development—from the feasibility study through the breakeven point—the usual techniques of financial analysis do not apply, since the major criterion for financial evaluation of preoperational status is whether there will be sufficient assets to carry the plan through to the breakeven point. Thus, the critical analysis depends on whether the sources of assets (capital, long-term debt, trade credit, gifts, and grants) are large enough to support the operation until revenues are generated from operations and then, together with operating revenues, whether they are large enough to meet cash requirements until breakeven. After breakeven, the normal techniques of analysis can be used (i.e., do revenues cover the expense of operation with adequate surplus or profit?).

Two major indicators of performance during the critical period before breakeven are the following ratios:

1. *Budget to sources of funds* (flow-of-funds analysis): If the budget is less than or equal to the sources of funds, then the plan appears to be adequately funded for the prebreakeven period. A ratio of 1:1 or less (i.e., 0.8:1) would indicate that the plan was satisfactory in this regard.

2. *Financial ratios:* These ratios compare performance to preestablished normative values to determine whether the plans have developed financial programs that allow them sufficient working capital and financial strength to operate. Ratio values for five HMOs that were in

operation for several years are provided in Table 49 and may be of value in establishing benchmark values for the operational stages of HMOs.

TABLE 49   HMO Prototype Ratio Analysis

Ratio Name	Year	CHC	GHA	GHC	CHP	KAI-OAK
		HMO Prototypes				
Current Assets/	1967	4.0	1.9	1.7	3.6	1.04
Current Liabilities	1968	1.6	1.8	1.9	3.0	1.04
	1969	1.6	1.6	1.5	2.2	.93
	1970	0.89	—	1.2	1.3	.97
Acid Test	1967	4.0	1.3	1.5	3.5	—
	1968	1.6	1.5	1.7	2.9	—
	1969	1.6	1.2	1.3	2.1	—
	1970	0.84	—	1.0	1.3	.77
Accounts Receivable	1967	16.0	7.8	15.4	—	29.8
Turnover	1968	8.0	6.5	13.6	6.0	28.2
	1969	10.0	6.7	13.0	6.0	31.3
	1970	11.0	—	14.0	5.0	—
Fixed Assets/	1967	17.0	8.8	2.1	—	2.2
Long-Term Debt	1968	17.0	8.5	1.9	1.7	2.5
	1969	(no debt)	9.2	2.3	5.6	2.7
	1970	4.4	—	1.8	1.1	2.2
Return on Investment	1967	0.09	0.02	0.06	—	—
(percentage)	1968	—	0.02	0.07	0.17	—
	1969	—	0.02	0.07	(−0.06)	—
	1970	—	—	0.05	0.04	—
Accounts Payable/	1967	—	6.4	2.3	6.8	—
Inventory	1968	—	7.7	1.7	7.6	—
	1969	—	8.6	2.3	7.0	—
	1970	—	—	1.8	14.6	—
Debt/Equity	1967	0.04	0.06	0.7	0.3	0.7
	1968	0.04	0.05	0.7	0.2	0.6
	1969	(no debt)	0.06	0.7	0.3	0.9
	1970	0.03	—	1.2	2.2	0.8
Administrative	1967	—	—	0.04	0.01	0.04
Expense/Total Expense	1968	—	—	0.03	0.01	0.04
(percentage)	1969	—	—	0.03	0.01	0.03
	1970	—	—	0.04	0.01	0.03
Profit Margin	1967	0.01	0.01	0.05	0.11	0.02
(percentage)	1968	—	0.01	0.04	0.06	0.01
	1969	—	0.01	0.05	—	—
	1970	—	—	0.04	0.08	—
Bad Debts/Accounts	1967	0.56	0.03	0.08	—	—
Receivable	1968	0.56	0.04	0.08	—	—
(percentage)	1969	0.62	0.04	0.08	—	—
	1970	0.65	—	1.05	—	—

TABLE 49 (continued)

Key: CHC = Community Health Center, Two Harbors, Minnesota
     GHA = Group Health Association, Washington, D.C.
     GHC = Group Health Cooperative of Puget Sound, Seattle, Washington
     GHP = Group Health Plan, St. Paul, Minnesota
     KAI-OAK = Kaiser Foundation Health Plan, Oakland, California
     — = Data not available.

Source: Adapted from Leon Gintzig and Robert G. Shouldice. "Prepaid Group Practice: An Analysis as a Delivery System." Washington, D.C., The George Washington University, 1972, pp. 85–94. Mimeographed.

Summary

Financial management is the administrator's method of bringing together all the components of the health plan and the tools of financial management—budgeting, actuarial analysis, underwriting, cash flow analysis and ratio analysis—which allows the manager to control as well as to evaluate the HMO's activities. Initial activities in the development of a good financial model are described as the financial planning process. Parts of this process, which were described in Chapters 7 and 8 on HMO development and marketing, are tied together in this discussion.

Based on objectives established for the HMO, several financial planning assumptions must be developed for control of risk. These include decisions concerning staffing ratios; assumptions about the level, type, and sharing of risk; projected utilization rates; and assumptions concerning the local levels of morbidity, mortality, and disability. Underwriting rules must be developed to manage risk and govern selection concerning type of group, size of group, industry, composition of the group, location of risk, plan of insurance, cost sharing, and previous coverage and experience of the group.

Several models for financial planning are available. Simple approaches include the facility-focused and the physician-focused models, both of which use a rule-of-thumb ratio of either facility-to-population or physicians-to-population to project the demand and resource requirements of the plan. Because the projections are based on generally accepted but unsubstantiated ratios, the manager must use these approaches with caution. They do provide crude estimates of demand in rural areas where unfulfilled demand is high.

The ambulatory-visit-focused model provides a demand statement of the number of ambulatory visits required by a population through the use of standard visit-to-population ratios. Although it uses rule-of-thumb ratios, these guidelines can be substantially refined. Thus, this method appears to be the basis of a useful model for financial planning.

The most useful models combined the three approaches. One such model is the comprehensive cost/income model, outlined by InterStudy, Inc. and the Division of Health Maintenance Organizations, DHEW. Costs are developed for major expense areas based on ratios. Revenues are then projected, and a funds flow analysis is prepared. A second combination approach is the comprehensive units-of-production model, developed for DHEW by the Boston Consulting Group, Inc. This model fully integrates the marketing aspects of population segmentation and penetration to develop a statement of demand; again, ratios of encounter-to-population are used to complete this first step. Plan capacity (staff, equipment, facilities, supplies) is then matched to the demand statement using consumption rates by resource. The final step is the application of a cost-per-unit of resource and a revenue-per-encounter to project a budget and a cash flow analysis. The model provides a highly sophisticated approach to demand, capacity, and financial estimation, but it also requires substantial data upon which to make these estimates. Because of possible limitations in data, and time and ability of managers to use this model, its usefulness may be clearly limited, although excellent results can be achieved through its use.

A final model, the comprehensive insurance underwriting model, is built around the insurance functions of risk taking, actuarial analysis, incentive/risk-sharing formulas, and rate making. This model, like the units-of-production model, segments the populations chosen and completes estimates of penetration. After data concerning the population are collected, underwriters are asked to analyze the population to determine the risk of providing services. Once risks are calculated that, in effect, describe the types and levels of services that will be required by the enrolled population, financial analysis can be completed on the basis of one of the other models.

In general, each model develops estimates of costs that include medical care, hospitalization, and administration. These costs are compared with revenue that will be generated from several sources—premiums, fees for service, copayments, sales of drugs and supplies, government payments, loans, grants, and so on. Cash flow analysis can then be completed to determine whether the program will be financially feasible. Adjustments are normally required to bring costs and revenues into alignment.

One of the major functions required in the financial planning process is risk management. Underwriting is the activity by which health plans evaluate and determine the risks of accepting populations as group enrollees. Several underwriting rules are followed that help define and place limitations on acceptability of groups, such as the type and size of the group, the industry, composition of the group, location, the plan of insurance, cost sharing, and previous coverage and experience of the group. Underwriting and enrollment of individuals follow more restrictive requirements than for groups because of the greater chance for adverse selection and billing difficulties.

Several mechanisms, in addition to placing restrictions on accepting certain high-risk groups, may be used to control risks. These include reinsurance and limitations on certain coverage, such as catastrophic illnesses, epidemics, or disasters. Good marketing analysis and underwriting (i.e., good management) may be the most important methods for handling risks.

Benefit packages are built around a basic set and an optional set of benefits. Generally, the programs offered to groups of enrollees are tailored to the needs of the group. Exclusions, limitations, and copayments may be included in the policy to limit or control risk and to prevent inappropriate use of services. Through the use of copayments, it is hoped that revenues from this source will help maintain low premium levels and control, to a certain extent, unnecessary utilization of physician services. Three basic models are followed in designing benefit packages—standard and supplementary sets of benefits, a totally custom-made package, and a standard plan to all subscribers.

Pricing of the benefit package (the premium) is traditionally the responsibility of an actuary, although many health maintenance organizations place this responsibility with the chief financial manager or the plan administrator. Rates for services to be included in the benefit package should be established so that the revenue from premiums will adequately cover total costs and allow for a surplus. Rates also must be equitable; in this regard two rate-making systems can be used—community and experience rating. Each system has its advantages and its drawbacks. In using either system, however, certain adjustments may be applied to the intermediate (capitation) rate, with the ultimate effect of adjusting the premium rate to reflect the risk level of the subscriber group.

Several approaches to rate making are used by HMOs. Commercial insurance companies have consistently used the "unit of exposure" approach. This method is built on the development of a manual of premium rates—charges for each benefit unit. Adjustments are then made, based on the experience of the group being underwritten. The "pragmatic approach" simply assumes that, at the breakeven population of 20,000 to 25,000 enrollees and a 1:1,100 physician-to-population ratio, the capitation rate can be found by dividing 1,100 by the average physician income and multiplying by two. A third method, the "traditional, standard, or budgetary approach," follows the financial planning "cost-income" model of identifying the costs of operation at a breakeven enrollment level and essentially dividing the total costs by the total enrollment level, then dividing by 12 to reflect a monthly capitation. Loading of the capitation rate to reflect various differences in groups produces the premium. A final rate-making approach is the "fee-for-service" approximation approach. Utilization rates per subscriber are determined, costs per unit of service are applied, and the capitation is then developed. Adjustments to the capitation produce the premium.

Capital for HMOs is a critical consideration in developing sources, including grants and loans from the federal HMO program, commercial banks, savings institutions, equity or long-term debt financing through bond issues, insurance companies, pension and welfare trust funds, major corporations, and charitable foundations. These sources, however, do not provide easy money to HMOs because of their relatively high risk status and lack of collateral. Well-prepared proposals facilitate the negotiations for funds.

A part of the overall financial management of the health plan is the administrator's use of performance operating statements, cash flow analysis, budgets, and accounting-ratio analysis. All these financial tools help the administrator guide the plan to success.

References

Boston Consulting Group, Inc. *Financial Planning in Ambulatory Health Programs.* Rockville, Md., National Center for Health Services Research and Development, Health Services and Mental Health Administration, U.S. Department of Health, Education, and Welfare, 1973. DHEW Publ. No. (HRA) 74-3027.

Health Insurance Association of America. *Principles of Group Health Insurance I.* Chicago, 1972.

Herbert, Michael E. *A Financial Guide for HMO Planners.* Minneapolis, Minn., InterStudy, 1974.

A. T. Kearney and Co., Inc. "Private Sector Financing and Development of Health Maintenance Organizations." New York, 1973. Unpublished paper prepared for the U.S. Department of Health, Education, and Welfare.

Kress, John R., and Singer, James. *HMO Handbook.* Rockville, Md., Aspen Systems Corporation, 1975, pp. 109–133.

LeCompte, Roger B. *Prepaid Group Practice: A Manual.* Chicago, Blue Cross Association, 1972, Chapter 2.

Medical Group Management Association. *Manual on Insurance.* Denver, Colo., 1974, pp. 65–76.

U.S. Department of Health, Education, and Welfare, Health Services and Mental Health Administration, Health Maintenance Organization Service. *Financial Planning Manual.* Rockville, Md., 1972. DHEW Publ. No. (HSM) 73-13007.

HMO Glossary

Actuarial Study—The calculation of risks and premiums and other statistical studies used in insurance underwriting.

Adverse Selection—Some population parameter, such as age (e.g., a much greater number of persons 65 years old or older in proportion to younger persons), that increases the potential for higher utilization than budgeted and increases costs above those covered by the capitation rate.

Algorithm—*See* **Protocol.**

Ambulatory Care—*See* **Outpatient Care.**

Assignment—(Also **Authorization to Pay Benefits**) A statement, usually included on a claim form, which permits the insured to authorize the insurance company to pay benefits directly to the provider of the services.

Authorization to Pay Benefits—*See* **Assignment.**

Beneficiary—(*See also* **Enrollee, Member;** also **Eligible Individual, Participant**) Any person eligible as either a subscriber or a dependent for service in accordance with a contract.

Benefit Package—A listing of specific services provided or assured by the HMO to enrollees.

Benefits—Specific areas of plan coverages or services provided, such as outpatient visits and hospitalization, that make up the range of medical services marketed by an HMO to its subscribers.

Blue Cross—A hospital insurance plan that provides benefits covering specified hospital-related services and pays member hospitals directly for services rendered.

Blue Laws—Medical and hospital service corporation laws that were originally enacted to regulate Blue Cross and Blue Shield plans. Under certain conditions, they may be used to describe the corporate form for an HMO or, in some states, may provide a mandatory form of incorporation. They generally are considered to limit the flexibility of the HMO organizational structure.

Blue Shield—A medical service insurance plan that provides benefits covering specific physician-rendered services and pays either the physician or patient.

345

Capitation/Capitation Fee/Capitation Payment—(Also **Per Capita**) The amount of money required per person by a health care vendor (or health insurance organization) to provide (insure) covered services to a person for a specific time (usually per month).

Carrier—An insurer; an underwriter of risk.

Case Unit Cost—An average cost for the treatment of illness usually derived by using the California Relative Value Study and making adjustment for the particular area.

Cash Indemnity Benefits—Amounts paid to the insured after he has received and filed a claim for a service. Such benefits may be received directly or may be assigned to the provider of service (e.g., the doctor) by the insured.

Certificate Holder—*See* **Subscriber.**

Clinic—(Also **Health Center**) A facility for the provision of preventive, diagnostic, and treatment services to ambulatory patients, in which patient care is under the professional supervision of persons licensed to practice medicine in the political jurisdiction where the facility is located.

Closed-Panel Practice—The group practice of medicine in which admission to the group is controlled by the group membership. Medical group practices are closed-panel practices versus IPAs and foundations, which are open to all members of the medical society and, thus, are open-panel practices.

Coinsurance—Policy provision under which insured pays or shares part of medical bill, usually according to a fixed percentage. Major medical expense policies usually provide for coinsurance, deductibles, and corridors. Coinsurance in most instances is 20 to 25 percent of amount deemed eligible for major medical benefits.

Community Corporation—An organization that has been developed by a community interest group or that provides for meaningful community input through board participation or input to the board.

Community-Rated Premium—The practice by some prepayment plans whereby net rates or premiums for plan subscribers are reasonably uniform and not dependent on individual claim experience or the experience of any one group. (For contrast, *see* **Experience-Rated Premium.**)

Community Rating—The rating system by which a plan or an indemnity carrier takes the total experience of the subscribers and uses this to determine a capitation rate that is common for all groups regardless of the individual claims experience of any one group.

Community-Wide Plans—Those in which the membership is open to qualified groups or individuals in the community, rather than limited to members of specified unions or employees of specified industries.

Composite Rating—A method of developing a rate structure in which the capitation rates for single and single/spouse member units include some of the medical care costs developed for a family unit. Composite rating also makes possible the development of rates for families of more than four people.

Comprehensive Benefits, Insurance Industry—Includes under one policy, in addition to the basic benefits, some or all of the following services outside the hospital: diagnostic services, preventive services, treatment in doctor's office or patient's home, and so forth. Used sometimes synonymously with "Major Medical Expense Benefits."

Comprehensive Care—Provision of a broad spectrum of health services, including physicians' services and hospitalization, that are required to prevent, diagnose, and treat physical and mental illnesses and to maintain health.

Comprehensive Medical Care Plans—Plans providing a wide range of care, including physicians' services in the home, in the office or clinic, and in the hospital. The benefits typically include hospitalization.

Contract Group—(*See also* **Enrolled Group**) A specific group of persons who are to be provided a particular program of benefits (e.g., a union local; a co-op group; federal employees).

Contributory—A term used to describe a group insurance plan under which the insured (subscriber) shares in the cost of the plan with the policyholder (in the HMO field, normally an employer).

Conversion Privilege—The provision that allows a member enrolled through a group to convert, regardless of age or physical condition, to a direct-pay program at the time of retirement or other separation from the group.

Copayment—A payment by the insured of a fee per day or per service specified within a contractual agreement and in addition to an insurance premium.

Cost Centers—Functional areas that generate the basic costs incurred in providing the plan's range of benefits.

Coverage—In general, the services or benefits provided, arranged, or paid for through a health insurance plan (a package of specified benefits); or the people eligible for care under such a plan.

Deductibles—Amounts required to be paid by the insured under a health insurance contract, before benefits become payable (similar to waiting periods of cash sickness insurance). Intended as a deterrent to overuse. In some major medical expense insurance, it is the difference between cost for service (e.g., $100 for a private hospital room) and fixed benefits by the carrier (e.g., $50 or $75 toward the private room cost).

Dependents—Generally the spouse and children, as defined in a contract, of a person or subscriber covered by a health insurance plan. Under some contracts, coverage may include parents and others.

Direct Payment Subscribers—(Also **Individual Coverage**) Persons enrolled in a prepayment plan who make individual premium payments directly to the plan rather than through a group. Rates of payment are generally higher and benefits may not be as extensive as for the subscriber enrolled and paying as a member of a group.

Direct Service Benefits—*See* **Service Benefits.**

Direct Service Plan—*See* **Group Health Plan.**

Dual Choice—(Also **Multiple Choice**) An option offered individuals in a group; the choice between two or more different arrangements for prepaying medical care, that is, indemnity insurance versus a group health plan.

Eligible Individual—*See* **Beneficiary.**

Emergency Care Benefits—Benefits for care received from nonplan doctors and nonplan facilities in the event of accident or emergency illness, whether in or out of the plan's service area.

Enrolled Group—(*See also* **Contract Group**) A group of persons with the same employer or with membership in common in an organization, who are enrolled in a health plan. Usually there are stipulations regarding the minimum size of the group and the minimum percentage of the group that must enroll before the coverage is available.

Enrollee—(*See also* **Beneficiary, Member;** also **Eligible Individual, Participant**) Any person eligible for service, as either a subscriber or a dependent, in accordance with a contract.

Enrollment—The process by which an individual becomes a subscriber for himself and/or his dependents for coverage in a health plan. This may be done either through an actual signing up of the individual, or by virtue of his collective bargaining agreement on his employer's conditions of employment. The result, therefore, is that the health plan is aware of its entire population of beneficiary eligibles. As a usual practice, it is incumbent on the individual to notify the health plan of any changes in family status that affect enrollment of dependents.

Expense Ratio—Ratio of HMO total expenses to earned premiums.

Experience-Rated Premium—A premium that is based on the anticipated claims experience of, or utilization of service by, a contract group according to its age, sex constitution, and any other attributes expected to affect its health services utilization, and that is subject to periodic adjustment in line with actual claims or utilization experience. (For contrast, *see* **Community-Rated Premium.**)

Experience Rating—A rating system by which a plan determines the capitation rate by the experience of the individual group enrolled. Each group will have a different capitation rate based on utilization. This system tends to increase the premiums required of small groups with high utilization.

Fee for Service—With respect to the physician or other supplier of service, this refers to payment of specific amounts for specific services rendered on a service unit basis— as opposed to retainer, salary, or other contract arrangements. In relation to the patient, it refers to payment in specific amounts for specific services received on a service unit basis, in contrast to the advance payment of an insurance premium or membership fee for coverage under which the services or payment to the supplier are provided.

Fee Schedule—A listing of accepted fees or established allowances for specified medical procedures. As used in medical care plans, it usually represents the maximum amounts the program will pay for the specified procedures.

FEHBP—Federal Employees Health Benefits Plan, also referred to as Federal Employees Plan or FEP.

Fixed Costs—Costs that do not change with fluctuations in enrollment or in utilization of services.

Foundation/Foundation for Medical Care—(*See also* **Individual Practice Association**) An association of physicians that organizes and develops a management and fiscal structure and sets a fee schedule for individual physicians who join the foundation. Foundations usually market the plan to subscribers, provide peer review, arrange claims payments, and set rates for subscribers.

Group Health Plan—(Also **Direct Service Plan, Group Practice Prepayment Plan, Prepaid Care Plan**) A plan that provides health services to persons covered by a prepayment program through a group of physicians usually working in a group clinic or center.

Group Practice—(Also **Medical Group Practice**) The definition adopted by the American Medical Association and most commonly used is ''Group medical practice is the application of medical service by a number of physicians working in systematic association with the joint use of equipment and technical personnel and with centralized administration and financial organization.'' (For contrast, *see* **Solo Practice.**)

Group Practice Prepayment Plan—*See* **Group Health Plan.**

Health and Welfare Fund—*See* **Welfare Fund.**

Health Center—*See* **Clinic.**

Health Plan—*See* **Group Health Plan.**

HMO—(Health Maintenance Organization) The term is specifically defined in the Health Maintenance Act of 1973 (P.L. 93-222) and its amendments (P.L. 94-460) as a legal entity or organized system of health care that provides directly or arranges for a comprehensive range of basic and supplemental health care services to a voluntarily enrolled population in a geographic area on a primarily prepaid and fixed periodic basis.

HMOS—Health Maintenance Organization Service of the Department of Health, Education, and Welfare. This service is now titled the Office of Health Maintenance Organizations (DHEW). HMOS is used in this text to refer to the federal DHEW agency responsible for HMO activities (see p. 62).

Hospital Affiliation—Hospitals with which the plan contracts to provide the hospital benefits of the plan.

Incentives—As related to medical-care delivery, this term refers to economic incentives for hospitals by means of third-party reimbursement formulas to motivate efficiency in management; or economic incentives for physicians that encourage decreased hospital utilization, promote judicious use of all resources, and increase delivery of preventive health services.

Indemnify—To compensate for damages, loss sustained, or expense incurred; to recompense for hardship.

Indemnity—Protection or security against damages or loss. Benefits are in the form of cash payments rather than services.

Indemnity Carrier—Usually an insurance company or insurance group that provides marketing, management, claims payment and review, and agrees to assume risk for its subscribers at some predetermined level.

Indemnity Health Insurance—(*See* **Indemnity Plan**)

Indemnity Plan—(Also **Indemnity Health Insurance**) A plan that reimburses physicians for services performed, or beneficiaries for medical expenses incurred. Such plans are contrasted with group health plans, which provide service benefits through group medical practice. (For contrast, *see* **Service Plan**.)

Individual Coverage—*See* **Direct Payment Subscribers**.

Individual Practice Association (IPA)—(*See also* **Foundation/Foundation for Medical Care**) A medical management organization engaged in arranging for the coordinated delivery of all or part of health care services to members enrolled in an HMO. The IPA enters into a service arrangement with persons licensed to provide health services who are practicing on an individual basis rather than on a group or salaried basis.

Inpatient Care—Care given a registered bed patient in a hospital, nursing home, or other medical or psychiatric institution.

IPA—*See* **Individual Practice Association**.

Loading—(*See also* **Risk Load**) Used, in conjunction with discounting, to adjust rates for individuals and groups. Loading is an integral part of experience rating but is not used in community rating. A factor that is multiplied into the rate to offset some adverse parameter in the group to which the HMO is delivering care, the risk load provides more money in reserves to offset expected deficits.

Loss Ratio—Ratio of HMO actual incurred expenses to total premiums; the relationship between money paid out for service and the amount collected in premiums.

Manual Rates—Commercial insurer's standard rate tables included in its rate manual or underwriter's manual and used to develop premium rates.

Medical Group—(*Also* **Medical Group Practice**) A group of physicians organized to provide medical services to members of a group health plan under a specified contract. Medical group in prepaid group practice includes a broad range of medical specialties, with capability for meeting most needs for medical diagnosis and treatment, including both primary care and specialty care (with the ability to purchase service beyond its capabilities on a fee-for-service basis); operates under common employment, or with a common financial interest, under a capitation arrangement or some system for payment other than fee for service; has available group offices and facilities, equipment, and the services of paramedical personnel and nonmedical assistance; and has responsibility for the care of a defined group of enrolled participants.

Medical Group Practice—*See* **Group Practice, Medical Group**.

Member—(*See also* **Beneficiary**) Individual enrolled for health care or benefits under a contract.

Multiple Choice—*See* **Dual Choice.**

Network—An arrangement of several delivery points (i.e., medical group practices) affiliated with a prepaid health plan/HMO; an arrangement of HMOs (either autonomous and separate legal entities, or subsidiaries of a large corporation) using one common insuring mechanism such as Blue Cross/Blue Shield; a broker organization (health plan) that arranges with physician groups, carriers, payer agencies, consumer groups, and others for services to be provided to enrollees.

Noncontributory Arrangement—An arrangement under which the employer, union, or other third party pays the full premium.

Nonprofit Plan—A term applied to a prepaid health plan under which no part of the net earnings accrues, or may lawfully accrue, to the benefit of any private shareholder or individual.

Office Visit—A formal face-to-face contact between the physician and the patient in a health center, office, or hospital outpatient department.

Open Enrollment—A period during which subscribers in a dual choice (see definition) health benefit program have an opportunity to select the alternate health plan being offered to them. Most frequently, open enrollment periods are negotiated and held for one month every one or two years.

Open-Panel Practice—*See* **Closed-Panel Practice.**

Out-of-Area Benefits—Those benefits that the plan supplies to its subscribers when they are outside the geographical limits of the HMO. These benefits usually include emergency care benefits and stipulate that within-the-area services for emergency care will be provided until the subscriber can be returned to the plan for medical management of the case.

Outpatient Care—Care given a person who is not bedridden (i.e., hospitalized).

Participant—*See* **Beneficiary.**

Per Capita—*See* **Capitation/Capitation Fee/Capitation Payment.**

Physician's Services—Services involving a face-to-face contact with a physician.

Plan—*See* **Group Health Plan.**

Plan Administration—The management unit with responsibility to run and control the HMO plan—includes accounting, billing, personnel, marketing, legal services, purchasing, possibly underwriting, management information, facility maintenance, servicing of accounts. This group normally contracts for medical services and hospital care.

Plan Sponsorship—The group that organizes the plan, finances its facilities, and/or makes up its governing board.

Policyholder—Under a group purchase plan, the policyholder is the employer, labor union, or trustee to whom a group contract is issued and in whose name a policy is written. In a plan contracting directly with the individual or family, the policyholder is the individual to whom the contract is issued.

Preexisting Condition—A physical condition of an insured person that existed prior to the issuance of his policy or his enrollment in a plan, and that may result in a limitation in the contract on coverage or benefits.

Premium—A prospectively determined rate that a subscriber pays for specific health services. Generally, a comprehensive prepaid health plan will have a premium rate for single subscribers with dependents. In addition, separate premium rates may be established for optional health care coverage. It cannot be assumed that the premium for a family is a multiple of the individual rate.

Prepaid Care Plan—*See* **Group Health Plan.**

Prepaid Group Practice—Prepaid group practice plans involve multispecialty associations of physicians and other health professionals who contract to provide a wide range of preventive, diagnostic, and treatment services on a continuing basis for enrolled participants.

Prepaid Individual Practice—(*See also,* **Foundation/Foundations for Medical Care, Individual Practice Association**) Plans that use the services of individual solo physicians in their private offices. Most of these plans are included under the category of Foundations for Medical Care.

Prepayment—A method of providing in advance for the cost of predetermined benefits for a population group, through regular periodic payments in the form of premiums, dues, or contributions, including those contributions that are made to a health and welfare fund by employers on behalf of their employees.

Primary Care—Professional and related services administered by an internist, family practitioner, obstetrician/gynecologist, or pediatrician in an ambulatory setting, with referral to secondary care specialists as necessary.

Professional Standards Review Organization (PSRO)—Organization mandated by P.L. 92-603 through which practicing physicians assume responsibility for health care services in the local region.

Protocol—A decision tree which describes a course of treatment or established practice patterns.

Provider—A person or organization providing health care services.

Reciprocity—The right of a member of a group health plan, temporarily away from home, to receive necessary medical care from a group health plan in the area where he is a visitor.

Reinsurance—The dividing of risk through transfer of a portion of the risk of one carrier insurance company or other third party to another organization, company, or group. Reinsurance may also be used by carriers in lessening risks of catastrophic losses to health insurance plans.

Reserves—A fiscal method of withholding a certain percentage of premiums to provide a fund for committed but undelivered health care and such uncertainties as higher hospital utilization levels than expected, overutilization of referrals, accidental catastrophies, and the like.

Risk—Any chance of loss; or the possibility that revenues of the HMO will not be sufficient to cover expenditures incurred in the delivery of contractual services.

Risk Control Insurance—*See* **Stop Loss.**

Risk Load—(*See also* **Loading**) A factor that is multiplied into the rate to offset some adverse parameter in the group.

Self-Administered Plan—A plan administered by the employer or welfare fund without recourse to an intermediate insurance carrier. Some benefits may be insured or subcontracted while others are self-insured.

Service Area—The geographic area covered by the plan, within which it provides direct service benefits.

Service Benefits—(Also **Direct Service Benefits**) Benefits provided by the plan itself.

Service Charges—Any extra charges specified in the contract for certain services not fully covered through prepayment.

Service Plan—The plan which provides benefits in the form of medical care and services for a stated premium. (For contrast, *see* **Indemnity Plan.**)

Skilled Nursing Facility (SNF)—A nursing or convalescent home offering skilled nursing care and rehabilitation services.

Solo Practice—Individual practice of medicine by physician who does *not* practice in a group, or share personnel, facilities, or equipment with three or more physicians. (For contrast, *see* **Group Practice.**)

Stop Loss—(Also **Risk Control Insurance**; often incorrectly referred to as **Reinsurance**) Insuring with a third party against a risk that the plan cannot financially and totally manage. For example, a comprehensive prepaid health plan can self-insure hospitalization costs or it can insure hospitalization costs with one or more insurance carriers.

Straight Rating—A single rate multiplied by the total number of people in a family to give the family rate.

Subscriber—(Also **Certificate Holder**) The person in whose name an individual or family certificate is issued. Other family members are "dependents." Note that the subscriber can be, but need not be, the policyholder.

Third-Party Payment—The payment for health care when the beneficiary is not making payment, in whole or in part, in his own behalf.

Token Payment—A partial payment or copayment made for a service or supply item. For example, some comprehensive prepaid health plans charge $1 for each office visit. Sometimes also known as "nominal" or "hesitation" payments.

Transferability—The right of a member of a group health plan who changes his place of residency to receive medical services in a group health plan in his new place of residency, with benefits and obligations as defined under prior agreement between the plans.

Underwriting—The process by which an insurer determines whether or not and on what basis it will accept an application for insurance.

Union-Sponsored Plan—A program of health benefits developed by a union. The union may operate the program directly or may contract for benefits. Funds to finance the benefits are usually paid out of a welfare fund that receives its income from employer contributions, employer and union member contributions, or union members alone.

Utilization—The extent to which a given group uses specified services in a specific period of time. Usually expressed as the number of services used per year per 100 or per 1,000 persons eligible for the services; utilization rates may be expressed in other types of ratios, that is, per eligible person covered.

Voluntarily Enrolled Group—An enrolled group of persons, each of whom has exercised an option to join the program.

Welfare Fund—(Also **Health and Welfare Fund**) A fund into which employer and/or employee contributions for health care are placed and that is administered by a board, usually with equal representation from labor and management. When the welfare fund provides health benefits, it either pays directly, purchases insurance, or provides service benefits.

Working Capital—Refers to an institution's investment in short-term assets—cash, short-term securities, accounts receivable, and inventories. *Gross* working capital is defined as an institution's total current assets. *Net* working capital is defined as current assets minus current liabilities. If the term "working capital" is used without further qualification, it generally refers to net working capital.

Appendix 1

Public Law 93-222
93rd Congress, S. 14
December 29, 1973

An Act

87 STAT. 914

To amend the Public Health Service Act to provide assistance and encouragement for the establishment and expansion of health maintenance organizations, and for other purposes.

Be it enacted by the Senate and House of Representatives of the United States of America in Congress assembled,

SHORT TITLE AND TABLE OF CONTENTS

Health Maintenance Organization Act of 1973.

SECTION 1. This Act, with the following table of contents, may be cited as the "Health Maintenance Organization Act of 1973".

TABLE OF CONTENTS

HEALTH MAINTENANCE ORGANIZATIONS

SEC. 2. The Public Health Service Act is amended by adding after title XII the following new title:

Ante, p. 594.

"TITLE XIII—HEALTH MAINTENANCE ORGANIZATIONS

"REQUIREMENTS FOR HEALTH MAINTENANCE ORGANIZATIONS

"SEC. 1301. (a) For purposes of this title, the term 'health maintenance organization' means a legal entity which (1) provides basic and supplemental health services to its members in the manner prescribed by subsection (b), and (2) is organized and operated in the manner prescribed by subsection (c).

Definition.

26-286 (272) O

354

Basic health services.

"(b) A health maintenance organization shall provide, without limitations as to time or cost other than those prescribed by or under this title, basic and supplemental health services to its members in the following manner:

"(1) Each member is to be provided basic health services for a basic health services payment which (A) is to be paid on a periodic basis without regard to the dates health services (within the basic health services) are provided; (B) is fixed without regard to the frequency, extent, or kind of health service (within the basic health services) actually furnished; (C) is fixed under a community rating system; and (D) may be supplemented by additional nominal payments which may be required for the provision of specific services (within the basic health services), except that such payments may not be required where or in such a manner that they serve (as determined under regulations of the Secretary) as a barrier to the delivery of health services. Such additional nominal payments shall be fixed in accordance with the regulations of the Secretary.

"(2) For such payment or payments (hereinafter in this title referred to as 'supplemental health services payments') as the health maintenance organization may require in addition to the basic health services payment, the organization shall provide to each of its members each health service (A) which is included in supplemental health services (as defined in section 1302(2)), (B) for which the required health manpower are available in the area served by the organization, and (C) for the provision of which the member has contracted with the organization. Supplemental health services payments which are fixed on a prepayment basis shall be fixed under a community rating system.

"(3) The services of health professionals which are provided as basic health services shall be provided through health professionals who are members of the staff of the health maintenance organization or through a medical group (or groups) or individual practice association (or associations), except that this paragraph shall not apply in the case of (A) health professionals' services which the organization determines, in conformity with regulations of the Secretary, are unusual or infrequently used, or (B) any basic health service provided a member of the health maintenance organization other than by such a health professional because it was medically necessary that the service be provided to the member before he could have it provided by such a health

"Health professionals."

professional. For purposes of this paragraph, the term 'health professionals' means physicians, dentists, nurses, podiatrists. optometrists, and such other individuals engaged in the delivery of health services as the Secretary may by regulation designate.

"(4) Basic health services (and supplemental health services in. the case of the members who have contracted therefor) shall within the area served by the health maintenance organization be available and accessible to each of its members promptly as appropriate and in a manner which assures continuity, and when medically necessary be available and accessible twenty-four hours a day and seven days a week. A member of a health maintenance organization shall be reimbursed by the organization for his expenses in securing basic or supplemental health services other than through the organization if it was medically necessary that the services be provided before he could secure them through the organization.

"(c) Each health maintenance organization shall—

"(1) have a fiscally sound operation and adequate provision against the risk of insolvency which is satisfactory to the Secretary;

"(2) assume full financial risk on a prospective basis for the provision of basic health services, except that a health maintenance organization may obtain insurance or make other arrangements (A) for the cost of providing to any member basic health services the aggregate value of which exceeds $5,000 in any year, (B) for the cost of basic health services provided to its members other than through the organization because medical necessity required their provision before they could be secured through the organization, and (C) for not more than 90 per centum of the amount by which its costs for any of its fiscal years exceed 115 per centum of its income for such fiscal year;

· "(3) enroll persons who are broadly representative of the various age, social, and income groups within the area it serves, except that in the case of a health maintenance organization which has a medically underserved population located (in whole or in part) in the area it serves, not more than 75 per centum of the members of that organization may be enrolled from the medically underserved population unless the area in which such population resides is also a rural area (as designated by the Secretary);

"(4) have an open enrollment period of not less than thirty days at least once during each consecutive twelve-month period during which enrollment period it accepts, up to its capacity, individuals in the order in which they apply for enrollment, except that if the organization demonstrates to the satisfaction of the Secretary that—

    "(A) it has enrolled, or will be compelled to enroll, a disproportionate number of individuals who are likely to utilize its services more often than an actuarially determined average (as determined under regulations of the Secretary) and enrollment during an open enrollment period of an additional number of such individuals will jeopardize its economic viability, or

    "(B) if it maintained an open enrollment period it would not be able to comply with the requirements of paragraph (3),
the Secretary may waive compliance by the organization with the open enrollment requirement of this paragraph for not more than three consecutive twelve-month periods and may provide additional waivers to that organization if it makes the demonstration required by subparagraph (A) or (B);

"(5) not expel or refuse to re-enroll any member because of his health status or his requirements for health services;

"(6) be organized in such a manner that assures that (A) at least one-third of the membership of the policymaking body of the health maintenance organization will be members of the organization, and (B) there will be equitable representation on such body of members from medically underserved populations served by the organization;

"(7) be organized in such a manner that provides meaningful procedures for hearing and resolving grievances between the health maintenance organization (including the medical group or groups and other health delivery entities providing health services for the organization) and the members of the organization;

"(8) have organizational arrangements. established in accordance with regulations of the Secretary, for an ongoing quality assurance program for its health services which program (A) stresses health outcomes, and (B) provides review by physicians

87 STAT. 917   Pub. Law 93-222   December 29, 1973

and other health professionals of the process followed in the provision of health services;

"(9) provide medical social services for its members and encourage and actively provide for its members health education services, education in the appropriate use of health services, and education in the contribution each member can make to the maintenance of his own health;

"(10) provide, or make arrangements for, continuing education for its health professional staff; and

"(11) provide, in accordance with regulations of the Secretary (including safeguards concerning the confidentiality of the doctor-patient relationship), an effective procedure for developing, compiling, evaluating, and reporting to the Secretary, statistics and other information (which the Secretary shall publish and disseminate on an annual basis and which the health maintenance organization shall disclose, in a manner acceptable to the Secretary, to its members and the general public) relating to (A) the cost of its operations, (B) the patterns of utilization of its services, (C) the availability, accessibility, and acceptability of its services, (D) to the extent practical, developments in the health status of its members, and (E) such other matters as the Secretary may require.

"DEFINITIONS

"SEC. 1302. For purposes of this title:

"(1) The term 'basic health services' means—

"(A) physician services (including consultant and referral services by a physician);

"(B) inpatient and outpatient hospital services;

"(C) medically necessary emergency health services;

"(D) short-term (not to exceed twenty visits), outpatient evaluative and crisis intervention mental health services;

"(E) medical treatment and referral services (including referral services to appropriate ancillary services) for the abuse of or addiction to alcohol and drugs;

"(F) diagnostic laboratory and diagnostic and therapeutic radiologic services;

"(G) home health services; and

"(H) preventive health services (including voluntary family planning services, infertility services, preventive dental care for children, and children's eye examinations conducted to determine the need for vision correction).

If a service of a physician described in the preceding sentence may also be provided under applicable State law by a dentist, optometrist, or podiatrist, a health maintenance organization may provide such service through a dentist, optometrist, or podiatrist (as the case may be) licensed to provide such service. For purposes of this paragraph, the term 'home health services' means health services provided at a member's home by health care personnel, as prescribed or directed by the responsible physician or other authority designated by the health maintenance organization. A health maintenance organization is authorized, in connection with the prescription of drugs, to maintain, review, and evaluate (in accordance with regulations of the Secretary) a drug use profile of its members receiving such service, evaluate patterns of drug utilization to assure optimum drug therapy, and provide for instruction of its members and of health professionals in the use of prescription and non-prescription drugs.

"(2) The term 'supplemental health services' means—

"(A) services of facilities for intermediate and long-term care;

"(B) vision care not included as a basic health service under paragraph (1)(A) or (1)(H);

"(C) dental services not included as a basic health service under paragraph (1)(A) or (1)(H);

"(D) mental health services not included as a basic health service under paragraph (1)(D);

"(E) long-term physical medicine and rehabilitative services (including physical therapy); and

"(F) the provision of prescription drugs prescribed in the course of the provision by the health maintenance organization of a basic health service or a service described in the preceding subparagraphs of this paragraph.

If a service of a physician described in the preceding sentence may also be provided under applicable State law by a dentist, optometrist, or podiatrist, a health maintenance organization may provide such service through an optometrist, dentist, or podiatrist (as the case may be) licensed to provide such service. A health maintenance organization is authorized, in connection with the prescription or provision of prescription drugs, to maintain, review, and evaluate (in accordance with regulations of the Secretary) a drug use profile of its members receiving such services, evaluate patterns of drug utilization to assure optimum drug therapy, and provide for instruction of its members and of health professionals in the use of prescription and non-prescription drugs.

"(3) The term 'member' when used in connection with a health maintenance organization means an individual who has entered into a contractual arrangement, or on whose behalf a contractual arrangement has been entered into, with the organization under which the organization assumes the responsibility for the provision to such individual of basic health services and of such supplemental health services as may be contracted for.

"(4) The term 'medical group' means a partnership, association, or other group—

"(A) which is composed of health professionals licensed to practice medicine or osteopathy and of such other licensed health professionals (including dentists, optometrists, and podiatrists) as are necessary for the provision of health services for which the group is responsible;

"(B) a majority of the members of which are licensed to practice medicine or osteopathy; and

"(C) the members of which (i) as their principal professional activity and as a group responsibility engage in the coordinated practice of their profession for a health maintenance organization; (ii) pool their income from practice as members of the group and distribute it among themselves according to a prearranged salary or drawing account or other plan; (iii) share medical and other records and substantial portions of major equipment and of professional, technical, and administrative staff; (iv) utilize such additional professional personnel, allied health professions personnel, and other health personnel (as specified in regulations of the Secretary) as are available and appropriate for the effective and efficient delivery of the services of the members of the group; and (v) arrange for and encourage continuing education in the field of clinical medicine and related areas for the members of the group.

"(5) The term 'individual practice association' means a partnership, corporation, association, or other legal entity which has entered into a services arrangement (or arrangements) with persons who are licensed to practice medicine, osteopathy, dentistry, podiatry, optome-

try, or other health profession in a State and a majority of whom are
licensed to practice medicine or osteopathy. Such an arrangement
shall provide—

"(A) that such persons shall provide their professional services
in accordance with a compensation arrangement established by
the entity; and

"(B) to the extent feasible (i) that such persons shall utilize
such additional professional personnel, allied health professions
personnel, and other health personnel (as specified in regulations
of the Secretary) as are available and appropriate for the effective
and efficient delivery of the services of the persons who are parties
to the arrangement, (ii) for the sharing by such persons of medical and other records, equipment, and professional, technical,
and administrative staff, and (iii) for the arrangement and
encouragement of the continuing education of such persons in the
field of clinical medicine and related areas.

"(6) The term 'section 314(a) State health planning agency' means
the agency of a State which administers or supervises the administration of a State's health planning functions under a State plan approved
under section 314(a) (hereinafter in this title referred to as a 'section
314(a) plan'); and the term 'section 314(b) areawide health planning
agency' means a public or nonprofit private agency or organization
which has developed a comprehensive regional, metropolitan, or other
local area plan or plans referred to in section 314(b) (hereinafter in
this title referred to as a 'section 314(b) plan').

"(7) The term 'medically underserved population' means the population of an urban or rural area designated by the Secretary as an area
with a shortage of personal health services or a population group
designated by the Secretary as having a shortage of such services.
Such a designation may be made by the Secretary only after consideration of the comments (if any) of (A) each section 314(a) State
health planning agency whose section 314(a) plan covers (in whole
or in part) such urban or rural area or the area in which such population group resides, and (B) each section 314(b) areawide health
planning agency whose section 314(b) plan covers (in whole or in
part) such urban or rural area or the area in which such population
group resides.

"(8) The term 'community rating system' means a system of fixing
rates of payments for health services. Under such a system rates of
payments may be determined on a per-person or per-family basis and
may vary with the number of persons in a family, but except as otherwise authorized in the next sentence, such rates must be equivalent for
all individuals and for all families of similar composition. The following differentials in rates of payments may be established under such
system:

"(A) Nominal differentials in such rates may be established to
reflect the different administrative costs of collecting payments
from the following categories of members:
"(i) Individual members (including their families).
"(ii) Small groups of members (as determined under regulations of the Secretary).
"(iii) Large groups of members (as determined under regulations of the Secretary).

"(B) Differentials in such rates may be established for members enrolled in a health maintenance organization pursuant to a
contract with a governmental authority under section 1079 or
1086 of title 10, United States Code, or under any other governmental program (other than the health benefits program authorized by chapter 89 of title 5, United States Code) or any health

80 Stat. 1181.
42 USC 246.

80 Stat. 863.

5 USC 8901.

December 29, 1973   Pub. Law 93-222
                                                        87 STAT. 920

benefits program for employees of States, political subdivisions
of States, and other public entities.

"(9) The term 'non-metropolitan area' means an area no part of
which is within an area designated as a standard metropolitan statistical area by the Office of Management and Budget and which does not
contain a city whose population exceeds fifty thousand individuals.

"GRANTS AND CONTRACTS FOR FEASIBILITY SURVEYS

"SEC. 1303. (a) The Secretary may make grants to and enter into
contracts with public or nonprofit private entities for projects for
surveys or other activities to determine the feasibility of developing
and operating or expanding the operation of health maintenance
organizations.

"(b) An application for a grant or contract under this section
shall contain—

"(1) assurances satisfactory to the Secretary that, in conducting surveys or other activities with assistance under a grant or
contract under this section, the applicant will (A) cooperate with
the section 314(b) areawide health planning agency (if any)   80 Stat. 1181;
whose section 314(b) plan covers (in whole or in part) the area   84 Stat. 1304.
for which the survey or other activity will be conducted, and   42 USC 246.
(B) notify the medical society serving such area of such surveys
or other activities; and

"(2) such other information as the Secretary may by regulation prescribe.

"(c) In considering applications for grants and contracts under
this section, the Secretary shall give priority to an application which
contains or is supported by assurances satisfactory to the Secretary
that at the time the health maintenance organization for which such
application or proposal is submitted first becomes operational not less
than 30 per centum of its members will be members of a medically
underserved population.

"(d)(1) Except as provided in paragraph (2), the following limi-   Limitations.
tations apply with respect to grants and contracts made under this
section:

"(A) If a project has been assisted with a grant or contract
under subsection (a), the Secretary may not make any other grant
or enter into any other contract under this section for such project.

"(B) Any project for which a grant is made or contract entered
into must be completed within twelve months from the date the
grant is made or contract entered into.

"(2) The Secretary may make not more than one additional grant
or enter into not more than one additional contract for a project for
which a grant has previously been made or a contract previously
entered into, and he may permit additional time (up to twelve months)
for completion of the project if he determines that the additional
grant or contract (as the case may be), or additional time, or both, is
needed to adequately complete the project.

"(e) The amount to be paid by the United States under a grant
made, or contract entered into, under subsection (a) shall be determined by the Secretary, except that (1) the amount to be paid by the
United States under any single grant or contract for any project may
not exceed $50,000, and (2) the aggregate of the amounts to be paid
by the United States for any project under such subsection under
grants or contracts, or both, may not exceed the greater of (A) 90
per centum of the cost of such project (as determined under regulations of the Secretary), or (B) in the case of a project for a health
maintenahce organization which will serve a medically underserved

population, such greater percentage (up to 100 per centum) of such
cost as the Secretary may prescribe if he determines that the ceiling
on the grants and contracts for such project should be determined by
such greater percentage.

"(f) Payments under grants under this section may be made in
advance or by way of reimbursement and at such intervals and on
such conditions as the Secretary finds necessary.

"(g) Contracts may be entered into under this section without
regard to sections 3648 and 3709 of the Revised Statutes (31 U.S.C.
529; 41 U.S.C. 5).

Post, p.930.

"(h) Payments under grants and contracts under this section shall
be made from appropriations made under section 1309(a).

"(i) Of the sums appropriated for any fiscal year under section
1309(a) for grants and contracts under this section, not less than
20 per centum shall be set aside and obligated in such fiscal year
for projects (1) to determine the feasibility of developing and operating or expanding the operation of health maintenance organizations
which the Secretary determines may reasonably be expected to have
after their development or expansion not less than 66 per centum of
their membership drawn from residents of non-metropolitan areas,
and (2) the applications for which meet the requirements of this title
for approval. Sums set aside in the fiscal year ending June 30, 1974, or
June 30, 1975, for projects described in the preceding sentence but not
obligated in such fiscal year for grants and contracts under this section
because of a lack of applicants for projects meeting the requirements
of such sentence shall remain available for obligation under this section in the succeeding fiscal year for projects other than those described
in clause (1) of such sentence.

"GRANTS, CONTRACTS, AND LOAN GUARANTEES FOR PLANNING AND FOR
INITIAL DEVELOPMENT COSTS

"SEC. 1304. (a) The Secretary may—
    "(1) make grants to and enter into contracts with public or
nonprofit private entities for planning projects for the establishment of health maintenance organizations or for the significant
expansion of the membership of, or areas served by, health maintenance organizations; and
    "(2) guarantee to non-Federal lenders payment of the prin-
cipal of and the interest on loans made to private entities (other
than nonprofit private entities) for planning projects for the
establishment or expansion of health maintenance organizations
to serve medically underserved populations.
Planning projects assisted under this subsection shall include development of plans for the marketing of the services of the health maintenance organization.

"(b)(1) The Secretary may—
    "(A) make grants to and enter into contracts with public or
nonprofit private entities for projects for the initial development
of health maintenance organizations; and
    "(B) guarantee to non-Federal lenders payment of the princi-
pal of and the interest on loans made to any private entity (other
than a nonprofit private entity) for a project for the initial development of a health maintenance organization which will serve a
medically underserved population.

"Initial
development."

"(2) For purposes of this section, the term 'initial development'
when used to describe a project for which assistance is authorized by
this subsection includes significant expansion of the membership of,
or the area served by, a health maintenance organization. Funds under

grants and contracts under this subsection and under loans guaranteed under this subsection may only be utilized for such purposes as the Secretary may prescribe in regulations. Such purposes may include

(A) the implementation of an enrollment campaign for such an organization, (B) the detailed design of and arrangements for the health services to be provided by such an organization, (C) the development of administrative and internal organizational arrangements, including fiscal control and fund accounting procedures, and the development of a capital financing program, (D) the recruitment of personnel for such an organization and the conduct of training activities for such personnel, and (E) the payment of architects' and engineers' fees.

"(3) A grant or contract under this subsection may only be made or entered into for initial development costs in the one-year period beginning on the first day of the first month in which such grant or contract is made or entered into. The number of grants made for any initial development project under this subsection when added to the number of contracts entered into for such project under this subsection may not exceed three. A loan guarantee under this subsection may only be made for a loan (or loans) for such costs incurred in a period not to exceed three years.

"(c)(1) An application for a grant, contract, or loan guarantee under subsection (a) for a planning project shall contain assurances satisfactory to the Secretary that in carrying out the planning project for which the grant, contract, or loan guarantee is sought, the applicant will (A) cooperate with the section 314(b) areawide health planning agency (if any) whose section 314(b) plan covers (in whole or in part) the area proposed to be served by the health maintenance organization for which the planning project will be conducted, and (B) notify the medical society serving such area of the planning project.

80 Stat. 1181;
84 Stat. 1304.
42 USC 246.

"(2) If the Secretary makes a grant or loan guarantee or enters into a contract under subsection (a) for a planning project for a health maintenance organization, he may, within the period in which the planning project must be completed, make a grant or loan guarantee or enter into a contract under subsection (b) for the initial development of that health maintenance organization; but no grant or loan guarantee may be made or contract entered into under subsection (b) for initial development of a health maintenance organization unless the Secretary determines that (A) sufficient planning for its establishment or expansion (as the case may be) has been conducted by the applicant for the grant, contract, or loan guarantee, and (B) the feasibility of establishing and operating, or of expanding, the health maintenance organization has been established by the applicant.

"(d) In considering applications for grants and contracts under this section, the Secretary shall give priority to an application which contains or is supported by assurances satisfactory to the Secretary that at the time the health maintenance organization for which such application is submitted first becomes operational not less than 30 per centum of its members will be members of a medically underserved population.

"(e)(1) Except as provided in paragraph (2), the following limitations apply with respect to grants, loan guarantees, and contracts made under subsection (a) of this section:

Limitations.

"(A) If a planning project has been assisted with grant, loan guarantee, or contract under subsection (a), the Secretary may not make any other planning grant or loan guarantee or enter into any other planning contract for such project under this section.

"(B) Any project for which a grant or loan guarantee is made or contract entered into must be completed within twelve months from the date the grant or loan guarantee is made or contract entered into.

"(2) The Secretary may not make more than one additional grant or loan guarantee or enter into not more. than one additional contract for a planning project for which a grant or loan guarantee has previously been made or a contract previously entered into, and he may permit additional time (up to twelve months) for completion of the project if he determines that the additional grant, loan guarantee, or contract (as the case may be), or additional time, or both, is needed to adequately complete the project.

"(f)(1) The amount to be paid by the United States under a grant made, or contract entered into, under subsection (a) for a planning project, and (except as provided in paragraph (3) of this subsection) the amount of principal of a loan for a planning project which may be guaranteed under such subsection, shall be determined by the Secretary, except that (A) the amount to be paid by the United States under any single grant or contract, and the amount of principal of any single loan guaranteed under such subsection, may not exceed $125,000, and (B) the aggregate of the amounts to be paid for any project by the United States under grants or contracts, or both, under such subsection, and the aggregate amount of principal of loans guaranteed under such subsection for any project, may not exceed the greater of (i) 90 per centum of the cost of such project (as determined under regulations of the Secretary), or (ii) in the case of a project for a health maintenance organization which will serve a medically underserved population, such greater percentage (up to 100 per centum) of such cost as the Secretary may prescribe if he determines that the ceiling on the grants, contracts, and loan guarantees (or any combination thereof) for such project should be determined by such greater percentage.

"(2) The amount to be paid by the United States under a grant made, or contract entered into, under subsection (b) for an initial development project, and (except as provided in paragraph (3) of this subsection) the amount of principal of a loan for an initial development project which may be guaranteed under such subsection, shall be determined by the Secretary; except that the amounts to be paid by the United States for any initial development project under grants or contracts, or both, under such subsection, and the aggregate amount of principal of loans guaranteed under such subsection for any project, may not exceed the lesser of—

"(A) $1,000,000, or

"(B) an amount equal to the greater of (i) 90 per centum of the cost of such project (as determined under regulations of the Secretary), or (ii) in the case of a project for a health maintenance organization which will serve a medically underserved population, such greater percentage (up to 100 per centum) of such cost as the Secretary may prescribe if he determines that the ceiling on the grants, contracts, and loan guarantees (or any combination thereof) for such project should be determined by such greater percentage.

"(3) The cumulative total of the principal of the loans outstanding at any time with respect to which guarantees have been issued under this section may not exceed such limitations as may be specified in appropriation Acts.

"(g) Payments under grants under this section may be made in advance or by way of reimbursement and at such intervals and on such conditions as the Secretary finds necessary.

"(h) Contracts may be entered into under this section without regard to sections 3648 and 3709 of the Revised Statutes (31 U.S.C. 529; 41 U.S.C. 5).

"(i) Payments under grants and contracts under this section shall Post, p. 930. be made from appropriations under section 1309(a).

"(j) Loan guarantees under subsection (a)(2) for planning projects may be made through the fiscal year ending June 30, 1976; and loan guarantees under subsection (b)(1)(B) for initial development projects may be made through the fiscal year ending June 30, 1977.

"(k)(1) Of the sums appropriated for any fiscal year under section 1309(a) for grants and contracts under subsection (a) of this section, not less than 20 per centum shall be set aside and obligated in such fiscal year for projects (A) to plan the establishment or expansion of health maintenance organizations which the Secretary determines may reasonably be expected to have after their establishment or expansion not less than 66 per centum of their membership drawn from residents of non-metropolitan areas, and (B) the applications for which meet the requirements of this title for approval. Sums set aside in the fiscal year ending June 30, 1974, or June 30, 1975, for projects described in the preceding sentence but not obligated in such fiscal year for grants and contracts under subsection (a) of this section because of a lack of applicants for projects meeting the requirements of such sentence shall remain available for obligation under such subsection in the succeeding fiscal year for projects other than those described in clause (A) of such sentence.

"(2) Of the sums appropriated for any fiscal year under section 1309(a) for grants and contracts under subsection (b) of this section, not less than 20 per centum shall be set aside and obligated in such fiscal year for projects (A) for the initial development of health maintenance organizations which the Secretary determines may reasonably be expected to have after their initial development not less than 66 per centum of their membership drawn from residents of non-metropolitan areas, and (B) the applications for which meet the requirements of this title for approval. Sums set aside in the fiscal year ending June 30, 1974, or in either of the next two fiscal years for projects described in the preceding sentence but not obligated in such fiscal year for grants and contracts under subsection (b) of this section because of a lack of applicants for projects meeting the requirements of such sentence shall remain available for obligation under such subsection in the succeeding fiscal year for projects other than those described in clause (A) of such sentence.

"LOANS AND LOAN GUARANTEES FOR INITIAL OPERATION COSTS

"Sec. 1305. (a) The Secretary may—

"(1) make loans to public or nonprofit private health maintenance organizations to assist them in meeting the amount by which their operating costs in the period of the first thirty-six months of their operation exceed their revenues in that period;

"(2) make loans to public or nonprofit private health maintenance organizations to assist them in meeting the amount by which their operating costs, which the Secretary determines are attributable to significant expansion in their membership or area served and which are incurred in the period of the first thirty-six months of their operation after such expansion, exceed their revenues in that period which the Secretary determines are attributable to such expansion; and

"(3) guarantee to non-Federal lenders payment of the principal Non-Federal lenders, guaranteed payment, condition. of and the interest on loans made to any private health maintenance organization (other than a private nonprofit health maintenance organization) for the amounts referred to in paragraph (1) or (2), but only if such health maintenance organization will serve a medically underserved population.

87 STAT. 925

No loan or loan guarantee may be made under this subsection for the operating costs of a health maintenance organization unless the Secretary determines that the organization has made all reasonable attempts to meet such costs.

Limitations.

"(b)(1) Except as provided in paragraph (2), the principal amount of any loan made or guaranteed under subsection (a) in any fiscal year for a health maintenance organization may not exceed $1,000,000 and the aggregate amount of principal of loans made or guaranteed, or both, under this section for a health maintenance organization may not exceed $2,500,000.

"(2) The cumulative total of the principal of the loans outstanding at any time which have been directly made, or with respect to which guarantees have been issued, under subsection (a) may not exceed such limitations as may be specified in appropriation Acts.

Post, p. 930.

"(c) Loans under this section shall be made from the fund established under section 1308(e).

"(d) A loan or loan guarantee may be made under this section through the fiscal year ending June 30, 1978.

"(e) Of the sums used for loans under this section in any fiscal year from the loan fund established under section 1308(e), not less than 20 per centum shall be used for loans for projects (1) for the initial operation of health maintenance organizations which the Secretary determines have not less than 66 per centum of their membership drawn from residents of nonmetropolitan areas, and (2) the applications for which meet the requirements of this title for approval.

"APPLICATION REQUIREMENTS

"SEC. 1306. (a) No grant, contract, loan, or loan guarantee may be made under this title unless an application therefor has been submitted to, and approved by, the Secretary.

"(b) The Secretary may not approve an application for a grant, contract, loan, or loan guarantee under this title unless—

Ante, pp. 920, 921.

"(1) in the case of an application for assistance under section 1303 or 1304, such application meets the application requirements of such section and in the case of an application for a loan or loan guarantee, such application meets the requirements of section 1308;

"(2) he determines that the applicant making the application would not be able to complete the project or undertaking for which the application is submitted without the assistance applied for;

"(3) the application contains satisfactory specification of the existing or anticipated (A) population group or groups to be served by the proposed or existing health maintenance organization described in the application, (B) membership of such organization, (C) methods, terms, and periods of the enrollment of members of such organization, (D) estimated costs per member of the health and educational services to be provided by such organization and the nature of such costs, (E) sources of professional services for such organization, and organizational arrangements of such organization for providing health and educational services, (F) organizational arrangements of such organization for an ongoing quality assurance program in conformity with the

Ante, p.914.

requirements of section 1301(c), (G) sources of prepayment and other forms of payment for the services to be provided by such organization, (H) facilities, and additional capital investments and sources of financing therefor, available to such organization to provide the level and scope of services proposed, (I) administrative, managerial, and financial arrangements and capabilities of such organization, (J) role for members in the planning and policymaking for such organization, (K) grievance procedures for members of such organization, and (L) evaluations of the support for and acceptance of such organization by the population to be served, the sources of operating support, and the professional groups to be involved or affected thereby;

"(4) contains or is supported by assurances satisfactory to the Secretary that the applicant making the application will, in accordance with such criteria as the Secretary shall by regulation prescribe, enroll, and maintain an enrollment of the maximum number of members that its available and potential resources (as determined under regulations of the Secretary) will enable it to effectively serve;

"(5) the section 314(b) areawide health planning agency whose section 314(b) plan covers (in whole or in part) the area to be served by the health maintenance organization for which such application is submitted, or if there is no such agency, the section 314(a) State health planning agency whose section 314(a) plan covers (in whole or in part) such area, has, in accordance with regulations of the Secretary under subsection (c) of this section, been provided an opportunity to review the application and to submit to the Secretary for his consideration its recommendations respecting approval of the application or if under applicable State law such an application may not be submitted without the approval of the section 314(b) areawide health planning agency or the section 314(a) State health planning agency, the required approval has been obtained;

80 Stat. 1181;
84 Stat. 1304.
42 USC 246.

"(6) in the case of an application made for a project which previously received a grant, contract, loan, or loan guarantee under this title, such application contains or is supported by assurances satisfactory to the Secretary that the applicant making the application has the financial capability to adequately carry out the purposes of such project and has developed and operated such project in accordance with the requirements of this title and with the plans contained in previous applications for such assistance; and

"(7) the application is submitted in such form and manner, and contains such additional information, as the Secretary shall prescribe in regulations.

An organization making multiple applications for more than one grant, contract, loan, or loan guarantee under this title, simultaneously or over the course of time, shall not be required to submit duplicate or redundant information but shall be required to update the specifications (required by paragraph (3)) respecting the existing or proposed health maintenance organization in such manner and with such frequency as the Secretary may by regulation prescribe.

Multiple applications.

"(c) The Secretary shall by regulation establish standards and procedures for section 314(b) areawide health planning agencies and section 314(a) State health planning agencies to follow in reviewing and commenting on applications for grants, contracts, loans, and loan guarantees under this title.

"ADMINISTRATION OF ASSISTANCE PROGRAMS

"SEC. 1307. (a)(1) Each recipient of a grant, contract, loan, or loan guarantee under this title shall keep such records as the Secretary shall prescribe, including records which fully disclose the amount and disposition by such recipient of the proceeds of the grant, contract, or

Record-keeping.

Pub. Law 93-222   December 29, 1973
87 STAT. 927

loan (directly made or guaranteed), the total cost of the undertaking in connection with which such assistance was given or used, the amount of that portion of the cost of the undertaking supplied by other sources, and such other records as will facilitate an effective audit.

"(2) The Secretary, or any of his duly authorized representatives, shall have access for the purpose of audit and examination to any books, documents, papers, and records of the recipients of a grant, contract, loan, or loan guarantee under this title which relate to such assistance.

Report to
Secretary of
H.E.W.

"(b) Upon expiration of the period for which a grant, contract, loan, or loan guarantee was provided an entity under this title, such entity shall make a full and complete report to the Secretary in such manner as he may by regulation prescribe. Each such report shall contain, among such other matters as the Secretary may by regulation require, descriptions of plans, developments, and operations relating to the matters referred to in section 1306(b)(3).

Ante, p. 925.

Post, p. 930.

"(c) If in any fiscal year the funds appropriated under section 1309 are insufficient to fund all applications approved under this title for that fiscal year, the Secretary shall, after applying the applicable priorities under sections 1303 and 1304, give priority to the funding of applications for projects which the Secretary determines are the most likely to be economically viable.

"(d) An entity which provides health services to a defined population on a prepaid basis and which has members who are entitled to insurance benefits under title XVIII of the Social Security Act or to medical assistance under a State plan approved under title XIX of such Act may be considered as a health maintenance organization for purposes of receiving assistance under this title if—

79 Stat. 291;
86 Stat. 1370.
42 USC 1395.
42 USC 1396.

"(1) with respect to its members who are entitled to such insurance benefits or to such medical assistance it (A) provides health services in accordance with section 1301(b), except that (i) it does not furnish to those members the health services (within the basic health services) for which it may not be compensated under such title XVIII or such State plan, and (ii) it does not fix the basic or supplemental health services payment for such members under a community rating system, and (B) is organized and operated in the manner prescribed by section 1301(c), except that it does not assume full financial risk on a prospective basis for the provision to such members of basic or supplemental health services with respect to which it is not required under such title XVIII or such State plan to assume such financial risk; and

"(2) with respect to its other members it provides health services in accordance with section 1301(b) and is organized and operated in the manner prescribed by section 1301(c).

"(e) In any fiscal year no loan guarantee may be made under this title if the making of such guarantee would cause the cumulative total of the principal of the loans guaranteed under this title in such fiscal year to exceed the amount of grant and contract funds obligated under this title in such fiscal year: except that this subsection shall not apply if the amount of grant and contract funds obligated under this title in such fiscal year equals the sums appropriated under section 1309 for grants and contracts for such fiscal year.

"GENERAL PROVISIONS RELATING TO LOAN GUARANTEES AND LOANS

"SEC. 1308. (a)(1) The Secretary may not approve an application for a loan guarantee under this title unless he determines that (A) the terms, conditions, security (if any), and schedule and amount of repayments with respect to the loan are sufficient to protect the financial interests of the United States and are otherwise reasonable, including a determination that the rate of interest does not exceed such per centum per annum on the principal obligation outstanding as the Secretary determines to be reasonable, taking into account the range of interest rates prevailing in the private market for similar loans and the risks assumed by the United States, and (B) the loan would not be available on reasonable terms and conditions without the guarantee under this title.

"(2)(A) The United States shall be entitled to recover from the applicant for a loan guarantee under this title the amount of any payment made pursuant to such guarantee, unless the Secretary for good cause waives such right of recovery; and, upon making any such payment, the United States shall be subrogated to all of the rights of the recipient of the payments with respect to which the guarantee was made.

"(B) To the extent permitted by subparagraph (C), any terms and conditions applicable to a loan guarantee under this title (including terms and conditions imposed under subparagraph (D)) may be modified by the Secretary to the extent he determines it to be consistent with the financial interest of the United States.

"(C) Any loan guarantee made by the Secretary under this title shall be incontestable (i) in the hands of an applicant on whose behalf such guarantee is made unless the applicant engaged in fraud or misrepresentation in securing such guarantee, and (ii) as to any person (or his successor in interest) who makes or contracts to make a loan to such applicant in reliance thereon unless such person (or his successor in interest) engaged in fraud or misrepresentation in making or contracting to make such loan.

"(D) Guarantees of loans under this title shall be subject to such further terms and conditions as the Secretary determines to be necessary to assure that the purposes of this title will be achieved.

"(b)(1) The Secretary may not approve an application for a loan under this title unless—   *Application requirements.*

    "(A) the Secretary is reasonably satisfied that the applicant therefor will be able to make payments of principal and interest thereon when due, and

    "(B) the applicant provides the Secretary with reasonable assurances that there will be available to it such additional funds as may be necessary to complete the project or undertaking with respect to which such loan is requested.

"(2) Any loan made under this title shall (A) have such security, (B) have such maturity date, (C) be repayable in such installments, (D) bear interest at a rate comparable to the current rate of interest prevailing, on the date the loan is made, with respect to loans guaranteed under this title, and (E) be subject to such other terms and conditions (including provisions for recovery in case of default), as the Secretary determines to be necessary to carry out the purposes of this title while adequately protecting the financial interests of the United States.

"(3) The Secretary may, for good cause but with due regard to the financial interests of the United States, waive any right of recovery which he has by reason of the failure of a borrower to make payments of principal of and interest on a loan made under this title, except that if such loan is sold and guaranteed, any such waiver shall have no effect upon the Secretary's guarantee of timely payment of principal and interest.   *Right of recovery, waiver.*

"(c)(1) The Secretary may from time to time, but with due regard to the financial interests of the United States, sell loans made by him under this title.   *Sale of loans.*

87 STAT. 929

"(2) The Secretary may agree, prior to his sale of any such loan, to guarantee to the purchaser (and any successor in interest of the purchaser) compliance by the borrower with the terms and conditions of such loan. Any such agreement shall contain such terms and conditions as the Secretary considers necessary to protect the financial interests of the United States or as otherwise appropriate. Any such agreement may (A) provide that the Secretary shall act as agent of any such purchaser for the purpose of collecting from the borrower to which such loan was made and paying over to such purchaser, any payments of principal and interest payable by such organization under such loan; and (B) provide for the repurchase by the Secretary of any such loan on such terms and conditions as may be specified in the agreement. The full faith and credit of the United States is pledged to the payment of all amounts which may be required to be paid under any guarantee under this paragraph.

"(3) After any loan under this title to a public health maintenance organization has been sold and guaranteed under this subsection, interest paid on such loan which is received by the purchaser thereof (or his successor in interest) shall be included in the gross income of the purchaser of the loan (or his successor in interest) for the purpose of chapter 1 of the Internal Revenue Code of 1954.

68A Stat. 3.
26 USC 1
et seq.

"(4) Amounts received by the Secretary as proceeds from the sale of loans under this subsection shall be deposited in the loan fund established under subsection (e).

Loan guarantee
fund.
Establishment.

"(d)(1) There is established in the Treasury a loan guarantee fund (hereinafter in this subsection referred to as the 'fund') which shall be available to the Secretary without fiscal year limitation, in such amounts as may be specified from time to time in appropriation Acts, to enable him to discharge his responsibilities under loan guarantees issued by him under this title. There are authorized to be appropriated from time to time such amounts as may be necessary to provide the sums required for the fund. To the extent authorized in appropriation Acts, there shall also be deposited in the fund amounts received by the Secretary in connection with loan guarantees under this title and other property or assets derived by him from his operations respecting such loan guarantees, including any money derived from the sale of assets.

"(2) If at any time the sums in the funds are insufficient to enable the Secretary to discharge his responsibilities under guarantees issued by him under this title, he is authorized to issue to the Secretary of the Treasury notes or other obligations in such forms and denominations, bearing such maturities, and subject to such terms and conditions, as may be prescribed by the Secretary with the approval of the Secretary of the Treasury. Such notes or other obligations shall bear interest at a rate determined by the Secretary of the Treasury, taking into consideration the current average market yield on outstanding marketable obligations of the United States of comparable maturities during the month preceding the issuance of the notes or other obligations. The Secretary of the Treasury shall purchase any notes and other obligations issued under this paragraph and for that purpose he may use as a public debt transaction the proceeds from the sale of any securities issued under the Second Liberty Bond Act, and the purposes for which the securities may be issued under that Act are extended to include any purchase of such notes and obligations. The Secretary of the Treasury may at any time sell any of the notes or other obligations acquired by him under this paragraph. All redemptions, purchases, and sales by the Secretary of the Treasury of such notes or other obligations shall be treated as public debt transactions of the United States. Sums borrowed under this paragraph shall be deposited in the fund

40 Stat. 288.
31 USC 774.

87 STAT. 930

and redemption of such notes and obligations shall be made by the Secretary from the fund.

"(e) There is established in the Treasury a loan fund (hereinafter in this subsection referred to as the 'fund') which shall be available to the Secretary without fiscal year limitation, in such amounts as may be specified from time to time in appropriation Acts, to enable him to make loans under this title. There shall also be deposited in the fund amounts received by the Secretary as interest payments and repayment of principal on loans made under this title and other property or assets derived by him from his operations respecting such loans, from the sale of loans under subsection (c) of this section, or from the sale of assets.

Loan fund. Establishment.

"AUTHORIZATIONS OF APPROPRIATIONS

"SEC. 1309. (a) For the purpose of making payments under grants and contracts under sections 1303, 1304(a), and 1304(b), there are authorized to be appropriated $25,000,000 for the fiscal year ending June 30, 1974, $55,000,000 for the fiscal year ending June 30, 1975, and $85,000,000 for the fiscal year ending June 30, 1976; and for the purpose of making payments under grants and contracts under section 1304(b) for the fiscal year ending June 30, 1977, there is authorized to be appropriated $85,000,000.

"(b) There is authorized to be appropriated to the loan fund established under section 1308(e) $75,000,000 in the aggregate for the fiscal years ending June 30, 1974, and June 30, 1975.

"EMPLOYEES' HEALTH BENEFITS PLANS

"SEC. 1310. (a) Each employer which is required during any calendar quarter to pay its employees the minimum wage specified by section 6 of the Fair Labor Standards Act of 1938 (or would be required to pay his employees such wage but for section 13(a) of such Act), and which during such calendar quarter employed an average number of employees of not less than twenty-five, shall, in accordance with regulations which the Secretary shall prescribe, include in any health benefits plan offered to its employees in the calendar year beginning after such calendar quarter the option of membership in qualified health maintenance organizations which are engaged in the provision of basic and supplemental health services in the areas in which such employees reside.

52 Stat. 1062; 77 Stat. 56; 80 Stat. 838. 29 USC 201. 75 Stat. 71; 80 Stat. 833; 86 Stat. 375. 29 USC 213.

"(b) If there is more than one qualified health maintenance organization which is engaged in the provision of basic and supplemental health services in the area in which the employees of an employer subject to subsection (a) reside and if—

"(1) one or more of such organizations provides basic health services through professionals who are members of the staff of the organization or a medical group (or groups), and

"(2) one or more of such organizations provides such services through an individual practice association (or associations), then of the qualified health maintenance organizations included in a health benefits plan of such employer pursuant to subsection (a) at least one shall be an organization which provides basic health services as described in clause (1) and at least one shall be an organization which provides basic health services as described in clause (2).

"(c) No employer shall be required to pay more for health benefits as a result of the application of this section than would otherwise be required by any prevailing collective bargaining agreement or other legally enforceable contract for the provision of health benefits between the employer and its employees. Failure of any employer to

Pub. Law 93-222   December 29, 1973

52 Stat. 1068;
63 Stat. 919.
29 USC 215.
"Qualified
health
maintenance
organization."

comply with the requirements of subsection (a) shall be considered a willful violation of section 15 of the Fair Labor Standards Act of 1938.

"(d) For purposes of this section, the term 'qualified health maintenance organization' means (1) a health maintenance organization which has provided assurances satisfactory to the Secretary that it provides basic and supplemental health services to its members in the manner prescribed by section 1301(b) and that it is organized and operated in the manner prescribed by section 1301(c), and (2) an entity which proposes to become a health maintenance organization and which the Secretary determines will when it becomes operational provide basic and supplemental health services to its members in the manner prescribed by section 1301(b) and will be organized and operated in the manner prescribed by section 1301(c).

"RESTRICTIVE STATE LAWS AND PRACTICES

"SEC. 1311. (a) In the case of any entity—

"(1) which cannot do business as a health maintenance organization in a State in which it proposes to furnish basic and supplemental health services because that State by law, regulation, or otherwise—

"(A) requires as a condition to doing business in that State that a medical society approve the furnishing of services by the entity,

"(B) requires that physicians constitute all or a percentage of its governing body,

"(C) requires that all physicians or a percentage of physicians in the locale participate or be permitted to participate in the provision of services for the entity, or

"(D) requires that the entity meet requirements for insurers of health care services doing business in that State respecting initial capitalization and establishment of financial reserves against insolvency, and

"(2) for which a grant, contract, loan, or loan guarantee was made under this title or which is a qualified health maintenance organization for purposes of section 1310 (relating to employees' health benefits plans),

such requirements shall not apply to that entity so as to prevent it from operating as a health maintenance organization in accordance with section 1301.

"(b) No State may establish or enforce any law which prevents a health maintenance organization for which a grant, contract, loan, or loan guarantee was made under this title or which is a qualified health maintenance organization for purposes of section 1310 (relating to employees' health benefits plans), from soliciting members through advertising its services, charges, or other nonprofessional aspects of its operation. This subsection does not authorize any advertising which identifies, refers to, or makes any qualitative judgment concerning, any health professional who provides services for a health maintenance organization.

"CONTINUED REGULATION OF HEALTH MAINTENANCE ORGANIZATIONS

"SEC. 1312. (a) If the Secretary determines that an entity which received a grant, contract, loan, or loan guarantee under this title as a health maintenance organization or which was included in a health benefits plan offered to employees pursuant to section 1310—

"(1) fails to provide basic and supplemental services to its members,

"(2) fails to provide such services in the manner prescribed by section 1301(b), or

"(3) is not organized or operated in the manner prescribed by section 1301(c),

the Secretary may, in addition to any other remedies available to him, bring a civil action in the United States district court for the district in which such entity is located to enforce its compliance with any assurances it furnished him respecting the provision of basic and supplemental health services or its organization or operation, as the case may be, which assurances were made under section 1310 or when application was made under this title for a grant, contract, loan, or loan guarantee.

"(b) The Secretary, through the Assistant Secretary for Health, shall administer subsection (a) in the Office of the Assistant Secretary for Health.

"LIMITATION ON SOURCE OF FUNDING FOR HEALTH MAINTENANCE ORGANIZATIONS

"SEC. 1313. No funds appropriated under any provision of this Act other than this title may be used—

"(1) for grants or contracts for surveys or other activities to determine the feasibility of developing or expanding health maintenance organizations or other entities which provide, directly or indirectly, health services to a defined population on a prepaid basis;

"(2) for grants or contracts, or for payments under loan guarantees, for planning projects for the establishment or expansion of such organizations or entities;

"(3) for grants or contracts, or for payments under loan guarantees, for projects for the initial development or expansion of such organizations or entities; or

"(4) for loans, or for payments under loan guarantees, to assist in meeting the costs of the initial operation after establishment or expansion of such organizations or entities.

"PROGRAM EVALUATION

"SEC. 1314. (a) The Comptroller General shall evaluate the operations of at least fifty of the health maintenance organizations for which assistance was provided under section 1303, 1304, or 1305. The period of operation of such health maintenance organizations which shall be evaluated under this subsection shall be not less than thirty-six months. The Comptroller General shall report to the Congress the results of the evaluation not later than ninety days after at least fifty of such health maintenance organizations have been in operation for at least thirty-six months. Such report shall contain findings— *Report to Congress.*

"(1) with respect to the ability of the organizations evaluated to operate on a fiscally sound basis without continued Federal financial assistance,

"(2) with respect to the ability of such organizations to meet the requirements of section 1301(c) respecting their organization and operation,

"(3) with respect to the ability of such organizations to provide basic and supplemental health services in the manner prescribed by section 1301(b),

"(4) with respect to the ability of such organizations to include indigent and high-risk individuals in their membership, and

"(5) with respect to the ability of such organizations to provide services to medically underserved populations.

87 STAT. 933

Study.

"(b) The Comptroller General shall also conduct a study of the economic effects on employers resulting from their compliance with the requirements of section 1310. The Comptroller General shall report to the Congress the results of such study not later than thirty-six months after the date of the enactment of this title.

Report to
Congress.

"(c) The Comptroller General shall evaluate (1) the operations of distinct categories of health maintenance organizations in comparison with each other, (2) health maintenance organizations as a group in comparison with alternative forms of health care delivery, and (3) the impact that health maintenance organizations, individually, by category, and as a group, have on the health of the public. The Comptroller General shall report to the Congress the results of such evaluation not later than thirty-six months after the date of the enactment of this title.

"ANNUAL REPORT

Review, report
to Congress.

"SEC. 1315. (a) The Secretary shall periodically review the programs of assistance authorized by this title and make an annual report to the Congress of a summary of the activities under each program. The Secretary shall include in such summary—

"(1) a summary of each grant, contract, loan, or loan guarantee made under this title in the period covered by the report and a list of the health maintenance organizations which during such period became qualified health maintenance organizations for purposes of section 1310;

"(2) the statistics and other information reported in such period to the Secretary in accordance with section 1301(c)(11);

"(3) findings with respect to the ability of the health maintenance organizations assisted under this title—

"(A) to operate on a fiscally sound basis without continued Federal financial assistance,

"(B) to meet the requirements of section 1301(c) respecting their organization and operation,

"(C) to provide basic and supplemental health services in the manner prescribed by section 1301(b),

"(D) to include indigent and high-risk individuals in their membership, and

"(E) to provide services to medically underserved populations; and

"(4) findings with respect to—

"(A) the operation of distinct categories of health maintenance organizations in comparison with each other,

"(B) health maintenance organizations as a group in comparison with alternative forms of health care delivery, and

"(C) the impact that health maintenance organizations, individually, by category, and as a group, have on the health of the public.

Review,

"(b) The Office of Management and Budget may review the Secretary's report under subsection (a) before its submission to the Congress, but the Office may not revise the report or delay its submission,

Comments, submittal to Congress,

and it may submit to the Congress its comments (and those of other departments or agencies of the Government) respecting such report."

QUALITY ASSURANCE

58 Stat. 691;
85 Stat. 65.
42 USC 241.

SEC. 3. Title III of the Public Health Service Act is amended by adding at the end thereof the following new part:

87 STAT. 934

"Part K—Quality Assurance

"QUALITY ASSURANCE

"SEC. 399c. (a)(1) The Secretary, through the Assistant Secretary for Health, shall conduct research and evaluation programs respecting the effectiveness, administration, and enforcement of quality assurance programs. Such research and evaluation programs shall be carried out in cooperation with the entity within the Department which administers the programs of assistance under section 304. *Research and evaluation programs.*

"(2) For the purpose of carrying out paragraph (1), there are authorized to be appropriated $4,000,000 for the fiscal year ending June 30, 1974, $8,000,000 for the fiscal year ending June 30, 1975, $9,000,000 for the fiscal year ending June 30, 1976, $9,000,000 for the fiscal year ending June 30, 1977, and $10,000,000 for the fiscal year ending June 30, 1978. *81 Stat. 534. 42 USC 242b. Appropriation.*

"(b) The Secretary shall make an annual report to the Congress and the President on (1) the quality of health care in the United States, (2) the operation of quality assurance programs, and (3) advances made through research and evaluation of the effectiveness, administration, and enforcement of quality assurance programs. The first annual report under this subsection shall be made with respect to calendar year 1974 and shall be submitted not later than March 1, 1975. The Office of Management and Budget may review the Secretary's report under this subsection before its submission to the Congress, but the Office may not revise the report or delay its submission to the Congress, and it may submit to the Secretary and the Congress its comments (and those of other departments and agencies of the Government) with respect to such report." *Annual report to President and Congress.*

HEALTH CARE QUALITY ASSURANCE PROGRAMS STUDY

SEC. 4. (a) The Secretary of Health, Education, and Welfare shall contract, in accordance with subsection (b), for the conduct of a study to—

(1) analyze past and present mechanisms (both required by law and voluntary) to assure the quality of health care, identify the strengths and weaknesses of current major prototypes of health care quality assurance systems, and identify on a comparable basis the costs of such prototypes;

(2) provide a set of basic principles to be followed by any effective health care quality assurance system, including principles affecting the scope of the system, methods for assessing care, data requirements, specifications for the development of criteria and standards which relate to desired outcomes of care, and means for assessing the responsiveness of such care to the needs and perceptions of the consumers of such care;

(3) provide an assessment of programs for improving the performance of health practitioners and institutions in providing high-quality health care, including a study of the effectiveness of sanctions and educational programs;

(4) define the specific needs for a program of research and evaluation in health care quality assurance methods, including the design of prospective evaluations protocols for health care quality assurance systems; and

(5) provide methods for assessing the quality of health care from the point of view of consumers of such care.

(b) The Secretary shall contract for the conduct of the study required by subsection (a) with a nonprofit private organization which— *Contract with private organization.*

(1) has a national reputation for objectivity in the conduct of studies for the Federal Government;

(2) has the capacity to readily marshall the widest possible range of expertise and advice relevant to the conduct of such study;

(3) has a membership and competent staff which have backgrounds in government, the health sciences, and the social sciences;

(4) has a history of interest and activity in health policy issues related to such study; and

(5) has extensive existing contracts with interested public and private agencies and organizations.

The Secretary shall enter into such contract within 90 days of the date of the enactment of the first Act making an appropriation under subsection (d).

Reports to congressional committees.

(c) An interim report providing a plan for the study required by subsection (a) shall be submitted by the organization conducting the study to the Committee on Interstate and Foreign Commerce of the House of Representatives and the Committee on Labor and Public Welfare of the Senate by June 30, 1974; and a final report giving the results of the study and providing specifications for an effective quality assurance system shall be submitted by such organization to the Committee on Interstate and Foreign Commerce of the House of Representatives and the Committee on Labor and Public Welfare of the Senate by January 31, 1976.

Appropriation.

(d) There is authorized to be appropriated $10,000,000, which shall be available without fiscal year limitation, for the conduct of the study required by subsection (a).

REPORTS RESPECTING MEDICALLY UNDERSERVED AREAS AND POPULATION GROUPS AND NON-METROPOLITAN AREAS

Reports to Congress.

Ante, p. 917.

SEC. 5. Within three months of the date of the enactment of this Act, the Secretary of Health, Education, and Welfare shall report to the Congress the criteria used by him in the designation of medically underserved areas and population groups for the purposes of section 1302(7) of the Public Health Service Act. Within one year of such date, the Secretary shall report to the Congress (1) the areas and population groups designated by him under such section 1302(7) as having a shortage of personal health services, (2) the comments (if any) submitted by State and areawide comprehensive health planning agencies under such section with respect to any such designation, and (3) the areas which meet the definitional standards under section 1302(9) of such Act for non-metropolitan areas. The Office of Management and Budget may review the Secretary's report under this section before its submission to the Congress, but the Office may not revise the report or delay its submission beyond the date prescribed for its submission, and it may submit to Congress its comments (and those of other departments and agencies of the Government) respecting such report.

Review.

Comments, submittal to Congress.

HEALTH SERVICES FOR INDIANS AND DOMESTIC AGRICULTURAL MIGRATORY AND SEASONAL WORKERS

68 Stat. 674.

SEC. 6. (a) The first section of the Act of August 5, 1954 (42 U.S.C. 2001), is amended by inserting "(a)" after "That" and by adding at the end thereof the following new subsection:

"(b) In carrying out his functions, responsibilities, authorities, and duties under this Act, the Secretary is authorized, with the consent of the Indian people served, to contract with private or other non-

December 29, 1973   Pub. Law 93-222
                                                    87 STAT. 936

Federal health agencies or organizations for the provision of health
services to such people on a fee-for-service basis or on a prepayment
or other similar basis.".
    (b) The Secretary of Health, Education, and Welfare, in connec-
tion with existing authority (except section 310 of the Public Health   76 Stat. 592.
Service Act) for the provision of health services to domestic agricul-   42 USC 242h.
tural migratory workers, to persons who perform seasonal agricultural
services similar to the services performed by such workers, and to the
families of such workers and persons, is authorized to arrange for the
provision of health services to such workers and persons and their
families through health maintenance organizations. In carrying out
this subsection the Secretary may only use sums appropriated after
the date of the enactment of this Act.

                        CONFORMING AMENDMENTS

    SEC. 7. (a) Section 1 of the Public Health Service Act is amended   58 Stat. 682;
to read as follows: 86 Stat. 137.
                                                                         42 USC 201 not
                           "SHORT TITLE

    "SECTION 1. This Act may be cited as the 'Public Health Service
Act'."
    (b) Title XIII of the Act of July 1, 1944 (58 Stat. 682) (as so   Repeal.
designated by section 2(b) of the Emergency Medical Services Systems Act of 1973 (Public Law 93-154)) is repealed.   Ante, p. 604.
    (c) Section 306(g) of the Federal National Mortgage Association
Act (12 U.S.C. 1721(g)) is amended by inserting ", or which are   82 Stat. 542.
guaranteed under title XIII of the Pubic Health Service Act" after
"chapter 37 of title 38, United States Code".   38 USC 1801.
Approved December 29, 1973.

LEGISLATIVE HISTORY:

HOUSE REPORTS: No. 93-451 accompanying H. R. 7974 (Comm. on
               Interstate and Foreign Commerce) and No. 93-714
               (Comm. of Conference).
SENATE REPORTS: No. 93-129 (Comm. on Labor and Public Welfare) and
               No. 93-621 (Comm. of Conference).
CONGRESSIONAL RECORD, Vol. 119 (1973):
    May 14, 15, considered and passed Senate.
    Sept. 12, considered and passed House, amended, in lieu of
        H. R. 7974.
    Dec. 18, House agreed to conference report.
    Dec. 19, Senate agreed to conference report.
WEEKLY COMPILATION OF PRESIDENTIAL DOCUMENTS, Vol. 10, No. 1 (1974):
    Dec. 29, 1973, Presidential statement.

                              O

Appendix 2

Public Law 94-460
94th Congress

An Act

To amend title XIII of the Public Health Service Act to revise and extend the program for the establishment and expansion of health maintenance organizations.

Oct. 8, 1976
[H.R. 9019]

Be it enacted by the Senate and House of Representatives of the United States of America in Congress assembled,

SHORT TITLE; REFERENCE TO ACT

SECTION 1. (a) This Act may be cited as the "Health Maintenance Organization Amendments of 1976".

(b) Whenever in title I an amendment or repeal is expressed in terms of an amendment to, or repeal of, a section or other provision, the reference shall be considered to be made to a section or other provision of the Public Health Service Act.

Health Maintenance Organization Amendments of 1976.
42 USC 300e note.

42 USC 201 note.

TITLE I—AMENDMENTS TO TITLE XIII OF THE PUBLIC HEALTH SERVICE ACT

SUPPLEMENTAL HEALTH SERVICES

SEC. 101. (a) Section 1301(b)(1) is amended by adding at the end the following: "A health maintenance organization may include a health service, defined as a supplemental health service by section 1302(2), in the basic health services provided its members for a basic health services payment described in the first sentence.".

(b) The first sentence of section 1301(b)(2) is amended by striking out "the organization shall provide" and all that follows in that sentence and substituting "the organization may provide to each of its members any of the health services which are included in supplemental health services (as defined in section 1302(2)).".

(c) Section 1301(b)(4) is amended by striking out "and supplemental health services in the case of the members who have contracted therefor" and substituting "and only such supplemental health services as members have contracted for".

42 USC 300e.

42 USC 300e-1.

STAFFING

SEC. 102. (a)(1) The first sentence of section 1301(b)(3) is amended (A) by striking out "or through" and by substituting ", through", (B) by striking out "(or groups) or" and substituting "(or groups), through an", and (C) by inserting after "(or associations)" the following: ", through health professionals who have contracted with the health maintenance organization for the provision of such services, or through any combination of such staff, medical group (or groups), individual practice association (or associations), or health professionals under contract with the organization".

(2) Section 1301(b)(3) is amended by adding after the first sentence the following: "A health maintenance organization may also, during the thirty-six month period beginning with the month follow-

42 USC 300e.

42 USC 300e-9.

42 USC 300e-1.

ing the month in which the organization becomes a qualified health maintenance organization (within the meaning of section 1310(d)), provide basic and supplemental health services through an entity which but for the requirement of section 1302(4)(C)(i) would be a medical group for purposes of this title. After the expiration of such period, the organization may provide basic or supplemental health services through such an entity only if authorized by the Secretary in accordance with regulations which take into consideration the unusual circumstances of such entity. A health maintenance organization may not, in any of its fiscal years, enter into contracts with health professionals or entities other than medical groups or individual practice associations if the amounts paid under such contracts for basic and supplemental health services exceed fifteen percent of the total amount to be paid in such fiscal year by the health maintenance organization to physicians for the provision of basic and supplemental health services, or, if the health maintenance organization principally serves a rural area, thirty percent of such amount, except that this sentence does not apply to the entering into of contracts for the purchase of basic and supplemental health services through an entity which but for the requirements of section 1302(4)(C)(i) would be a medical group for purposes of this title. Contracts between a health maintenance organization and health professionals for the provision of basic and supplemental health services shall include such provisions as the Secretary may require (including provisions requiring appropriate continuing education).".

42 USC 300e-1.

(b)(1) Section 1302(4)(C) is amended (A) by striking out clause (iv), (B) by redesignating clause (v) as clause (iv), and (C) by inserting "and" at the end of clause (iii).

(2) Section 1302(5)(B) is amended (A) by striking out clause (i), and (B) by redesignating clauses (ii) and (iii) as clauses (i) and (ii), respectively.

OPEN ENROLLMENT

42 USC 300e.

SEC. 103. (a) Section 1301(c) is amended by amending paragraph (4) to read as follows:

"(4) have an open enrollment period in accordance with the provisions of subsection (d) ;".

(b) Section 1301 is amended by adding at the end thereof the following:

"(d)(1)(A) A health maintenance organization which—

"(i) has for at least 5 years provided comprehensive health services on a prepaid basis, or

"(ii) has an enrollment of at least 50,000 members,

shall have at least once during each fiscal year next following a fiscal year in which it did not have a financial deficit an open enrollment period (determined under subparagraph (B)) during which it shall accept individuals for membership in the order in which they apply for enrollment and, except as provided in paragraph (2), without regard to preexisting illness, medical condition, or degree of disability.

"(B) An open enrollment period for a health maintenance organization shall be the lesser of—

"(i) 30 days, or

"(ii) the number of days in which the organization enrolls a number of individuals at least equal to 3 percent of its total net increase in enrollment (if any) in the fiscal year preceding the fiscal year in which such period is held.

For the purpose of determining the total net increase in enrollment in a health maintenance organization, there shall not be included any individual who is enrolled in the organization through a group which had a contract for health care services with the health maintenance organization at the time that such health maintenance organization was determined to be a qualified health maintenance organization under section 1310.

42 USC 300e–9.

"(2) Notwithstanding the requirements of paragraph (1) a health maintenance organization shall not be required to enroll individuals who are confined to an institution because of chronic illness, permanent injury, or other infirmity which would cause economic impairment to the health maintenance organization if such individual were enrolled.

"(3) A health maintenance organization may not be required to make the effective date of benefits for individuals enrolled under this subsection less than 90 days after the date of enrollment.

"(4) The Secretary may waive the requirements of this subsection for a health maintenance organization which demonstrates that compliance with the provisions of this subsection would jeopardize its economic viability in its service area.".

Waiver.

DEFINITION OF SERVICES

SEC. 104. (a)(1) Paragraph (1)(H) of section 1302 is amended to read as follows:

42 USC 300e–1.

"(H) preventive health services (including (i) immunizations, (ii) well-child care from birth, (iii) periodic health evaluations for adults, (iv) voluntary family planning services, (v) infertility services, and (vi) children's eye and ear examinations conducted to determine the need for vision and hearing correction).".

(2) Paragraph (1) of section 1302 is amended by striking out "or podiatrist" each place it occurs and substituting "podiatrist, or other health care personnel".

(b) Paragraph (2) of such section is amended—

(1) by striking out "under paragraph (1)(A) or (1)(H)" in subparagraphs (B) and (C);

(2) by striking out "and" at the end of subparagraph (E), by striking out the period at the end of subparagraph (F) and substituting "; and", and by adding after subparagraph (F) the following:

"(G) other health services which are not included as basic health services and which have been approved by the Secretary for delivery as supplemental health services.";

(3) by striking out "or podiatrist" each place it occurs and substituting "podiatrist, or other health care personnel".

COMMUNITY RATING

SEC. 105. (a)(1) Section 1301(b)(1) is amended by adding at the end thereof the following new sentence: "In the case of an entity which before it became a qualified health maintenance organization (within the meaning of section 1310(d)) provided comprehensive health services on a prepaid basis, the requirement of clause (C) shall not apply to such entity until the expiration of the forty-eight month period beginning with the month following the month in which the entity became such a qualified health organization.".

42 USC 300e.

42 USC 300e.

(2) The last sentence of section 1301(b)(2) is amended by inserting before the period the following: "except that, in the case of an entity which before it became a qualified health maintenance organization

42 USC 300e–9.

(within the meaning of section 1310(d)) provided comprehensive health services on a prepaid basis, the requirement of this sentence shall not apply to such entity during the forty-eight month period beginning with the month following the month in which the entity became such a qualified health maintenance organization".

42 USC 300e–5.

(3) Section 1306(b) is amended (A) by striking out "and" at the end of paragraph (6), (B) by redesignating paragraph (7) as paragraph (8), and (C) by inserting after paragraph (6) the following new paragraph:

"(7) the application contains such assurances as the Secretary may require respecting the intent and the ability of the applicant to meet the requirements of paragraphs (1) and (2) of section 1301(b) respecting the fixing of basic health services payments and supplemental health services payments under a community rating system; and"

42 USC 300e–1.

(b) Section 1302(8)(A) is amended by inserting "differences in marketing costs and" after "reflect".

(c) Subparagraph (B) of section 1302(8) is redesignated as subparagraph (C) and the following new subparagraph is inserted after subparagraph (A):

"(B) Nominal differentials in such rates may be established to reflect the compositing of the rates of payment in a systematic manner to accommodate group purchasing practices of the various employers.".

MEDICAL GROUP REQUIREMENTS

42 USC 300e–1.

SEC. 106. (a) Section 1302(4)(C) is amended by striking out "(i) as their principal professional activity and as a group responsibility engage in the coordinated practice of their profession for a health maintenance organization" and substituting "(i) as their principal professional activity engage in the coordinated practice of their profession and as a group responsibility have substantial responsibility for the delivery of health services to members of a health maintenance organization".

(b) Section 1302(4)(C)(ii) is amended by striking out "plan" and substituting "similar plan unrelated to the provision of specific health services".

(c) 1302(4)(C) (as amended by section 102(b)(1)) is amended by—

(1) striking "and" before "(iv)", and

(2) striking the period at the end of subparagraph (C) and substituting "; and (v) establish an arrangement whereby a member's enrollment status is not known to the health professional who provides health services to the member.".

INCREASE IN LIMITS ON ASSISTANCE FOR FEASIBILITY SURVEYS, PLANNING, INITIAL DEVELOPMENT, AND INITIAL OPERATION

42 USC 300e–2.

SEC. 107. (a) Section 1303(e) is amended by striking "$50,000" and substituting "$75,000".

42 USC 300e–3.

(b)(1) Section 1304(f)(1)(A) is amended by striking "$125,000" and substituting "$200,000".

(2) Section 1304(f)(2)(A) is amended by inserting after "$1,000,000" the following: "or, in the case of a project for a health maintenance organization which will provide services to an additional

service area (as defined by the Secretary) or which will provide services in one or more areas which are not contiguous, $1,600,000".

(c) Section 1305(a) is amended by striking out "first thirty-six months" each place it occurs and substituting "first sixty months".

42 USC 300e-4.

LOAN GUARANTEES FOR PRIVATE ENTITIES

SEC. 108. (a) Section 1304(a)(2) is amended to read as follows:
"(2) guarantee to non-Federal lenders payment of the principal of and the interest on loans made to—
"(A) nonprofit private entities for planning projects for the establishment or expansion of health maintenance organizations, or
"(B) other private entities for such projects for health maintenance organizations which will serve medically underserved populations.".

42 USC 300e-3.

(b) Section 1304(b)(1)(B) is amended to read as follows:
"(B) guarantee to non-Federal lenders payment of the principal of and the interest on loans made to—
"(i) nonprofit private entities for projects for the initial development of health maintenance organizations, or
"(ii) other private entities for such projects for health maintenance organizations which will serve medically underserved populations.".

(c) Section 1305(a)(3) is amended to read as follows:
"(3) guarantee to non-Federal lenders payment of the principal of and the interest on loans made to—
"(A) nonprofit private health maintenance organizations for the amounts referred to in paragraph (1) or (2), or
"(B) other private health maintenance organizations for such amounts but only if the health maintenance organization will serve a medically underserved population.".

42 USC 300e-4.

(d) (1) Section 1304(d) is amended by adding at the end the following new sentence: "In considering applications for loan guarantees under this section, the Secretary shall give special consideration to applications for projects for health maintenance organizations which will serve medically underserved populations.".

Special consideration.

(2) Section 1305 is amended by adding at the end thereof the following new subsection:
"(f) In considering applications for loan guarantees under this section, the Secretary shall give special consideration to applications for health maintenance organizations which will serve medically underserved populations.".

MISCELLANEOUS AMENDMENTS

SEC. 109. (a)(1) Section 1305(a) is amended by striking out "in the period of" in paragraphs (1) and (2) and substituting "during a period not to exceed".

42 USC 300e-4.

(2) The last sentence of 1305(b)(1) is amended to read as follows: "In any fiscal year the amount disbursed to a health maintenance organization under this section (either directly by the Secretary or by an escrow agent under the terms of an escrow agreement or by a lender under a loan guaranteed under this section) may not exceed $1,000,000.".

Limitation.

42 USC 300e-6.   (b) (1) Section 1307 (e) is amended—
                        (A) by inserting "for a private health maintenance organiza-
                    tion (other than a private nonprofit health maintenance organiza-
                    tion)" after "may be made", and
                        (B) by inserting "for private health maintenance organizations
                    (other than private nonprofit health maintenance organizations)"
                    after "guaranteed".
42 USC 300e-7.   (2) Section 1308 (c) is amended by adding after paragraph (4) the
                    following new paragraph:
                        "(5) Any reference in this title (other than in this subsection and
                    in subsection (d)) to a loan guarantee under this title does not include
                    a loan guarantee made under this subsection.".
                        (c) (1) Section 1308 (a) (1) (A) is amended by striking out "for
                    similar loans" and substituting "for loans with similar maturities,
                    terms, conditions, and security".
                        (2) Section 1308 (b) (2) (D) is amended by striking out "loans guar-
                    anteed under this title" and substituting "marketable obligations of
                    the United States of comparable maturities, adjusted to provide for
                    appropriate administrative charges".
42 USC 300e-2.   (d) (1) The last sentence of section 1303 (i) is amended—
                        (A) by striking "the fiscal year ending June 30, 1974, or
                    June 30, 1975," and substituting "any fiscal year"; and
                        (B) by striking "for projects other than those described in
                    clause (1) of such sentence" and substituting "for any project,
                    with priority being given to projects described in clause (1) of
                    such sentence".
42 USC 300e-3.   (2) The last sentence of section 1304 (k) (1) is amended—
                        (A) by striking "the fiscal year ending June 30, 1974, or
                    June 30, 1975," and substituting "any fiscal year"; and
                        (B) by striking "for projects other than those described in
                    clause (A) of such sentence" and substituting "for any project,
                    with priority being given to projects described in clause (A) of
                    such sentence".
                        (3) The last sentence of section 1304 (k) (2) is amended—
                        (A) by striking "the fiscal year ending June 30, 1974, or in
                    either of the next two fiscal years" and substituting "any fiscal
                    year"; and
                        (B) by striking "for projects other than those described in
                    clause (A) of such sentence" and substituting "for any project,
                    with priority being given to projects described in clause (A) of
                    such sentence".
                        (e) Section 1304 (b) (2) (D) is amended by striking out "for such
                    an organization" and substituting "who will engage in practice
                    principally for the health maintenance organization".

                            EMPLOYEE HEALTH BENEFITS PLANS

42 USC 300e-9.   SEC. 110. (a) Section 1310 is amended—
                        (1) by amending subsection (a) to read as follows:
                    "SEC. 1310. (a) (1) In accordance with regulations which the
                    Secretary shall prescribe—
                        "(A) each employer—
                        "(i) which is now or hereafter required during any
                    calendar quarter to pay its employees the minimum wage
                    prescribed by section 6 of the Fair Labor Standards Act of
29 USC 206.   1938 (or would be required to pay its employees such wage
29 USC 213.   but for section 13 (a) of such Act), and

"(ii) which during such calendar quarter employed an average number of employees of not less than 25,

shall include in any health benefits plan, and

"(B) any State and each political subdivision thereof which during any calendar quarter employed an average number of employees of not less than 25, as a condition of the payment to the State of funds under section 314(d), 317, 318, 1002, 1525, or 1613, shall include in any health benefits plan,

42 USC 246, 247b, 247c, 300a, 300m-4, 300p-3.

offered to such employees in the calendar year beginning after such calendar quarter the option of membership in qualified health maintenance organizations which are engaged in the provision of basic health services in health maintenance organization service areas in which at least 25 of such employees reside.

"(2) If any of the employees of an employer or State or political subdivision thereof described in paragraph (1) are represented by a collective bargaining representative or other employee representative designated or selected under any law, offer of membership in a qualified health maintenance organization required by paragraph (1) to be made in a health benefits plan offered to such employees (A) shall first be made to such collective bargaining representative or other employee representative, and (B) if such offer is accepted by such representative, shall then be made to each such employee.";

(2) by amending paragraphs (1) and (2) of subsection (b) to read as follows:

"(1) one or more of such organizations provides basic health services (A) without the use of an individual practice association and (B) without the use of contracts (except for contracts for unusual or infrequently used services) with health professionals, and

"(2) one or more of such organizations provides basic health services through (A) an individual practice association (or associations), (B) health professionals who have contracted with the health maintenance organization for the provision of such services, or (C) a combination of such association (or associations) or health professionals under contract with the organization,";

(3) by striking out the last sentence of subsection (c); and

(4) by adding after subsection (d) the following new subsections:

Civil penalty.

"(e)(1) Any employer who knowingly does not comply with one or more of the requirements of subsection (a) shall be subject to a civil penalty of not more than $10,000. If such noncompliance continues, a civil penalty may be assessed and collected under this subsection for each thirty-day period such noncompliance continues. Such penalty may be assessed by the Secretary and collected in a civil action brought by the United States in a United States district court.

"(2) In any proceeding by the Secretary to assess a civil penalty under this subsection, no penalty shall be assessed until the employer charged shall have been given notice and an opportunity to present its views on such charge. In determining the amount of the penalty, or the amount agreed upon in compromise, the Secretary shall consider the gravity of the noncompliance and the demonstrated good faith of the employer charged in attempting to achieve rapid compliance after notification by the Secretary of a noncompliance.

"(3) In any civil action brought to review the assessment of a civil penalty assessed under this subsection, the court shall, at the request of any party to such action, hold a trial de novo on the assessment of such civil penalty and in any civil action to collect such a civil penalty, the court shall, at the request of any party to such action, hold a trial de novo on the assessment of such civil penalty unless in a prior civil action to review the assessment of such penalty the court held a trial de novo on such assessment.

"Employer."

"(f) For purposes of this section, the term 'employer' does not include (1) the Government of the United States, the government of the District of Columbia or any territory or possession of the United States, a State or any political subdivision thereof, or any agency or instrumentality (including the United States Postal Service and Postal Rate Commission) of any of the foregoing; or (2) a church, convention or association of churches, or any organization operated, supervised or controlled by a church, convention or association of churches which organization (A) is an organization described in section 501(c)(3) of the Internal Revenue Code of 1954, and (B) does not discriminate (i) in the employment, compensation, promotion, or termination of employment of any personnel, or (ii) in the extension of staff or other privileges to any physician or other health personnel, because such persons seek to obtain or obtained health care, or participate in providing health care, through a health maintenance organization.

26 USC 501.

Notice, hearing.

"(g) If the Secretary, after reasonable notice and opportunity for hearing to a State, finds that it or any of its political subdivisions has failed to comply with one or more of the requirements of subsection (a), the Secretary shall terminate payments to such State under sections 314(d), 317, 318, 1002, 1525, and 1613 and notify the Governor of such State that further payments under such sections will not be made to the State until the Secretary is satisfied that there will no longer be any such failure to comply.

42 USC 246, 247b, 247c, 300a, 300m-4 300p-3.

"(h) The duties and functions of the Secretary, insofar as they involve making determinations as to whether an organization is a qualified health maintenance organization within the meaning of subsection (d), shall be administered through the Assistant Secretary for Health and in the Office of the Assistant Secretary for Health, and the administration of such duties and functions shall be integrated with the administration of section 1312(a).".

42 USC 300e-11.

(b) Section 8902 of title 5, United States Code, relating to Federal employee health insurance, is amended by adding at the end thereof the following new subsection:

"(l) The Commission shall contract under this chapter for a plan described in section 8903(4) of this title with any qualified health maintenance carrier which offers such a plan. For the purpose of this subsection, 'qualified health maintenance carrier' means any qualified carrier which is a qualified health maintenance organization within the meaning of section 1310(d)(1) of title XIII of the Public Health Service Act (42 U.S.C. 300c-9(d)).".

"Qualified health maintenance carrier."
42 USC 300e-9.

ENFORCEMENT REQUIREMENTS

42 USC 300e-11.

SEC. 111. (a) Section 1312(a) is amended by striking out all of the section following paragraph (3) and substituting the following: "the Secretary may take the action authorized by subsection (b)."

(b) Section 1312(b) is amended to read as follows:

Determination, notification.

"(b)(1) If the Secretary makes, with respect to any entity which provided assurances to the Secretary under section 1310(d)(1), a determination described in subsection (a), the Secretary shall notify the entity in writing of the determination. Such notice shall specify the manner in which the entity has not complied with such assurances

PUBLIC LAW 94-460—OCT. 8, 1976   90 STAT. 1953

and direct that the entity initiate (within 30 days of the date the notice
is issued by the Secretary or within such longer period as the Secretary determines is reasonable) such action as may be necessary to
bring (within such period as the Secretary shall prescribe) the entity
into compliance with the assurances. If the entity fails to initiate   Notification.
corrective action within the period prescribed by the notice or fails
to comply with the assurances within such period as the Secretary
prescribes (A) the entity shall not be a qualified health maintenance
organization for purposes of section 1310 until such date as the Sec-   42 USC 300e-9.
retary determines that it is in compliance with the assurances, and (B)
each employer which has offered membership in the entity in compliance with section 1310, each lawfully recognized collective bargaining representative or other employee representative which represents
the employees of each such employer, and the members of such entity
shall be notified by the entity that the entity is not a qualified health
maintenance organization for purposes of such section. The notice
required by clause (B) of the preceding sentence shall contain, in
readily understandable language, the reasons for the determination
that the entity is not a qualified health maintenance organization. The   Publication in
Secretary shall publish in the Federal Register each determination   Federal Register.
referred to in this paragraph.

"(2) If the Secretary makes, with respect to an entity which has
received a grant, contract, loan, or loan guarantee under this title, a
determination described in subsection (a), the Secretary may, in addition to any other remedies available to him, bring a civil action in the
United States district court for the district in which such entity is
located to enforce its compliance with the assurances it furnished
respecting the provision of basic and supplemental health services or
its organization or operation, as the case may be, which assurances
were made in connection with its application under this title for the
grant, contract, loan, or loan guarantee.".

(c) Section 1312 is amended by adding at the end the following new   42 USC 300e-
subsection: 11.

"(c) The Secretary, acting through the Assistant Secretary for   Administration.
Health, shall administer subsections (a) and (b) in the Office of the
Assistant Secretary for Health.".

HMO'S AND FEDERAL HEALTH BENEFITS PROGRAMS

SEC. 112. Section 1307(d) is amended by adding after and below   42 USC 300e-6.
paragraph (2) the following new sentence: "An entity which provides
health services to a defined population on a prepaid basis and which
has members who are enrolled under the health benefits program
authorized by chapter 89 of title 5, United States Code, may be con-   5 USC 8901
sidered as a health maintenance organization for purposes of receiving   *et seq.*
assistance under this title if with respect to its other members it provides health services in accordance with section 1301(b) and is   42 USC 300e.
organized and operated in the manner prescribed by section 1301(c).".

EXTENSIONS AND AUTHORIZATIONS

SEC. 113. (a) Section 1304(j) is amended (1) by striking out   42 USC 300e-3.
"September 30, 1976" and substituting "September 30, 1978", and (2)
by striking out "September 30, 1977" and substituting "September 30,
1979".

(b) Subsection (d) of section 1305 is amended to read as follows: 42 USC 300e-4.
"(d) No loan may be made or guaranteed under this section after
September 30, 1980.".

42 USC 300e–8.

(c) Section 1309(a) is amended—
    (1) by striking out "and" after "1975,",
    (2) by inserting after "1976" the following: ", $45,000,000 for
the fiscal year ending September 30, 1977, and $45,000,000 for the
fiscal year ending September 30, 1978",
    (3) by striking out "ending June 30, 1977" and substituting
"ending September 30, 1977", and
    (4) by striking out "$85,000,000" the first time it occurs and
substituting "$40,000,000", and by striking out "$85,000,000" the
second time it occurs and substituting "$50,000,000".

RESTRICTIVE STATE LAWS

42 USC 300e–
10.
Digest.

SEC. 114. Section 1311 is amended by adding at the end the following new subsection:
    "(c) The Secretary shall, within 6 months after the date of the
enactment of this subsection, develop a digest of State laws, regulations, and practices pertaining to development, establishment, and
operation of health maintenance organizations which shall be updated
at least quarterly and relevant sections of which shall be provided to
the Governor of each State annually. Such digest shall indicate which
State laws, regulations, and practices appear to be inconsistent with the
operation of this section. The Secretary shall also insure that appropriate legal consultative assistance is available to the States for the
purpose of complying with the provisions of this section."

PROGRAM EVALUATION BY THE COMPTROLLER GENERAL

42 USC 300e–
13.

SEC. 115. So much of section 1314(a) as precedes paragraph (1)
thereof is amended to read as follows:

42 USC 300e–
2–300e–4.
Report to
Congress.

    "SEC. 1314. (a) The Comptroller General shall evaluate the opera-
tions of at least ten or one-half (whichever is greater) of the health
maintenance organizations for which assistance was provided under
sections 1303, 1304, and 1305, and which, by December 31, 1976, have
been designated by the Secretary under section 1310(d) as qualified
health maintenance organizations. The Comptroller General shall
report to the Congress the results of the evaluation by June 30, 1978.
Such report shall contain findings—".

ADMINISTRATION OF PROGRAMS

SEC. 116. Title XIII is amended by adding after section 1315 the
following new section:

"ADMINISTRATION OF PROGRAM

42 USC 300e–
15.
42 USC 300e–9,
300e–11.

    "SEC. 1316. The Secretary shall administer this title (other than
sections 1310 and 1312) through a single identifiable administrative
unit of the Department.".

CONFORMING AMENDMENTS

42 USC 300n–1.

SEC. 117. (a) Section 1532(c) is amended by adding the following
sentence at the end thereof: "The criteria established by any health
systems agency or State Agency under paragraph (8) shall be consistent with the standards and procedures established by the Secretary

42 USC 300e–5.

under section 1306(c) of this Act.".

PUBLIC LAW 94-460—OCT. 8, 1976　　　90 STAT. 1955

(b)(1) Paragraph (6) of section 1302 is amended to read as follows:
"(6) The term 'health systems agency' means an entity which is designated in accordance with section 1515 of this Act.".

42 USC 300e-1.
"Health systems agency."
42 USC 300*l*-4.

(2) Paragraph (7) of section 1302 is amended by—
　(A) striking "section 314(a) State health planning agency whose section 314(a) plan" and substituting "State health planning and development agency which"; and
　(B) striking "section 314(b) areawide health planning agency whose section 314(b) plan", and substituting "health systems agency designated for a health service area which".

(3) Paragraph (1) of section 1303(b) is amended by striking "section 314(b) areawide health planning agency (if any) whose section 314(b) plan" and substituting "each health systems agency designated for a health service area which".

42 USC 300e-2.

(4) Paragraph (1) of section 1304(c) is amended by striking "section 314(b) areawide health planning agency (if any) whose section 314(b) plan" and substituting "each health systems agency designated for a health service area which".

42 USC 300e-3.

(5) Section (b)(5) of section 1306 is amended to read as follows:
"(5) each health systems agency designated for a health service area which covers (in whole or in part) the area to be served by the health maintenance organization for which such application is submitted :".

42 USC 300e-5.

(6) Subsection (c) of section 1306 is amended by striking "section 314(b) areawide health planning agencies and section 314(a) State health planning agencies" and substituting "health systems agencies".

EFFECTIVE DATES

SEC. 118. (a) Except as provided in subsection (b), the amendments made by this title shall take effect on the date of the enactment of this Act.

42 USC 300e note.

(b)(1) The amendments made by sections 101, 102, 103, 104, and 106 shall (A) apply with respect to grants, contracts, loans, and loan guarantees made under sections 1303, 1304, and 1305 of the Public Health Service Act for fiscal years beginning after September 30, 1976, (B) apply with respect to health benefit plans offered under section 1310 of such Act after such date, and (C) for purposes of section 1312 take effect October 1, 1976.

42 USC 300e-2–300e-4.
42 USC 300e-9.
42 USC 300e-11.
42 USC 300e.

(2) Subsection (d) of section 1301 of the Public Health Service Act (added by section 103(b) of this Act) shall take effect with respect to fiscal years of health maintenance organizations beginning on or after the date of the enactment of this Act.

(3) The amendments made by section 107 shall apply with respect to grants, contracts, loans, and loan guarantees made under sections 1303, 1304, and 1305 of the Public Health Service Act for fiscal years beginning after September 30, 1976.

(4) The amendments made by sections 109(a)(1) and 109(c) shall apply with respect to loan guarantees made under section 1305 of the Public Health Service Act after September 30, 1976.

(5) The amendment made by section 109(e) shall apply with respect to projects assisted under section 1304 of the Public Health Service Act after September 30, 1976.

(6) The amendments made by paragraphs (1) and (2) of section 110(a) shall apply with respect to calendar quarters which begin after the date of the enactment of this Act.

90 STAT. 1956   PUBLIC LAW 94-460—OCT. 8, 1976

42 USC 300e-9.

42 USC 300e-11.

(7) The amendments made by paragraphs (3) and (4) of section 110 shall apply with respect to failures of employers to comply with section 1310(a) of the Public Health Service Act after the date of the enactment of this Act.

(8) The amendment made by section 111 shall apply with respect to determinations of the Secretary of Health, Education, and Welfare described in section 1312(a) of the Public Health Service Act and made after the date of the enactment of this Act.

TITLE II—AMENDMENTS TO SOCIAL SECURITY ACT

MEDICARE AMENDMENTS

42 USC 1395mm.

"Health maintenance organization."

42 USC 1395x.

42 USC 300e.

"Basic health services."

Administration.

SEC. 201. (a) Section 1876(b) of the Social Security Act is amended to read as follows:

"(b)(1) The term 'health maintenance organization' means a legal entity which provides health services on a prepayment basis to individuals enrolled with such organizations and which—

"(A) provides to its enrollees who are insured for benefits under parts A and B of this title or for benefits under part B alone, through institutions, entities, and persons meeting the applicable requirements of section 1861, all of the services and benefits covered under such parts (to the extent applicable under subparagraph (A) or (B) of subsection (a)(1)) which are available to individuals residing in the geographic area served by the organization;

"(B) provides such services in the manner prescribed by section 1301(b) of the Public Health Service Act, except that solely for the purposes of this section—

"(i) the term 'basic health services' and references thereto shall be deemed to refer to the services and benefits included under parts A and B of this title;

"(ii) the organization shall not be required to fix the basic health services payment under a community rating system;

"(iii) the additional nominal payments authorized by section 1301(b)(1)(D) of such Act shall not exceed the limits applicable under subsection (g) of this section; and

"(iv) payment for basic health services provided by the organization to its enrollees under this section or for services such enrollees receive other than through the organization shall be made as provided for by this title;

"(C) is organized and operated in the manner prescribed by section 1301(c) of the Public Health Service Act, except that solely for the purposes of this section—

"(i) the term 'basic health services' and references thereto shall be deemed to refer to the services and benefits included under parts A and B of this title;

"(ii) the organization shall not be reimbursed for the cost of reinsurance except as permitted by subsection (i) of this section; and

"(iii) the organization shall have an open enrollment period as provided for in subsection (k) of this section.

"(2)(A) The duties and functions of the Secretary, insofar as they involve making determinations as to whether an organization is a 'health maintenance organization' within the meaning of paragraph (1), shall be administered through the Assistant Secretary for Health and in the Office of the Assistant Secretary for Health, and the administration of such duties and functions shall be integrated with the administration of section 1312 (a) and (b) of the Public Health Service Act.

42 USC 300e-11.

"(B) Except as provided in subparagraph (A), the Secretary shall administer the provisions of this section through the Commissioner of Social Security.".

(b) Section 1876(h) of such Act is amended to read as follows:

42 USC 1395mm.

"(h)(1) Except as provided in paragraph (2), each health maintenance organization with which the Secretary enters into a contract under this section shall have an enrolled membership at least half of which consists of individuals who have not attained age 65.

"(2) The Secretary may waive the requirement imposed in paragraph (1) for a period of not more than three years from the date a health maintenance organization first enters into an agreement with the Secretary pursuant to subsection (i), but only for so long as such organization demonstrates to the satisfaction of the Secretary by the submission of its plan for each year that it is making continuous efforts and progress toward compliance with the provisions of paragraph (1) within such three-year period.".

Waiver.

(c) Section 1876(i)(6)(B) of such Act is amended by striking out "(other than those with respect to out-of-area services)" and inserting in lieu thereof "(other than costs with respect to out-of-area services and, in the case of an organization which has entered into a risk-sharing contract with the Secretary pursuant to paragraph (2)(A), the cost of providing any member with basic health services the aggregate value of which exceeds $5,000 in any year)".

(d) Section 1876 is amended by adding at the end thereof the following—

"(k) Each health maintenance organization with which the Secretary enters into a contract under this section shall have an open enrollment period at least every year under which it accepts up to the limits of its capacity and without restrictions, except as may be authorized in regulations, individuals who are eligible to enroll under subsection (d) in the order in which they apply for enrollment (unless to do so would result in failure to meet the requirements of subsection (h)) or would result in enrollment of enrollees substantially nonrepresentative, as determined in accordance with regulations of the Secretary, of the population in the geographic area served by such health maintenance organization.".

Open enrollment period.

(e) The amendments made by this section shall be effective with respect to contracts entered into between the Secretary and health maintenance organizations under section 1876 of the Social Security Act on and after the first day of the first calendar month which begins more than 30 days after the date of enactment of this Act.

Effective date. 42 USC 1395mm note.

MEDICAID AMENDMENTS

SEC. 202. (a) Section 1903 of the Social Security Act is amended by adding at the end thereof the following new subsection:

42 USC 1396b.

"(m)(1)(A) The term 'health maintenance organization' means a legal entity which provides health services to individuals enrolled in such organization and which—

"Health maintenance organization."

"(i) provides to its enrollees who are eligible for benefits under this title the services and benefits described in paragraphs (1), (2), (3), (4)(C), and (5) of section 1905, and, to the extent required by section 1902(a)(13)(A)(ii) to be provided under a State plan for medical assistance, the services and benefits described in paragraph (7) of section 1905(a);

42 USC 1396d. 42 USC 1396a.

"Basic health
services."
42 USC 300e.

"(ii) provides such services and benefits in the manner prescribed in section 1301(b) of the Public Health Service Act (except that, solely for purposes of this paragraph, the term 'basic health services' and references thereto, when employed in such section, shall be deemed to refer to the services and benefits described in paragraphs (1), (2), (3), (4)(C), and (5) of section 1905(a), and, to the extent required by section 1902(a)(13)(A)(ii) to be provided under a State plan for medical assistance, the services and benefits described in paragraph (7) of section 1905 (a)); and

42 USC 1396d.
42 USC 1396a.

"(iii) is organized and operated in the manner prescribed by section 1301(c) of the Public Health Service Act (except that solely for purposes of this paragraph, the term 'basic health services' and references thereto, when employed in such section shall be deemed to refer to the services and benefits described in section 1905 (a) (1), (2), (3), (4)(C), and (5), and to the extent required by section 1902(a)(13)(A)(ii) to be provided under a State plan for medical assistance, the services and benefits described in paragraph (7) of section 1905(a)).

Administration.

"(B) The duties and functions of the Secretary, insofar as they involve making determinations as to whether an organization is a health maintenance organization within the meaning of subparagraph (A), shall be administered through the Assistant Secretary for Health and in the Office of the Assistant Secretary for Health, and the administration of such duties and functions shall be integrated with the administration of section 1312 (a) and (b) of the Public Health Service Act.

42 USC 300e-
11.

"(2)(A) Except as provided in subparagraphs (B) and (C), no payment shall be made under this title to a State with respect to expenditures incurred by it for payment for services provided by any entity—

"(i) which is responsible for the provision of—

"(I) inpatient hospital services and any other service described in paragraph (2), (3), (4), (5), or (7) of section 1905(a), or

"(II) any three or more of the services described in such paragraphs,

when payment for such services is determined under a prepaid capitation risk basis or under any other risk basis;

"(ii) which the Secretary (or the State as authorized by paragraph (3)) has not determined to be a health maintenance organization as defined in paragraph (1); and

"(iii) more than one-half of the membership of which consists of individuals who are insured under parts A and B of title XVIII or recipients of benefits under this title.

"(B) Subparagraph (A) does not apply with respect to payments under this title to a State with respect to expenditures incurred by it for payment for services provided by an entity which—

42 USC 247d,
254c.

"(i)(I) received a grant of at least $100,000 in the fiscal year ending June 30, 1976, under section 319(d)(1)(A) or 330(d)(1) of the Public Health Service Act, and (II) for the period beginning July 1, 1976, and ending on the expiration of the period for which payments are to be made under this title has been the recipient of a grant under either such section; and

PUBLIC LAW 94–460—OCT. 8, 1976   90 STAT. 1959

"(II) provides to its enrollees, on a prepaid capitation risk basis or on any other risk basis, all of the services and benefits described in paragraphs (1), (2), (3), (4) (C), and (5) of section 1905(a) and, to the extent required by section 1902(a) (13) (A) (ii) to be provided under a State plan for medical assistance, the services and benefits described in paragraph (7) of such section; or

42 USC 1396d.
42 USC 1396a.

"(ii) is a nonprofit primary health care entity located in a rural area (as defined by the Appalachian Regional Commission)—

"(I) which received in the fiscal year ending June 30, 1976, at least $100,000 (by grant, subgrant, or subcontract) under the Appalachian Regional Development Act of 1965, and

40 USC app. 1.

"(II) for the period beginning July 1, 1976, and ending on the expiration of the period for which payments are to be made under this title either has been the recipient of a grant, subgrant, or subcontract under such Act or has provided services under a contract (initially entered into during a year in which the entity was the recipient of such a grant, subgrant, or subcontract) with a State agency under this title on a prepaid capitation risk basis or on any other risk basis; or

"(iii) which has contracted with the single State agency for the provision of services (but not including inpatient hospital services) to persons eligible under this title on a prepaid risk basis prior to 1970.

"(C) Subparagraph (A)(iii) shall not apply with respect to payments under this title to a State with respect to expenditures incurred by it for payment for services by an entity during the three-year period beginning on the date of enactment of this subsection or beginning on the date the entity enters into a contract with the State under this title for the provision of health services on a prepaid risk basis, whichever occurs later, but only if the entity demonstrates to the satisfaction of the Secretary by the submission of plans for each year of such three-year period that it is making continuous efforts and progress toward achieving compliance with subparagraph (A)(iii).

"(3) A State may, in the case of an entity which has submitted an application to the Secretary for determination that it is a health maintenance organization within the meaning of paragraph (1) and for which no such determination has been made within 90 days of the submission of the application, make a provisional determination for the purposes of this title that such entity is such a health maintenance organization. Such provisional determination shall remain in force until such time as the Secretary makes a determination regarding the entity's qualification under paragraph (1).".

(b) The amendment made by subsection (a) shall apply with respect to payments under title XIX of the Social Security Act to States for services provided—

42 USC 1396b note.
42 USC 1396.

(1) after the date of enactment of subsection (a) under contracts under such title entered into or renegotiated after such date, or

(2) after the expiration of the 1-year period beginning on such date of enactment,

whichever occurs first.

90 STAT. 1960   PUBLIC LAW 94-460—OCT. 8, 1976

TITLE III—MISCELLANEOUS AMENDMENTS

CENTER FOR HEALTH SERVICES POLICY ANALYSIS

? USC 247c.
SEC. 301. Section 305(d)(1) of the Public Health Service Act is amended (1) by striking out "two national special emphasis centers" and substituting "three national special emphasis centers", (2) by striking out "and one" and substituting "one", and (3) by inserting before the last close parenthesis a semicolon and the following: "and one of which (to be designated as the Health Services Policy Analysis Center) shall focus on the development and evaluation of national policies with respect to health services, including the development of health maintenance organizations and other forms of group practice, with a view toward improving the efficiencies of the health services delivery system".

HOME HEALTH EXTENSION

42 USC 1395x note.
SEC. 302. (a) Section 602(a)(5) of Public Law 94-63 is amended by inserting ", $2,000,000 for the period July 1, 1976, through September 30, 1976, $8,000,000 for the fiscal year ending September 30, 1977" after "1976".

(b) Section 602(b)(4) of Public Law 94-63 is amended by inserting ", $1,000,000 for the period July 1, 1976, through September 30, 1976, and $4,000,000 for the fiscal year ending September 30, 1977" after "1976".

EXTENSION OF REPORTING DATE

42 USC 289k-2.
SEC. 303. Section 603(b) of Public Law 94-63 is amended by striking "Within one year" and substituting "Not later than 2 years".

TECHNICAL

21 USC 360d.
SEC. 304. Section 514(a) of the Federal Food, Drug, and Cosmetic Act is amended by redesignating paragraphs (4) and (5) as paragraphs (3) and (4), respectively.

Approved October 8, 1976.

LEGISLATIVE HISTORY:

HOUSE REPORTS: No. 94-518 (Comm. on Interstate and Foreign Commerce) and
No. 94-1513 (Comm. of Conference).
SENATE REPORT: No. 94-844 accompanying S. 1926 (Comm. on Labor and Public
Welfare).
CONGRESSIONAL RECORD:
Vol. 121 (1975): Nov. 7, considered and passed House.
Vol. 122 (1976): June 14, considered and passed Senate, amended, in lieu of
S. 1926.
Sept. 16, Senate agreed to conference report.
Sept. 23, House agreed to conference report.
WEEKLY COMPILATION OF PRESIDENTIAL DOCUMENTS:
Vol. 12, No. 42 (1976): Oct. 9, Presidential statement.

O

Appendix 3

RULES AND REGULATIONS

Title 42—Public Health

CHAPTER I—PUBLIC HEALTH SERVICE, DEPARTMENT OF HEALTH, EDUCATION, AND WELFARE

SUBCHAPTER J—HEALTH CARE DELIVERY SYSTEMS

PART 110—HEALTH MAINTENANCE ORGANIZATIONS

Interim Regulations

AGENCY: Public Health Service, HEW.

ACTION: Interim regulations.

SUMMARY: These regulations implement certain aspects of Title XIII of the Public Health Service Act, "Health Maintenance Organizations" (42 U.S.C. 300e et seq.), as amended by the Health Maintenance Organization Amendments of 1976 (Pub. L. 94–460). Included are regulations which set forth requirements regarding the organization and operation of qualified health maintenance organizations (Subpart A), requirements for entities requesting Federal financial assistance for the development and initial operation of health maintenance organizations (Subparts B, C, D, and E), and requirements for entities seeking a determination by the Secretary that they are qualified health maintenance organizations under Title XIII (Subpart F).

EFFECTIVE DATE: June 8, 1977.

FOR FURTHER INFORMATION CONTACT:

Frank H. Seubold, Ph. D., Director, Division of Health Maintenance Organizations, 5600 Fishers Lane, Parklawn Building, Room 12–05, Rockville, Maryland 20857 (301–443–4106) or

Mr. William J. McLeod, Director, Office of Health Maintenance Organizations Qualification and Compliance, 5600 Fishers Lane, Parklawn Building, Room 14A–35, Rockville, Maryland 20857 (301–443–2778).

SUPPLEMENTARY INFORMATION: Regulations to implement certain provisions of Title XIII of the Public Health Service Act were published in the FEDERAL REGISTER on October 18, 1974, (39 FR 37308–37323; Subparts A, B, C, D, E, and G) and on August 8, 1975, (40 FR 33520–33524; Subpart F). With respect to Subpart F, certain provisions were proposed to be amended in a Notice of Proposed Rulemaking published on September 17, 1976, in the FEDERAL REGISTER

(41 FR 40292). The Assistant Secretary for Health of the Department of Health, Education, and Welfare, with the approval of the Secretary of Health, Education, and Welfare hereby amends the regulations cited above by deleting all provisions that are inconsistent with the Health Maintenance Organization Amendments of 1976 (Pub. L. 94–460) and by adding, as appropriate, the text of the statutory amendments. In addition, it was necessary in certain instances to add clarifying language which will allow the activities of the health maintenance organization program to be administered under the authority of the 1976 amendments.

For reasons set out below, the Secretary has determined that public participation in rulemaking prior to issuance of these regulations and a delay in their effective date would be impractical and contrary to the public interest, and, accordingly, that good cause exists for making these regulations effective immediately on June 8, 1977. Because the new law moderates certain restrictive provisions of the original Act, there is an urgent need to revise the current regulations as soon as possible so that organizations may qualify under the amended law. In addition, applicants for grants and loans will benefit substantially from the less restrictive provisions of the new law, and, with only a two year extension of the financial assistance programs, revised regulations are urgently needed.

Following the issuance of these interim regulations, the Department intends to issue a Notice of Proposed Rulemaking which would propose to revise these regulations by implementing all of the provisions of the Health Maintenance Organization Amendments of 1976, except for the amendments to Titles XVIII (Medicare) and XIX (Medicaid) of the Social Security Act. The public would be given 60 days to comment on these proposed regulations, including the amendments made in these interim regulations.

Set forth below is a summary of the amendments made by these interim regulations.

A.—DISCUSSION OF THE HEALTH MAINTENANCE ORGANIZATION AMENDMENTS OF 1976

Attention is called to features of the

amended law which required either deleting inconsistent provisions in the current regulations or adding the text of the statutory amendments. Provisions of the 1976 amendments included in the interim regulations are:

1.—SUPPLEMETAL HEALTH SERVICES

Allows inclusion of supplemental health services in the basic health services which a health maintenance organization provides its members for a basic health services payment.

Makes the offer of supplemental health services optional for the health maintenance organization.

2.—STAFFING

Permits the health maintenance organization to provide the services of health professionals which are provided as basic health services through any combination of staff, medical group, individual practice association, or health professionals under contract.

Broadens the range of personnel who may be utilized to provide basic health services.

Limits extent of direct contracting between a health maintenance organization and health professionals for the provision of basic health services to 15 percent (30 percent for a health maintenance organization serving a rural area) of the total compensation paid to physicians for the provision of basic and supplemental health services.

3.—OPEN ENROLLMENT

Requires open enrollment to be offered only by a health maintenance organization which did not incur a deficit in its most recent fiscal year and

a. Has provided comprehensive health care services on a prepaid basis for at least 5 years, or

b. Has an enrollment of 50,000.

Provides that the open enrollment period is the lesser of 30 days or the period within which the health maintenance organization enrolls a number of individuals at least equal to 3 percent of its net increase in enrollment during the prior year, excluding any increase in enrollment under contracts which were in effect prior to qualification. The health maintenance organization may not be required to enroll individuals who are confined to an institution because of chronic illness, permanent injury, or other infirmity which would cause economic impairment to the health maintenance organization.

Provides that the health maintenance organization may not be required to make the effective date for benefits less than 90 days after the date of enrollment.

Permits the Secretary to waive the open enrollment requirement if the health maintenance organization demonstrates that its economic viability would be jeopardized by compliance with the requirement.

4.—DEFINITION OF SERVICES

Eliminates preventive dental care for children from the list of required basic health services.

Defines preventive health services to include immunizations, well-child care from birth, periodic health examinations for adults, voluntary family planning services, services for infertility, and children's eye and ear examinations.

5.—COMMUNITY RATING

Permits health maintenance organizations which provided comprehensive health services on a prepaid basis at the time of qualification as a health maintenance organization 48 months to meet the requirement that payments for basic and certain supplemental health services be fixed under a community rating system.

Requires applications for assistance to include an additional assurance with respect to the fixing of basic health services payments and supplemental health services payments under a community rating system.

Adds difference in marketing costs to the nominal differentials allowable under a community rating system.

Allows nominal differentials in rates to accommodate the group purchasing practices of employers under the community rating system.

6.—MEDICAL GROUP REQUIREMENTS

Partially relieves the requirement that the "principal" practice activity of the medical group must be for the health maintenance organization, by requiring the group to have a "substantial" responsibility for delivery of health services to health maintenance organization members.

Provides that payment to group members is to be unrelated to the frequency of services performed.

Requires that the health maintenance organization member's enrollment status is not to be made known to the health professional providing services to the member.

7.—INCREASE IN LIMITS ON ASSISTANCE FOR

FEASIBILITY SURVEYS, PLANNING, INITIAL DEVELOPMENT, AND INITIAL OPERATION

Increases feasibility grant limit from $50,000 to $75,000.

Increases planning grant limit from $125,000 to $200,000.

Allows up to $1,600,000 for the initial development of certain health maintenance organizations which will undertake to expand or will serve non-contiguous services areas.

Extends period for use of loan funds (time to reach break even) from 36 months to 60 months; maximum loan remains at $2,500,000.

8.—LOAN GUARANTEES FOR PRIVATE ENTITIES

Permits guarantee of private loans to non-profit private entities.

Provides for special consideration for applicants which will serve medically underserved populations.

9.—MISCELLANEOUS AMENDMENTS

Extends the period of loan assistance from 36 to 60 months and permits the health maintenance organization to break even in less than 60 months without being required immediately to repay part of the loan.

Facilitates the administration of the loan program by revising language relating to the interest rate for loans.

Permits use of initial development grant funds to recruit physicians who will engage in practice principally for the health maintenance organization.

10.—HEALTH MAINTENANCE ORGANIZATIONS AND FEDERAL EMPLOYEE HEALTH BENEFITS PROGRAM

Provides that an entity serving Federal employees under contract with the Civil Service Commission can be considered a qualified health maintenance organization if it meets all the requirements of the Health Maintenance Organization Act with respect to its other enrollees.

11.—CONFORMING AMENDMENTS

Changes references in the original Act to "the section 314(a) State health planning agency" and "the section 314 (b) areawide health planning agency" to read "State health planning and development agency" and "health systems agency", respectively.

B.—CLARIFYING LANGUAGE ADDED

In certain cases, clarifying language was necessary and has been added to the interim regulations as follows:

1. The term "comprehensive health services" was defined by listing the services set forth at § 110.603(b), which describes a transitionally qualified health maintenance organization (§ 110.101(s)).

2. A specific "use of funds" statement was added to the requirements for feasibility surveys and planning and initial development projects (§§ 110.305 (c) and 110.405(a)(3) and (b)(4)).

3. The definition of the term "operating cost" was expanded to include the use of Federal funds for restricted reserve accounts required by State authority (§ 110.501(a)).

4. In the case of applicants for qualification which have regional components (see § 110.101(1)(4)), the regulations now provide that the applicant may be considered to be a transitionally qualified health maintenance organization for those regional components which have signed the assurances required for transitional qualification. However, if all of the regional components have not signed these assurances within one year or if any of the components fails to comply with the applicable time-phased plan for becoming an operational qualified health maintenance organization, the qualification of the entire entity will be terminated (§ 110.603(b)(3)).

C.—PROCEDURAL CHANGES IN QUALIFICATION APPLICATION REQUIREMENTS

Certain procedural changes have been made with respect to qualification application requirements. The application requirements for qualification applicants previously contained in § 110.604(b), (c), and (d), have been deleted from the interim regulations and will be revised and set forth in a separate application form provided by the Secretary. Application forms and instructions may be obtained by writing the Office of Health Maintenance Organizations Qualification and Compliance, Assistant Secretary for Health, Department of Health, Education, and Welfare, 5600 Fishers Lane, Rockville, Maryland 20857 or the Regional Health Administrator in the appropriate Regional Office of the Department of Health, Education, and Welfare at the addresses set forth at 45 CFR 5.31(b).

NOTE.—The Department of Health, Education, and Welfare has determined that this document does not contain a major proposal requiring preparation of an Inflation Impact Statement under Executive Order 11821 and OMB Circular A-107.

Dated: April 8, 1977.

JAMES F. DICKSON,

*Acting Assistant Secretary
for Health.*

Approved: May 28, 1977.
JOSEPH A. CALIFANO, JR.,
Secretary.

AUTHORITY: Sec. 215, 58 Stat. 690, (42 U.S.C. 216); secs. 1301–1316, as amended, 90 Stat. 1945–1960 (42 U.S.C. 300e–15).

Subpart A—Requirements for a Health Maintenance Organization

§ 110.101   Definitions.

As used in this part:

(a) "Health maintenance organization" means a legal entity which provides or arranges for the provision of basic and supplemental health services to its members in the manner prescribed by, is organized and operated in the manner prescribed by, and otherwise meets the requirements of, section 1301 of the Act and the regulations under this subpart.

(b) "Basic health services" means:

(1) Physicians services (including consultant and referral services by a physician);

(2) Outpatient services and inpatient hospital services;

(3) Medically necessary outpatient and inpatient emergency health services;

(4) Short-term (not to exceed twenty visits), outpatient evaluative, and crisis intervention mental health services;

(5) Medical treatment and referral services (including referral services to appropriate ancillary services) for the abuse of or addiction to alcohol and drugs;

(6) Diagnostic laboratory and diagnostic and therapeutic radiologic services;

(7) Home health services; and

(8) Preventive health services (including (i) immunizations, (ii) well-child care from birth, (iii) periodic health evaluation for adults, (iv) voluntary family planning services, (v) services for infertility, and (vi) children's eye and ear examinations conducted to determine the need for vision and hearing correction).

(c) "Supplemental health services" means:

(1) Services of facilities for intermediate and long-term care;

(2) Vision care not included as a basic health service;

(3) Dental services;

(4) Mental health services not in-

cluded as a basic health service;

(5) Long-term physical medicine and rehabilitative services (including physical therapy); and

(6) The provision of prescription drugs prescribed in the delivery of a basic health service or a supplemental health service provided by the health maintenance organization.

(d) "In-area" means the geographical area defined by the health maintenance organization as its service area in which it provides health services to its members directly through its own resources or through arrangements with other providers in the area.

(e) "Out-of-area" means that area outside of the geographical area defined by the health maintenance organization as its service area.

(f) "Member", when used in connection with a health maintenance organization, means an individual who has entered into a contractual arrangement, or on whose behalf a contractual arrangement has been entered into, with the organization under which the organization assumes the responsibility for the provision to such individual of basic health services and of such supplemental health services as may be contracted for.

(g) "Subscriber" means a member who has entered into a contractual relationship with the health maintenance organization.

(h) (1) "Health professionals" means physicians, dentists, nurses, podiatrists, optometrists, physicians' assistants, clinical psychologists, social workers, pharmacists, nutritionists, occupational therapists, physical therapists, and other professionals engaged in the delivery of health services who are licensed, practice under an institutional license, are certified, or practice under authority of the health maintenance organization, a medical group, individual practice association, or other authority consistent with State law.

(2) "Physician" means a doctor of medicine or a doctor of osteopathy.

(i) "Medical group" means a partnership, association, corporation, or other entity:

(1) Which is composed of health professionals licensed to practice medicine or osteopathy and of such other licensed health professionals (including dentists, optometrists, and podiatrists) as are necessary for the provision of health services for which the group is responsible;

(2) A majority of the members of which are licensed to practice medicine or osteopathy; and

(3) The members of which

(i) As their principal professional activity (over 50 percent individually) and as a group responsibility engage in the coordinated practice of their profession and as a group have substantial responsibility (over 35 percent in the aggregate of their professional activity) for the delivery of health services to members of a health maintenance organization or present a time phased plan, which is acceptable to the Secretary and to which they are committed, to meet this requirement within 3 years from the date the health maintenance organization is found by the Secretary to be a qualified health maintenance organization. Following the expiration of such 3 year period, the Secretary may waive the requirement that over 35 percent of the activity of a medical group be for members of a health maintenance organization.

(ii) Pool their income from practice as members of the group and distribute it among themselves according to a prearranged salary or drawing account or other similar plan unrelated to the provision of specific health services;

(iii) Share health (including medical) records and substantial portions of major equipment and of professional, technical, and administrative staff;

(iv) Establish an arrangement whereby a member's enrollment status is not known to the health professional who provides health services to the member; and

(v) Arrange for and encourage continuing education in the field of clinical medicine and related areas for the members of the group; and

(4) Which has a written services agreement with a health maintenance organization to provide services to members of the health maintenance organization.

(j) "Individual practice association" means a partnership, corporation, association, or other entity: (1) Which has as its primary objective the delivery or arrangements for the delivery of health services and which has entered into a written service arrangement or arrangements with health professionals, a majority of whom are licensed to practice medicine or osteopathy. Such written services arrangement shall provide:

(i) That such persons shall provide their professional services in accordance with a compensation arrangement established by the entity; and

(ii) To the extent feasible:

(A) For the sharing by such persons

of health (including medical) and other records, equipment, and professional, technical, and administrative staff; and

(B) For the arrangement and encouragement of the continuing education of such persons in the field of clinical medicine and related areas; and

(2) Which has a written services agreement with a health maintenance organization to arrange for the provision of services to members of the health maintenance organization.

(k) "Medically underserved population" means the population of an urban or rural area designated by the Secretary as an area with a shortage of personal health services. Designations with respect to such urban or rural areas will be made by the Secretary as described in § 110.203(g).

(l) "Community rating system" (community rate) means a system of fixing rates of payments for health services. Under such a system rates of payments may be determined on a per-person or per-family basis and may vary with the number of persons in a family, but except as otherwise authorized in this paragraph, such rates must be equivalent for all individuals and for all families of similar composition. This does not preclude changes in the rates of payments for health services based on a community rating system which are established for new enrollments or reenrollments and which changes do not apply to existing contracts until the renewal of such contracts. Only the following differentials in rates of payments may be established under such system:

(1) Nominal differentials in such rates may be established to reflect differences in marketing costs and the different administrative costs of collecting payments from the following categories of subscribers:

(i) Individual (non-group) subscribers (including their families),

(ii) Small groups of subscribers (100 subscribers or less),

(iii) Large groups of subscribers (over 100 subscribers).

(2) Nominal differentials in such rates may be established to reflect the compositing of the rates of payment in a systematic manner to accommodate group purchasing practices of the various employers.

(3) Differentials in such rates may be established for subscribers enrolled in a health maintenance organization: (i) Under a contract with a governmental authority under section 1079 ("Contracts for Medical Care for Spouses and Children: Plans") or section 1086 ("Contracts for Health Benefits for Certain Members, Former Members and their Dependents") of Title 10 ("Armed Forces"), United States Code; or (ii) Under any other governmental program (other than the health benefits program authorized by chapter 89 ("Health Insurance"), of Title 5 ("Government Organization and Employees"), United States Code); or (iii) Under any health benefits program for employees of States, political subdivisions of States, and other public entities.

(4) A health maintenance organization may establish a separate community rate for separate regional components of the organization upon satisfactory demonstration to the Secretary of the following:

(i) Each such regional component is geographically distinct and separate from any other regional component;

(ii) Membership is established with respect to the individual regional component, rather than with respect to the parent health maintenance organization; and

(iii) Each such regional component provides substantially the full range of basic health services to its members, without extensive referral between components of the organization for such services, and without substantial utilization by any two such components of the same health care facilities. The separate community rate for each such regional component of the health maintenance organization must be based on the different costs of providing health services in such regions.

(m) "Nonmetropolitan area" means an area no part of which is within an area designated as a standard metropolitan statistical area by the Office of Management and Budget and which does not contain a city whose population exceeds fifty thousand individuals.

(n) "Rural area" means any area not listed as a place having a population of 2,500 or more in Document No. PC(1)–A, "Number of Inhabitants", Table VI, "Population of Places", and not listed as an urbanized area in Table XI, "Population of Urbanized Areas" of the same document (1970 Census, Bureau of the Census, U.S. Department of Commerce).

(o) "Non-Federal lender" means any lender other than an agency or instrumentality of the United States.

(p) "Act" means the Public Health Service Act.

(q) "Secretary" means the Secretary of Health, Education, and Welfare and any other officer or employee of the Department of Health, Education, and Welfare to whom the authority involved has been delegated.

(r) "Qualified health maintenance organization" means an entity which has been found by the Secretary to meet the applicable requirements of title XIII of the Act and the applicable regulations of this part.

(s) "Comprehensive health services" means health services which are provided or arranged for individuals or groups by a public or private organization and are health services which individuals might reasonably require in order to be maintained in good health. These health services include as a minimum the following services, which may be limited as to time and cost: Physician services (§ 110.102(a)(1)); outpatient services and inpatient hospital services (§ 110.102(a)(2)); medically necessary emergency health services (§ 110.102 (a)(3)); diagnostic laboratory and diagnostic and therapeutic radiologic services (§ 110.102(a)(6)).

§ 110.102   Health benefits plan; basic health services.

A health maintenance organization shall:

(a) Provide or arrange for the provision of basic health services to its members as needed and without limitations as to time and cost other than those prescribed in the Act and these regulations, as follows:

(1) Physician services (including consultant and referral services by a physician), which shall be provided by a licensed physician, or if a service of a physician may also be provided under applicable State law by other health professionals, a health maintenance organization may provide such service through such other health professionals;

(2) Outpatient services, which shall include diagnostic or treatment services or both for patients who are ambulatory and may be provided in a nonhospital based health care facility or at a hospital; inpatient hospital services, which shall include but not be limited to, room and board, general nursing care, meals and special diets when medically necessary, use of operating room and related facilities, intensive care unit and services, X-ray, laboratory, and other diagnostic tests, drugs, medications, biologicals, anesthesia and oxygen services, special duty nursing when medically necessary, physical therapy, radiation therapy, inhalation therapy, and administration of whole blood and blood plasma;

outpatient services and inpatient hospital services shall include short-term rehabilitation services as appropriate;

(3) Instructions to its members on procedures to be followed to secure in-area and out-of-area medically necessary emergency health services (see § 110.104(a)(2));

(4) At least 20 outpatient visits per member per year, as may be necessary and appropriate for short-term evaluative or crisis intervention mental health services, or both;

(5) Diagnosis, medical treatment and referral services (including referral services to appropriate ancillary services) for the abuse of or addiction to alcohol and drugs;

(i) Diagnosis and medical treatment shall include detoxification for alcoholism or drug abuse on either an outpatient or inpatient basis, whichever is medically determined to be appropriate, in addition to treatment for other medical conditions;

(ii) Referral services may be either for medical or for non-medical ancillary services. Medical services shall be a part of basic health services; non-medical ancillary services (such as vocational rehabilitation, employment counseling), need not be a part of basic health services;

(6) Diagnostic laboratory and diagnostic and therapeutic radiology services in support of basic health services;

(7) Home health services provided at a member's home by health care personnel, as prescribed or directed by the responsible physician or other authority designated by the health maintenance organization; and

(8) Preventive health services, which shall be made available to members and shall include at least the following:

(i) A broad range of voluntary family planning services;

(ii) Services for infertility;

(iii) Well-child care from birth and periodic health evaluations for adults.

(iv) Eye and ear examinations for children through age 17, to determine the need for vision and hearing correction; and

(v) Pediatric and adult immunizations, in accord with accepted medical practice.

(b) In addition, a health maintenance organization may include a health service defined as a supplemental health service by § 110.101(c) among the basic health services provided or arranged for its members for a basic health services payment.

(c) The following are not required to

be provided as basic health services:

(1) Corrective appliances and artificial aids;

(2) Mental health services, except as required under section 1302(1)(D) of the Act;

(3) Cosmetic surgery, unless medically necessary;

(4) Prescribed drugs and medicines incidental to outpatient care;

(5) Ambulance services, unless medically necessary;

(6) Treatment for chronic alcoholism and drug addiction, except as required by section 1302(1)(E) of the Act and paragraph (a)(5) of this section;

(7) Care for military service connected disabilities for which the member is legally entitled to services and for which facilities are reasonably available to this member;

(8) Care for conditions that State or local law requires be treated in a public facility;

(9) Dental services;

(10) Vision care;

(11) Custodial or domiciliary care;

(12) Experimental medical, surgical, or other experimental health care procedures unless approved as a basic health service by the policy making body of the health maintenance organization;

(13) Personal or comfort items and private rooms, unless medically necessary during inpatient hospitalization; and

(14) Whole blood and blood plasma.

§ 110.103 Health benefits plan: Supplemental health services.

(a) Each health maintenance organization may provide to each of its members any of the following health services which are included in supplemental health services (as defined in § 110.101(c)):

(i) Services of facilities for intermediate and long-term care;

(ii) Vision care not included as a basic health service;

(iii) Dental services not included as a basic health service;

(iv) Mental health services not included as a basic health service;

(v) Long-term physical medicine and rehabilitative services (including physical therapy);

(vi) Prescription drugs prescribed in the course of provision of basic outpatient or supplemental health services; and

(vii) Other health services which are not included as basic health services and which have been approved by the Secretary for delivery as supplemental health services.

(b) A health maintenance organization shall determine the level and scope of such supplemental health services included among basic health services provided to its members for a basic health services payment or such services offered to its members as supplemental health services.

(c) A health maintenance organization is authorized, if it so elects, in connection with the prescription or provision of prescription drugs, to maintain, review, and evaluate a drug use profile of its members receiving such services, evaluate patterns of drug utilization to assure optimum drug therapy, and provide for instruction of its members and of health professionals in the use of prescription and nonprescription drugs. Each health maintenance organization providing such services shall insure that:

(1) The program is developed jointly by the physicians and pharmacists associated with the health maintenance organization;

(2) The objectives of the program are explained to all health professionals and members of the health maintenance organization;

(3) Individual rights are protected and that all information regarding and identifying an individual is available only to appropriate health professionals of the health maintenance organization, and to the individual member at his request;

(4) The primary thrust of the program is optimum drug therapy for the individual member of the health maintenance organization; and

(5) The information obtained in drug utilization review is utilized in educational programs for professionals and members of the health maintenance organization.

§ 110.104 Providers of services.

(a) Basic health services shall be provided or arranged for through health professionals who are employed by the health maintenance organization as members of the staff of the health maintenance organization, through a medical group (or groups), which has contracted with the health maintenance organization, through an individual practice association (or associations), which has contracted with the health maintenance organization, through health professionals who have contracted with the health maintenance organization for the provision of such services, or through any combination of such staff, medical group (or groups), individual practice association (or associations), or health professionals under contract with the organization. Such contracts shall include the acceptance by the members of the medical groups or individual practice associations of effective incentives, such as risk sharing or other financial incentives, designed to avoid unnecessary or unduly costly utilization of health services. A health maintenance organization may not, in any of its fiscal years, enter into contracts with health professionals (other than as members of its staff) or entities other than medical groups or individual practice associations if the amounts paid under such contracts for basic and supplemental health services exceed fifteen percent of the total amount to be paid in such fiscal year by the health maintenance organization to physicians for the provision of basic and supplemental health services, or, if the health maintenance organization principally serves a rural area, thirty percent of such amount, except that this sentence does not apply to the entering into of contracts for the purchase of basic and supplemental health services through an entity which but for the requirements of § 110.101(1)(3)(i) would be a medical group for purposes of this subpart. Contracts between a health maintenance organization and health professionals for the provision of basic and supplemental health services shall include such provisions as the Secretary may require (including provisions requiring appropriate continuing education). Basic health services shall be so provided unless:

(1) The services are unusual or infrequently used services which do not warrant provision through staff of the health maintenance organization, or a medical group, or an individual practice association or any combination of the above as demonstrated by the health maintenance organization to the satisfaction of the Secretary. The provision of such services not provided through the staff of a health maintenance organization or through a medical group or an individual practice association shall be arranged for by the health maintenance organization with other providers in the area; or

(2) The services are medically necessary (i.e., are not provided for reasons of convenience) and are provided to a member other than through the health maintenance organization because the member's condition would be jeopardized before he could obtain such services through the health maintenance organization; or

(3) The services are provided as part of inpatient hospital services by employees or staff of a hospital.

(b) Each health maintenance organization shall pay the provider, or reimburse its members for the payment of, reasonable charges for basic health services or supplemental health services for which its members have contracted, which are medically necessary emergency services obtained within area or out-of-area, other than through the health maintenance organization. Each health maintenance organization shall adopt procedures to review promptly all claims from members for reimbursement for the provision of medically necessary health services, which procedures shall include the determination of the medical necessity for obtaining such services.

(c) Supplemental health services shall be provided or arranged for by the health maintenance organization and need not be provided by providers of basic health services under contract with the health maintenance organization.

§ 110.105 Payment for basic health services.

(a) Each health maintenance organization shall provide or arrange for the provision of basic health services for a basic health services payment which:

(1) Is to be paid on a periodic basis without regard to the dates such health services are provided;

(2) Is fixed without regard to the frequency, extent, or kind of such health services actually furnished;

(3) Is fixed under a community rating system, except as provided in paragraph (c) of this section; and

(4) May be supplemented by additional nominal copayments which may be required for the provision of specific basic health services. Each health maintenance organization may establish one or more copayment options, calculated on the basis of a community rating system.

(i) To insure that copayments are not a barrier to the utilization of health services or membership in the organization, a health maintenance organization shall not impose copayment charges that exceed 50 percent of the total cost of providing any single service to its members, nor in the aggregate more than 20 percent of the total cost of providing all basic health services.

(ii) No copayment may be imposed on any subscriber or members covered by his contract with the health maintenance organization in any calendar year, when the copayments made by such subscriber or members in such calendar year total

50 percent of the total annual premium cost which such subscriber or members would be required to pay if he or they were enrolled under an option with no copayments, if such subscriber or members demonstrates that copayments in that amount have been paid in such year.

(b) A health maintenance organization may include a health service defined as a supplemental health service by § 110.101(c) in the basic health services provided its members for a basic health services payment.

(c) In the case of an entity which before it became a qualified health maintenance organization (within the meaning of section 1310(d) of the Act) provided comprehensive health services on a prepaid basis, the requirement for community rating shall not apply to such entity until the expiration of the forty-eight month period beginning with the month following the month in which the entity became a qualified health maintenance organization.

(d) If, pursuant to workmen's compensation or employer's liability law or other legislation of similar purpose or import, a third party would be responsible for all or part of the cost of basic health services provided by the health maintenance organization if services had not been provided by the health maintenance organization, then the health maintenance organization may collect from the third party the portion of the cost of such services for which such third party would be so responsible.

§ 110.106 Payment for supplemental health services.

(a) A health maintenance organization may require supplemental health services payments, in addition to the basic health services payments, for the provision of each health service included in the supplemental health services set forth in § 110.103 for which subscribers have contracted.

(b) Supplemental health services payments may be made in any agreed upon manner, such as prepayment, or fee-for-service. Supplemental health services payments which are fixed on a prepayment basis, however, shall be fixed under a community rating system, except that, in the case of an entity which before it became a qualified health maintenance organization (within the meaning of section 1310(d) of the Act) provided comprehensive health services on a prepaid basis, the requirement of this sentence shall not apply to such an entity during the forty-eight month period beginning

with the month following the month in which the entity became such a qualified health maintenance organization.

(c) If, pursuant to any workmen's compensation or employer's liability law or other legislation of similar purpose or import, a third party would be responsible for all or part of the cost of supplemental health services provided by the health maintenance organization if services had not been provided by the health maintenance organization, then the health maintenance organization may collect from the third party the portion of the cost of such services for which such third party would be so responsible.

§ 110.107 Availability, accessibility, and continuity of basic and supplemental health services.

Within the area served by the health maintenance organization, basic health services and only such supplemental health services for which members have contracted shall:

(a) Be provided or arranged for by the health maintenance organization;

(b) Be available and accessible to each of the health maintenance organization's members promptly as appropriate with respect to:

(1) Its geographic location, hours of operation, and provisions for after-hours services (medically necessary emergency services must be available and accessible 24 hours a day, 7 days a week); and

(2) Staffing patterns within generally accepted norms for meeting the projected membership needs; and

(c) Be provided in a manner which assures continuity, including but not limited to:

(1) Provision of a health professional who is primarily responsible for coordinating the member's overall health care; and

(2) Development of a health (including medical) recordkeeping system through which all pertinent information relating to the health care of the patient is accumulated and is readily available to appropriate professionals.

§ 110.108 Organization and operation.

Each health maintenance organization shall—

(a) Have a fiscally sound operation, as demonstrated by a financial plan, satisfactory to the Secretary, which:

(1) Identifies the achievement and maintenance of a positive cash flow, including provisions for retirement of ex-

isting and proposed indebtedness;

(2) Demonstrates the ability to establish reserves in compliance with applicable State laws pertaining to fiscal responsibility or such reserves as the Secretary may determine necessary relative to repayment of principal and interest on loans made or guaranteed under this part;

(3) Demonstrates an approach to the risk of insolvency which allows for continuation of benefits for the duration of the contract period for which payment has been made, continuation of benefits to members who are confined on the date of insolvency in an inpatient facility until their discharge, and payments to unaffiliated providers for services rendered; and

(4) Demonstrates that the entity has procured and maintains in force a fidelity bond or bonds, in such amount, but not less than $100,000, as may be fixed by its Board of Directors or other policymaking body, covering every officer and employee entrusted with the handling of its funds. The bond may have reasonable deductibles, based upon the financial strength of the entity.

(b) Assume full financial risk on a prospective basis for the provision of basic health services, except that a health maintenance organization may obtain insurance or make other arrangements:

(1) For the cost of providing to any member basic health services the aggregate value of which exceeds $5,000 in any year;

(2) For the cost of basic health services provided to its members other than through the organization because medical necessity required their provision before they could be secured through the organization; and

(3) For not more than 90 percent of the amount by which its costs for any of its fiscal years exceed 115 percent of its income for such fiscal year;

(c) After full and fair disclosure of benefits, coverage, rates, grievance procedures, location, and hours of service, and a general description of participating providers, offer enrollment to persons who are broadly representative of the various age, social, and income groups within the area it serves except that in the case of a health maintenance organization which has a medically underserved population located (in whole or in part) in the area it serves, not more than 75 percent of the members of that organization may be enrolled from the medically underserved popula-

tion unless the area in which such population resides is also a rural area; and

(d) Have an open enrollment period as follows:

(1) (i) A health maintenance organization which—

(A) Has for at least 5 years provided comprehensive health services on a prepaid basis, or

(B) Has an enrollment of at least 50,000 members, shall have at least once during each fiscal year next following a fiscal year in which it did not have a financial deficit, as reported and certified by an independent Certified Public Account, an open enrollment period (determined under paragraph (d) (1) (ii) of this section) during which it shall accept individuals for membership in the order in which they apply for enrollment and, except as provided in paragraph (d) (2) of this section, without regard to preexisting illness, medical condition, or degree of disability.

(ii) An open enrollment period for a health maintenance organization shall be the lesser of—

(A) 30 days, or

(B) The number of days in which the organization enrolls a number of individuals at least equal to 3 percent of its total net increase in enrollment (if any) in the fiscal year preceding the fiscal year in which such period is held. For the purpose of determining the total net increase in enrollment in a health maintenance organization, there shall not be included any individual who is enrolled in the organization through a group which had a contract for health care services with the health maintenance organization at the time that such health maintenance organization was determined to be a qualified health maintenance organization under Subpart F of this part.

(2) Notwithstanding the requirements of paragraph (d) (1) of this section, a health maintenance organization shall not be required to enroll individuals who are confined to an institution because of chronic illness, permanent injury, or other infirmity which would cause economic impairment to the health maintenance organization, as demonstrated to the satisfaction of the Secretary, if such individuals were enrolled.

(3) A health maintenance organization may not be required to make the effective date of benefits for individuals enrolled under this subsection less than 90 days after the date of enrollment.

(4) The Secretary may waive the requirements of this paragraph for a health maintenance organization which demon-

strates that compliance with the provisions of this subsection would jeopardize its economic viability in its service area.

(e) In order to obtain a waiver under paragraph (d)(4) of this section of the annual open enrollment period required in paragraph (d) of this section, the applicant shall submit documentation that the health maintenance organization has prospectively determined on an actuarial basis, utilizing data available in the area or from similar organizations elsewhere, that the average utilization of services of potential individual members would so increase costs as to jeopardize the economic viability of the organization if it maintained an open enrollment period. The data concerning the prospective utilization of individual members need not be obtained by the health maintenance organization from actual individual cases in its area, but may be composite data from known experiences.

(f) Not expel or refuse to re-enroll any member because of his health status or his health care needs, nor refuse to enroll individual members of a group on the basis of the health status or health care needs of such individuals;

(g) Offer each subscriber leaving a group a membership agreement on the same terms and conditions as are available to a non-group subscriber;

(h) Be organized in such a manner that assures that:

(1) No later than one year after becoming operational as a qualified health maintenance organization, at least one-third of the membership of the Board of Directors of the health maintenance organization or in the absence of such, its equivalent policy-making body, will be members of the organization. No member having ownership or interest in, or employed by or gaining financing reward from direct dealings with, the health maintenance organization, or with a plan-affiliated institution or organization, and no members of his immediate family shall be included in the minimum one-third member representation on the Board or policy-making body; except that none of the foregoing shall prohibit the payment of directors' fees or other similar fees, or interest and dividends derived from membership in a cooperative, to persons serving on such Board or body; and

(2) There shall be equitable representation on the member portion of such policy-making body of members from the medically underserved populations in proportion to their enrollment relative to the entire enrollment; except that if the medically underserved membership is at least 5 percent of the total enrollment, then such population shall not be without representation;

(i) Be organized in such a manner that provides meaningful procedures for hearing and resolving grievances between the health maintenance organization (including the staff of the health maintenance organization, the medical group, and the individual practice association) and the members of the organization, which procedures will assure that grievances and complaints will be transmitted in a timely manner to appropriate decision-making levels within the organization which have authority to take corrective action;

(j) Have organizational arrangements, consistent with program emphasis on quality health care, for an ongoing quality assurance program for its health services which program:

(1) Stresses health outcomes to the extent consistent with the state of the art;

(2) Provides review by physicians and other health professionals of the process followed in the provision of health services;

(3) Utilizes systematic data collection of performance and patient results, provides interpretation of such data to the practitioners, and institutes needed change; and

(4) Is designed in such a manner as is likely to meet the standards established pursuant to section 1155(e) of the Social Security Act (i.e. Professional Standards Review) for services provided by hospitals and other operating health care facilities or organizations;

(k) Assure that the providers through which the health maintenance organization provides basic and supplemental health services are certified under Title XVIII of the Social Security Act (Medicare) in accordance with 20 CFR Part 405, or in accordance with the regulations governing participation of providers in the Medical Assistance Program under Title XIX of the Social Security Act (Medicaid): *Provided,* That clinical laboratories subject to section 353 of the Act (Clinical Laboratories Improvement Act) shall, unless exempted thereunder, be certified in accordance with regulations governing participation of such laboratories under such Titles XVIII and XIX;

(l) Provide, or make arrangements for, continuing education for its health professional staff;

(m) In support of the provision of health services, offer its members the following:

(1) Health education services and education in the appropriate use of health services and in the contribution each member can make to the maintenance of his own health;

(2) Instruction in personal health care measures;

(3) Information about its services, including recommendations on generally accepted medical standards for use and frequency of such services; and

(4) Nutritional education and counseling;

(n) In support of the provision of health services, offer its members medical social services, which shall include appropriate assistance in dealing with the physical, emotional and economic impact of illness and disability through services such as pre- and post-hospitalization planning, referral to services provided through community health and social welfare agencies, and related family counseling;

(o) Provide an effective procedure while safeguarding the confidentiality of the doctor-patient relationship, to develop, compile, evaluate, and report, at such times and in such manner as the Secretary may require, to the Secretary, to its members, and to the general public, statistics and other information relating to;

(1) The cost of its operations;

(2) The patterns of utilization of its services;

(3) The availability, accessibility, and acceptability of its services;

(4) To the extent practical, developments in the health status of its members; and

(5) Such other matters as the Secretary may require;

(p) Be organized and operated in a manner intended to preserve human dignity;

(q) Establish adequate procedures to insure confidentiality of its members' health (including medical) records; and

(r) Make arrangements with referral resources to assure that the health maintenance organization is kept informed about the services provided to its members.

§ 110.109   Special requirements: Titles XVIII and XIX of the Social Security Act.

(a) A health maintenance organization which otherwise complies with section 1301(b) and section 1301(c) of the Act, and with the applicable regulations of this part, and which enrolls members who are entitled to insurance benefits

under Title XVIII of the Social Security Act or to medical assistance under a State plan approved under Title XIX of such Act, may still be considered a qualified health maintenance organization, if with respect to its Title XVIII and Title XIX members:

(1) It provides, at a minimum, only those health services for which it will be compensated under Title XVIII or under the Title XIX State plan, and it does not require such members to obtain coverage of any health service for which it will not be compensated under Title XVIII or under Title XIX State plan;

(2) It fixes payments for any services paid for under Title XVIII or under a Title XIX State plan on a basis other than a community rating system;

(3) It assumes full financial risk for the provision of health services only as required under Title XVIII of the Social Security Act or under its contract with a State for services under the Title XIX State plan;

(4) With respect to health services provided which it is not required to provide or for which it is not compensated under Title XVIII or under the contract with a State for services under the Title XIX State plan, it fixes payments for such services on a community rating system, fee-for-service, or other basis; and

(5) It complies with the applicable reimbursement provisions authorized under Title XVIII or under the Title XIX State plan of the State with which it is contracting.

(b) A health maintenance organization which enters into a contract with the Secretary under Title XVIII of the Social Security Act or with a State under Title XIX of such Act shall comply with the applicable Title XVIII or Title XIX deductible and coinsurance requirements in accordance with the provisions of Title XVIII or the Title XIX State plan of the State with which it is contracting. Copayment options which are not in accordance with a Title XIX State plan may not be imposed on Title XIX enrollees.

(c) At no time shall the members of a qualified health maintenance organization who are entitled to insurance benefits under Title XVIII of the Social Security Act or to medical assistance under a State plan approved under Title XIX of the Social Security Act constitute more than 50 percent of the total membership unless for good cause shown the Secretary waives such requirement.

(d) Any grievance procedures authorized under Title XVIII or Title XIX of the Social Security Act are not super-seded by the provisions of § 110.108(1).

§ 110.110 Special requirements: Federal Employee Health Benefits Program.

(a) An entity which provides health services to a defined population on a pre-paid basis and which has members who are enrolled under the health benefits program authorized by chapter 89 of title 5, United States Code, may be considered as a health maintenance organization for purposes of receiving assistance under this part if with respect to its other members it provides health services in ac-cordance with section 1301(b) of the Act and the applicable regulations of this part and is organized and operated in the manner prescribed by section 1301(c) of the Act and the applicable regulations of this part.

Subpart B—Federal Financial Assistance: General

§ 110.201 Applicability.

The regulations of this subpart apply to the award of grants, loans, and loan guarantees to public or nonprofit pri-vate entities or private entities (other than nonprofit private entities) for proj-ects as authorized by sections 1303, 1304, and 1305 of the Act.

§ 110.202 Definitions.

(a) "Nonprofit" as applied to a private entity, agency, institution, or organiza-tion means a private entity, agency, in-stitution, or organization, no part of the net earnings of which inures, or may law-fully inure, to the benefits of any private shareholder or individual.

(b) The term "health system agency" means an entity which has been desig-nated in accordance with section 1515 of the Public Health Service Act; and the term "State health planning and de-velopment agency" means an agency which has been designated in accordance with section 1521 of the Act.

(c) "Significant expansion" means (1) a planned increase in membership, to be effected at a rate which exceeds the average growth rate (see §§ 110.303 (g), 110.403(h), and 110.404(f)) of the health maintenance organization and which will require an increase in the number of health professionals serving members of the health maintenance or-ganization or an expansion of the phys-ical capacity of the total health facili-ties; or (2) a planned expansion of the service area beyond the current service area which would be made possible by the addition of health service delivery facilities and health professionals to serve members at a new site or sites in areas previously without such service sites. Only organizations which have been found by the Secretary to be quali-fied health maintenance organizations are eligible to apply for assistance for expansion under sections 1303 and 1304 of the Act.

§ 110.203 Application requirements.

(a) An application for a grant, loan, or loan guarantee shall be submitted to the Secretary at such time and in such form and manner as the Secretary may prescribe.

(b) The application shall contain a budget and a narrative describing the manner in which the applicant intends to conduct the project and carry out the requirements of these regulations. The application must describe the project in sufficient detail to identify clearly the need for and nature, specific objectives, plan and methods of the project.

(c) The application must be executed by an individual authorized to act for the applicant and to assume in behalf of the applicant the obligations imposed by the statute, the regulations of this subpart, and any additional conditions of the award.

(d) Applicants must submit an au-dited full financial statement unless ex-empted by the Secretary. An applicant whose financial statement shows unobli-gated cash assets which presumably could be used to conduct all or part of the project or undertaking for which appli-cation is made must also submit a de-tailed statement satisfactory to the Sec-retary stating why the unobligated cash assets of the applicant (other than those to be used to meet the applicant's con-tribution requirements) are not avail-able or are inadequate for the planned project. An applicant for a loan or loan guarantee shall also submit a written verification from at least two public or two private lending agencies or institu-tions demonstrating that, after a formal request,

(1) Funds have been denied in the amount requested in the application, or

(2) Funds in the amount requested in the application are available only at an interest rate in excess of those currently in effect for the loan and loan guarantee program on the date of the application. On the basis of the information submit-ted, the Secretary will determine whether or not the applicant would not

be able to complete the project or undertaking for which the application is submitted without the assistance applied for.

(e) Each application must contain the following assurances, as appropriate:

(1) In the case of an application for assistance under section 1303 of the Act, if the survey or other activity supported demonstrates that the development and operation or the expansion of the operation of a health maintenance organization is feasible, the applicant will be, or will form, or expand the operation of, as the case may be, a health maintenance organization;

(2) In the case of an application for assistance under section 1304 of the Act, the applicant will develop and operate or expand the operation of, as the case may be, a health maintenance organization;

(3) When operational as a health maintenance organization, the applicant will (i) provide basic and supplemental health services to its members, (ii) provide such services in the manner prescribed by section 1301(b) of the Act and by the regulations of this part, and (iii) be organized and operated in the manner prescribed by section 1301(c) of the Act and by the regulations of this part;

(4) When operational as a health maintenance organization, the applicant will enroll, and maintain an enrollment of, the maximum number of members that its available and potential resources will enable it to serve effectively. Maximum number of members is defined as the actual or projected enrollment which the health maintenance organization can serve, considering the availability of the required health manpower in the area to be served by the organization and the capacity of the facilities of the organization; and

(5) A statement of intent (including a demonstration of the applicant's ability) to meet the requirements of paragraphs (1) and (2) of section 1301(b) of the Act and the applicable regulations of this part respecting the fixing of basic health services payments and such supplemental health services that the member has contracted for on a prepayment basis under a community rating system.

(f) Each application which evidences or projects an enrollment of at least 66 percent from a nonmetropolitan area shall identify the area in which such population resides and indicate the percent of anticipated enrollment to be drawn from such area.

(g) Each application which evidences, or projects an enrollment of at least 30 percent of its members from a medically underserved population when the health maintenance organization first receives financial assistance or becomes operational shall identify the area in which such population resides, the total population of that area, and the percent of anticipated enrollment to be drawn from that area. Medically underserved areas will be designated by the Secretary, taking into consideration the following factors, among others:

(1) Available health resources in relation to size of the area and its population, including appropriate ratios of primary care physicians (both doctors of medicine and doctors of osteopathy) in general or family practice, internal medicine, pediatrics, obstetrics and gynecology, or general surgery, to population;

(2) Health indices for the population of the area, such as infant mortality rate;

(3) Economic factors affecting the population's access to health services, such as percentage of the population with incomes below the poverty level; and

(4) Demographic factors affecting the population's need/demand for health services, such as percentage of the population age 65 or over.

The designation of such areas may be made by the Secretary only after consideration of the comments, if any, of the appropriate health systems agency or State health planning and development agency whose plan covers (in whole or in part) the area in which such population group resides.

(h) Each application must show that each health systems agency whose plan covers (in whole or in part) the area to be served by the health maintenance organization for which such application is submitted (or if there is no such agency, the State health planning and development agency whose State health plan covers, in whole or in part, such area) has been sent a copy of the application concurrent with its submission to the appropriate Regional Office of the Department of Health, Education, and Welfare. Such health systems agency or State health planning and development agency shall have 60 days in which to review and comment on the application, commencing on the day the application is received. The applicant shall request that the comments of such agencies be forwarded to the Secretary through the appropriate Department of Health, Education, and Welfare Regional Office not later than 60 days from the date the application is received.

(i) If under applicable State law, the application may not be submitted without the approval of the health systems agency, or State health planning and development agency, the applicant shall obtain such approval which must be included as a part of the application.

(j) The application shall provide written information describing the applicant's development and operation of any prior projects which were supported by funds or by loans or loan guarantees under Title XIII of the Act. Applicants must also describe projects for the planning or operation of health service delivery programs supported under any other titles of the Public Health Service Act, or for which applications under the Act are currently under consideration.

(k) Applicants for more than one grant, loan, or loan guarantee under Title XIII of the Act, simultaneously or over the course of time, shall not be required to duplicate information, but shall update such information with each subsequent application.

§ 110.204 Health systems agency or State health planning and development agency review and comments.

The appropriate health systems agency or State health planning and development agency should provide to the Secretary through the appropriate Department of Health, Education, and Welfare Regional Office comments and recommendations on approval, including the general bases for comments pertinent to inadequacies, if any, in the applications, with respect to the following:

(a) Compatibility of the proposed project with the area-wide or State plan for health services;

(b) Accuracy and thoroughness of the description of the medical services area in which the applicant proposes to develop, operate, or expand a health maintenance organization;

(c) Accuracy and thoroughness with which applicant has identified the population groups to be served by the proposed health maintenance organization as required by §§ 110.203(f) and 110.203 (g);

(d) Anticipated impact of the proposed project on the general accessibility and availability of care in the area, including:

(1) Whether the proposed project meets the needs of the community for health services in the proposed service area;

(2) Effects of offering an alternative form of health services to individuals or groups; and

(3) Identification of existing barriers to the effective delivery of health services, which may include geographic, economic, cultural and language barriers;

(e) Economic impact, including:

(1) Effects on existing health resources or facilities; and

(2) Potential of proposed project to draw new health resources into the area; and

(f) Agency cooperation, including:

(1) Applicant's statement of intent to work cooperatively with the appropriate health systems agency or State health planning and development agency; and

(2) The experience of the applicant, if any, in dealing with other segments of the health care community; and

(g) Whether arrangements for services appear realistic, achievable and appropriate, including, but not limited to:

(1) Potential for proposed project to be adequately staffed to accommodate enrolled members or anticipated membership;

(2) Potential for adequate provision of the services, considering availability of manpower and equipment, and success of previous attempts to recruit personnel;

(3) Availability of health professionals in the area, and adequate evidence of cooperative planning with these providers (including summaries of verbal contacts or copies of correspondence); and

(4) Reliability of evidence of support for and acceptance of the proposed project by the community.

§ 110.205 Records, reports, inspection, and audit.

(a) Each grant, loan, or loan guarantee awarded pursuant to this part shall be subject to the condition that the recipient shall maintain records which disclose the amount of disposition of the proceeds of the grant, or loan (directly made or guaranteed), the total cost of the undertaking in connection with which such assistance was given or used, the amount of that portion of the cost of the undertaking supplied by other sources, and such other records as will facilitate an effective audit.

(b) The Secretary and the Comptroller General of the United States, or any of their duly authorized representatives, shall have access for the purpose of audit, examination or evaluation to any books, documents, papers, and records of the recipients of a grant, loan or loan guarantee under Title XIII of the Act which relate to such assistance.

(c) A report shall be submitted to the Secretary by the recipient of a grant, loan, or loan guarantee under Title XIII of the Act not later than 60 days after the termination date of each project, describing existing and anticipated plans, developments and operations in accordance with information required under section 1306(b)(3) of the Act.

(d) Such other reports shall be submitted as the Secretary may require to meet the provisions of the Act and these regulations.

§ 110.206   Additional conditions.

The Secretary may, with respect to the approval of any grant, contract, loan, or loan guarantee, impose additional conditions prior to or at the time of any approval when, in his judgment, such conditions are necessary to assure or protect the advancement of the approved project, the interests of public health, or the conservation of project funds.

§ 110.207   Nondiscrimination.

Attention is called to the requirements of Title VI of the Civil Rights Act of 1964 (78 Stat. 252, 42 U.S.C. 2000d et seq.) and in particular section 601 of such Act which provides that no person in the United States shall on the grounds of race, color, or national origin be excluded from participation in, be denied the benefits of, or be subjected to discrimination under any program or activity receiving Federal financial assistance. A regulation implementing such title VI, which applied to all financial assistance under this part, has been issued by the Secretary of Health, Education, and Welfare with the approval of the President (45 CFR Part 80). In addition no person shall, on the grounds of sex, or creed (unless otherwise medically indicated) be excluded from participation in, be denied the benefits of, or be subjected to discrimination under any program or activity receiving Federal financial assistance. Nor shall any person be denied employment in or by such program or activity so receiving Federal financial assistance on the grounds of age, sex, creed, or marital status.

§ 110.208   Inventions or discoveries.

An award under this part is subject to the regulations of the Department of Health, Education, and Welfare as set forth in 45 CFR Parts 6, "Inventions and Patents (General)" and 8, "Inventions Resulting from Research Grants, Fellowship Awards, and Contracts for Research." Such regulations shall apply to any activity for which funds are in fact used whether within the scope of the project as approved or otherwise. Ap-

propriate measures shall be taken by the award recipient and by the Secretary to assure that no contracts, assignments or other arrangements inconsistent with the award obligations are continued or entered into and that all personnel involved in the supported activity are aware of and comply with such obligations. Laboratory notes, related technical data, and information pertaining to inventions and discoveries shall be maintained for such periods, and filed with or otherwise made available to the Secretary or those he may designate at such times and in such manner as he may determine necessary to carry out such Department regulations.

§ 110.209   Publications, copyright, and data.

(a)(1) Except as may otherwise be provided under the terms and conditions of the award, the applicant may copyright without prior approval any data developed or resulting from a project supported under this part, subject, however, to a royalty-free, non-exclusive, and irrevocable license or right in the Government to reproduce, translate, publish, use, disseminate, and dispose of such materials and to authorize others to do so.

(2) The government may use, duplicate, or disclose in any manner and for any purpose whatsoever, and have or permit others to do so, all data developed during the term of Federal financial assistance.

(3) Whenever any data is to be obtained from a contractor or subcontractor under the assisted projects, the applicant shall include this section (§ 110.209) in the contract or subcontract without alteration, making it applicable to the subject matter of the contract or subcontract, and no other clause shall be used to diminish the government's right in that contractor's or subcontractor's data.

(b) As used in this section, the term "data" means writings, films, sound recordings, pictorial reproductions. drawings, designs or other graphic representations, procedural manuals, forms, diagrams, work-flow charts, equipment descriptions, data files and data processing or computer programs, and works of any similar nature (whether or not copyrighted or copyrightable) which are developed during the term of Federal financial assistance.

§ 110.210   Confidentiality.

Each award is subject to the condition that all information obtained by the personnel of the project from participants in the project related to their examination, care, and treatment shall be held confidential, and shall not be divulged without the individual's informed consent except as may be required by law or as may be necessary to provide service to the individual or to the Secretary as part of his duties under the Act. Information may be disclosed in summary, statistical, or other form which does not identify particular individuals.

§ 110.211   Applicability of 45 CFR Part 74.

The provisions of 45 CFR Part 74, establishing uniform administrative requirements and cost principles, shall apply to all awards under this part to State and local governments as those terms are defined in Subpart A of that Part 74. The relevant provisions of the following subparts of Part 74 shall also apply to all other grantee organizations under this part:

Subpart:
  A—General.
  B—Cash Depositories.
  C—Bonding and Insurance.
  D—Retention and Custodial Requirements for Records.
  F—Grant-related Income.
  G—Matching and Cost Sharing.
  K—Grant Payment Requirements.
  I—Budget Revision Procedures.
  M—Grant Closeout, Suspension, and Termination.
  O—Property.
  Q—Cost Principles.

§ 110.212   Use of funds.

Any grants, loans, and loan guarantees awarded pursuant to this Part as well as other Federal funds to be used in the performance of the approved project shall be expended solely for carrying out the approved project in accordance with the statute, the regulations of this part, and the terms and conditions of the award or assistance.

§ 110.213   Grantee accountability.

(a) All payments made by the Secretary under grants awarded pursuant to sections 1303 and 1304 of the Act shall be recorded by the grantee in accounting records separate from the records of all other grant funds, including funds derived from other grant awards. With respect to each approved project the grantee shall account for the sum total of all amounts paid by presenting or otherwise making available evidence satisfactory to the Secretary of expenditures for direct and indirect costs meeting the requirements of this part: *Pro-*

vided, however, That when the amount awarded for indirect cost was based on a predetermined, fixed-percentage of estimated direct costs, the amount allowed for indirect costs shall be computed on the basis of such predetermined fixed-percentage rates applied to the total, or a selected element thereof, of the reimbursable direct costs incurred.

(b) (1) A grantee shall render, with respect to each approved project, a full account, as provided herein, as of date of the termination of grant support. The Secretary may require other special and periodic accounting.

(2) There shall be payable to the Federal Govrnment as final settlement with respect to each approved project the total sum of:

(i) Any amount not accounted for pursuant to paragraph (a) of this section;

(ii) Any other amounts due pursuant to Subparts F, M, and O of 45 CFR Part 74.

Such total sum shall constitute a debt owed by the grantee to the Federal Government and shall be recovered from the grantee or its successors or assignees by setoff or other action as provided by law.

§ 110.214   Continued support.

Neither the approval of any project nor any award of financial assistance shall commit or obligate the United States to make any additional, supplemental, continuation, or other award with respect to any approved project or portion thereof. For continuation support, applicants must make separate applications at such times and in such manner as the Secretary may direct.

Subpart C—Grants for Feasibility Surveys

§ 110.301   Applicability.

The regulations of this subpart, in addition to the regulations of Subpart B of this part, are applicable to grants awarded pursuant to section 1303 of the Act for projects to conduct surveys or other activities to determine the feasibility of developing and operating or expanding the operation of health maintenance organizations.

§ 110.302   Eligibility.

(a) *Eligible applicants.* Any public or private nonprofit entity which is or proposes to develop or become a health maintenance organization is eligible to apply for an award under this subpart, except that in the case of applications for support of expansion, only organizations which have been found by the Secretary to be qualified health maintenance organizations are eligible to apply.

(b) *Eligible projects.* Awards may be made pursuant to section 1303 of the Act, the regulations of Subpart B of this part, and this subpart, to eligible applicants to assist in conducting surveys or other activities to determine the feasibility of developing or expanding the operation of organizations which meet or propose to meet the requirements under subpart A of these regulations.

§ 110.303 Project elements.

An approvable application must provide:

(a) Statements which describe concisely:

(1) The goals and objectives for the proposed health maintenance organization;

(2) The administrative, managerial, and organizational arrangements and resources to be utilized to conduct the feasibility study;

(3) The proposed service area; and

(4) Intended financial participation of the applicant, specifying the type of contributions, such as cash or services, loans of full- or part-time staff, equipment, spaces, materials, or facilities or other contributions;

(b) An assurance that the applicant will cooperate with the appropriate health systems agency or State health planning and development agency;

(c) Written evidence of notification to the local medical societies of the applicant's intention to apply for assistance;

(d) Letters or other forms of evidence that there is general support for and acceptance of the proposed health maintenance organization by the community which the applicant proposes to serve;

(e) Concise plans for conducting the feasibility study, which must include, at a minimum, a description of tasks for each activity listed below, accompanied by a time-phased milestone chart indicating proposed funding and manpower to be allocated to each activity (where circumstances indicate that it would be appropriate and consistent with the intent of the Act, additional activities may be proposed in the application):

(1) Identify pertinent State laws, regulations, and practices relating to operating as a health maintenance organization;

(2) Identify population groups which would be sources of payment for services when the health maintenance organiza-

tion becomes operational;

(3) Identify potential providers or sources of providers of basic health services;

(4) Develop an estimate of the amount to be charged for basic health services when the proposed health maintenance organization becomes operational;

(5) Develop an estimate of the enrollment and funds required to reach the financial breakeven point; and

(6) Develop a preliminary estimate of the facilities required for operational status;

(f) In addition, in the case of an existing organization which provides health care services financed on a prepaid capitation basis to an enrolled population which is requesting assistance to become a health maintenance organization, identification of gaps between the applicant's current operation and the requirements of Subpart A of this part;

(g) In addition, in the case of qualified health maintenance organizations requesting assistance for significant expansion:

(1) Data on prepaid membership totals for annual intervals over the past five years, or if the health maintenance organization has not been operating for five years, such data on a quarterly basis for the time during which it has been in operation;

(2) The current enrollment figure;

(3) A description of the current health service delivery facilities, including an estimate of their capacity;

(4) The number and specialties of current health professionals serving its members; and

(5) The plans for the proposed significant expansion which demonstrate that the definition of significant expansion in § 110.202(c) will be met.

§ 110.304 Evaluation and award.

(a) Within the limits of funds available for such purpose, the Secretary may make awards to cover up to 90 percent of the cost of projects, or in the case of projects which will draw not less than 30 percent nor more than the appropriate percentage (as determined under § 110.-108(c) of its anticipated enrollment from medically underserved populations, up to 100 percent of the costs, to those applicants whose projects will, in his judgment best promote the purposes of section 1303 of the Act and the regulations of this subpart, taking into account:

(1) The degree to which the proposed project satisfactorily provides for elements set forth in § 110.303 above.

(2) The comments of the appropriate

health systems agency or State health planning and development agency.

(3) The degree to which the goals and objectives of the proposed project will promote the purposes of the Act and are consistent with the generally recognized capability of effectively organized and managed health maintenance organizations to reduce inappropriate hospital utilization, to contain health care costs, to use effectively medical and other health manpower, to emphasize early detection and treatment of illness, and to contribute to a better distribution and quality of health care.

(4) The capability of the applicant to organize and manage the project successfully.

(5) The soundness of the proposed plan for conducting the feasibility study and for assuring effective utilization of grant funds.

(6) The potential of the project to obtain indications of the willingness of basic medical and health care providers to participate in the operation of the health maintenance organization.

(7) The probability of financial viability based on potential sources of financial support for development and operations and potential sources of enrollment.

(8) The inclusion of medically underserved populations in the projected enrollment.

(9) Location relative to the number of organizations providing health services to a defined population on a prepaid capitation basis, which are already operating in the proposed geographic area.

(10) The percentage of total anticipated enrollment to be drawn from nonmetropolitan areas to be served.

(11) Evidence of the applicant's intended contribution to the project.

(12) In the case of an existing organization operating on a prepaid capitation basis, the applicant's potential for expeditious transition into a qualified health maintenance organization.

(13) In the case of expansion projects, the potential rate of increase of expansion, or the potential increase in the area to be served by the expanded health maintenance organization.

(b) In considering applications under this subpart, the Secretary will give priority to applications which contain assurances satisfactory to the Secretary that when the organizations become operational not less than 30 percent of their members will be members of a medically underserved population.

§ 110.305   Funding duration and limitation.

(a) The amount of any award shall be determined by the Secretary on the basis of his estimate of the sum necessary for project costs: *Provided, however,* That any single grant may not exceed $75,000.

(b) Feasibility survey applicants may propose that the award period be 12 months or less. Feasibility survey projects shall be completed within the period of the award. The Secretary may make not more than one additional grant for a project for a feasibility survey for which a grant has previously been made, and may permit additional time (up to 12 months) for completion of the project if he determines that the additional grant or additional time, or both, is needed to complete the project adequately.

(c) Funds under grants for feasibility surveys shall be used only for activites set forth in § 110.303(e) and for activities designed to fill the gaps referred to in § 110.303(f).

Subpart D—Grants and Loan Guarantees for Planning and Initial Development Costs

§ 110.401   Applicability.

The regulations of this subpart, in addition to the regulations of Subpart B of this part, are applicable to:

(a) Grants awarded pursuant to section 1304 of the Act for projects for planning, and initial development of health maintenance organizations or for significant expansion, as defined in § 110.202(c), of the membership of, or areas served, by qualified health maintenance organizations, and

(b) Guarantees made to non-Federal lenders of payment of the principal of and the interest on loans made to—

(1) Nonprofit private entities for such projects for the establishment or expansion of health maintenance organizations, or

(2) Private entities (other than nonprofit private entities) for such projects for health maintenance organizations which will serve medically underserved populations.

§ 110.402   Eligibility.

(a) *Eligible applicants.* (1) Any public entity which is or which proposes to become a health maintenance organization is eligible to apply for a grant under this subpart, except that in the case of applications for support of expansion, only organizations which have been found by the Secretary to be qualified health maintenance organizations are eligible to apply.

(2) Any nonprofit private entity which is or which proposes to become a health maintenance organization is eligible to apply for a grant or a loan guarantee under this subpart, except that in the case of applications for support of expansion, only organizations which have been found by the Secretary to be qualified health maintenance organizations are eligible to apply.

(3) Any private entity (other than a nonprofit private entity) which is or which proposes to become a health maintenance organization and which proposes to serve a medically underserved population is eligible to apply for a loan guarantee under this subpart, except that in the case of applications for support of expansion, only organizations which have been found by the Secretary to be qualified health maintenance organizations are eligible to apply.

(b) *Eligible projects*—(1) *Grants.* Awards of grants may be made pursuant to section 1304 of the Act and the regulations of Subpart B of this part and this subpart to eligible applicants for planning for the establishment of health maintenance organizations, or for the significant expansion of the membership of, or areas served by the health maintenance organizations meeting the requirements of Subpart A of this part, or for the initial development or actual expansion of such organizations;

(2) *Loan guarantees.* (i) In the case of nonprofit private entities, guarantees may be made pursuant to section 1304 of the Act and the regulations of Subpart B of this part and this subpart to eligible applicants for the payment of the principal of and the interest on loans for planning projects for the establishment of health maintenance organizations, or the significant expansion of existing organizations which have been found by the Secretary to meet the applicable requirements of Title XIII of the Act and the applicable regulations of this part, or for the initial development or actual expansion of such health maintenance organizations.

(ii) In the case of private entities (other than nonprofit private entities), guarantees may be made pursuant to section 1304 of the Act and the regulations of Subpart B of this part and this subpart to eligible applicants for the payment of the principal of and the interest on loans for planning projects for the establishment of health mainte-

nance organizations, or the significant expansion of existing organizations which have been found by the Secretary to meet the applicable requirements of Title XIII of the Act and the applicable regulations of this part, or for the initial development or actual expansion of such health maintenance organizations: *Provided,* That at least 30 percent of the projected members of such organizations are from medically underserved populations.

§ 110.403 **Project elements for planning.**

An approvable application must provide:

(a) Statements which describe in detail:

(1) The goals and objectives of the proposed health maintenance organization;

(2) The administrative, managerial, and organizational arrangements and resources to be utilized in the performance of the proposed activities;

(3) The proposed service area; and

(4) The intended financial participation of the applicant, specifying the type of contribution such as cash or services, loans of full- or part-time staff, equipment, space, materials, facilities, or other contributions.

(b) An assurance that the applicant will cooperate with the appropriate health systems agency or State health planning and development agency.

(c) Written evidence of notification to the local medical societies of the applicant's intention to apply for assistance.

(d) Letters or other forms of evidence that there is support for and acceptance of the project by organizations, institutions, and/or employer groups which may participate in the development of the proposed health maintenance organization.

(e) A detailed report of the results of the survey or study which established the feasibility of developing the health maintenance organization, as well as of any other activities relating to the development of the health maintenance organization undertaken prior to application for planning assistance. With regard to the report of the feasibility survey, information on the following must be included:

(1) Status of the applicant in terms of pertinent State laws, regulations, and practices relating to operating as a health maintenance organization;

(2) Organizational structure of the proposed health maintenance organization;

(3) Providers of basic health services
who have agreed or might reasonably be
expected to agree to provide health benefits;

(4) The types of population groups
which would be sources of prepayment
for an operational health maintenance
organization and other potential sources
of payment for services when operational;

(5) Sources of payment and operational support including:

(i) Preliminary estimate of the amount
to be charged for basic health benefits
when the proposed health maintenance
organization becomes operational; and

(ii) Estimate of enrollment and income required to reach the financial
breakeven point; and

(6) A preliminary estimate of facilities required for operational status.

(f) Concise plans for accomplishing
planning stage activities, which must include at a minimum, a description of
tasks for each activity listed below, accompanied by a time-phased milestone
chart indicating proposed funding and
manpower to be allocated to each such
activity (where circumstances indicate
that it would be appropriate and consistent with the intent of the Act, additional activities may be proposed):

(1) Recruit key project staff;

(2) Plan for and initiate appropriate
action relating to any State legal and/or
regulatory restrictions;

(3) Develop formal organization;

(4) Establish community support;

(5) Refine market estimate made in
feasibility survey;

(6) Develop health benefits plan;

(7) Develop premium structure;

(8) Develop plans for marketing of the
services and enrollment of members;

(9) Develop budget and financial plan;

(10) Identify providers of basic health
services and develop preliminary agreements to negotiate with these providers;
and

(11) Plan for necessary facilities and
equipment.

(g) In addition, in the case of an existing organization which provides
health care services financed on a prepaid capitation basis to an enrolled population which is requesting assistance to
become a qualified health maintenance
organization, an identification of gaps
between the applicant's current operation and the requirements of Subpart A
of this part.

(h) In addition, in the case of qualified health maintenance organizations

requesting assistance for significant
expansion:

(1) Data on prepaid membership totals for annual intervals over the past
five years, or if the health maintenance
organization has not been operating for
five years, such data on a quarterly basis
for the time during which it has been
in operation;

(2) The current enrollment figure;

(3) A description of the current health
service delivery facilities, including an
estimate of their capacity;

(4) The number and specialties of current health professionals serving its
members; and

(5) The detailed plans for the proposed significant expansion which demonstrate that the definition of significant expansion in § 110.202(c) will be
met.

§ 110.404 Project elements for initial
development.

An approvable application must
provide:

(a) Written evidence satisfactory to
the Secretary that the feasibility of the
establishment and operation or expansion has been established by the applicant and that sufficient planning for the
establishment or expansion has been
conducted by the applicant. In addition,
applicants must provide the information,
assurances and evidence required by
§ 110.403 (a), (b), (c), and (d) and must
report all other activities relating to the
development of the health maintenance
organization undertaken prior to application for initial development assistance.

(b) Detailed plans, which must include, at a minimum, tasks designed to
accomplish the activities listed below,
accompanied by a time-phased milestone
chart indicating proposed funding and
manpower to be allocated to each (where
circumstances indicate that it would be
appropriate and consistent with the intent of the Act, additional activities may
be proposed in the application):

(1) Develop a schedule to meet the requirements of Subpart A of this part;

(2) Complete activities related to resolving legal issues;

(3) Recruit and train personnel essential for operation as a health maintenance organization;

(4) Develop a comprehensive financial
plan;

(5) Organize physician and other basic
health services;

(6) Construct/renovate health maintenance organization facilities;

(7) Organize ambulatory care facility;

(8) Formalize contract arrangements;

(9) Initiate enrollment plan and implement a staffing plan that demonstrates compliance with the appropriate. 15 or 30 percent limitation on contracts for basic and supplemental health services under § 110.104(a); and

(10) Create any operating reserves required by State authorities.

(c) Signed letters from at least three physicians indicating that they intend or are willing to be employed by or to contract with the proposed health maintenance organization for the provision of basic health services to its members and, signed letters from one or more hospitals indicating that they intend to or are willing to negotiate an agreement to provide hospital services to members from the proposed health maintenance organization as necessary.

(d) In the case of an applicant which intends to serve Title XIX eligibles as part of the intended enrollment, evidence that the State Title XIX agency is willing to negotiate a prepaid capitation contract in the form of a letter or other document from the State Title XIX agency.

(e) In addition, in the case of an existing organization which provides health care services financed on a prepaid capitation basis to an enrolled population, which is requesting assistance to become a qualified health maintenance organization, and identification of gaps between the applicant's current operation and the requirements of Subpart A of this part.

(f) In addition, in the case of qualified health maintenance organizations requesting assistance for significant expansion:

(1) Data on prepaid membership totals for annual intervals over the past five years, such data on a quarterly basis for the total number of years during which it has been in operation;

(2) The current enrollment figure;

(3) A description of the current health service delivery facilities, including an estimate of their capacity;

(4) The number and specialties of current health professionals serving its members; and

(5) The plans for the proposed significant expansion which demonstrate that the definition of significant expansion in § 110.202(c) will be met.

§ 110.405 Funding duration and limitation.

(a) *Planning projects.* (1) The amount of any award shall be determined by the Secretary on the basis of his estimate of the sum necessary for project costs: *Provided*, That any single grant and the

amount of principal of any single loan guaranteed under section 1304 of the Act may not exceed $200,000.

(2) In considering applications under this subpart, the Secretary will give priority to applications which contain assurances satisfactory to the Secretary that when the organization becomes operational, not less than 30 percent of its members will be members of a medically underserved population. In considering applications for loan guarantees for planning projects under this subpart, the Secretary will give special consideration to applications for projects for health maintenance organizations which will serve medically underserved populations. Applicants may propose that the award period be for one year or less, as appropriate to the planning activities to be accomplished. Planning projects shall be completed within the period of the award. The Secretary may not make more than one additional grant or loan guarantee for a planning project for which a grant or loan guarantee has previously been made, and may permit additional time (up to 12 months) for completion of the project if he determines that the additional grant or loan guarantee (as the case may be) or additional time, or both, is needed to complete the project adequately.

(3) Funds under grants and loans guaranteed for planning projects shall be used only for the activities set forth in § 110.403(f) and for activities required to fill the gaps referred to in § 110.403(g).

(b) *Initial development projects.* (1) The amount of any award shall be determined by the Secretary on the basis of his estimate of the sums necessary for project costs: *Provided, however,* That the aggregate amount of loan guarantees and grants for any initial development project may not exceed $1,000,000 or, in the case of a project for a health maintenance organization which will provide services to an additional service area or which will provide services in two or more areas which are not contiguous, $1,600,000.

(2) Applicants may propose that the award period for initial development activities be one year or less, as appropriate to the initial development activities to be accomplished. Initial development projects shall be completed within the period of the award beginning on the first day of the month in which such award was made, and the number of grants made for any initial development project under section 1304 of the Act may not exceed a total of three. A loan

guarantee for an initial development project may only be made for a loan (or loans) for initial development costs incurred in a period not to exceed three years.

(3) In considering applications for loan guarantees for initial development projects under this subpart, the Secretary will give special consideration to applications for projects for health maintenance organizations which will serve medically underserved populations.

(4) Funds under grants and loans guaranteed for projects for initial development shall be used only for activities set forth in § 110.104(b) (except that such funds may not be used for the costs of construction or for recruitment of personnel who will not engage in practice principally for the health maintenance organization) and for activities required to fill gaps referred to in § 110.-404(e).

§ 110.406   Evaluation and award.

(a) Within the limits of funds available for such purpose, the Secretary may make awards to cover up to 90 percent of the cost of projects, or in the case of projects which will draw not less than 30 percent nor more than the appropriate percentage (as determined under § 110.108(c)) of its anticipated enrollment from medically underserved populations, up to 100 percent of the costs, to those applicants whose projects will, in his judgment, best promote the purposes of section 1304 of the Act and the regulations of this subpart, taking into account:

(1) The degree to which the proposed project satisfactorily provides for the elements set forth in § 110.403 or § 110.-404.

(2) The comments of the appropriate health systems agency or State health planning and development agency.

(3) Whether the feasibility of the project has been established, and in the case of initial development applications, whether all requirements of a planning application have been met.

(4) The appropriateness of the goals and objectives of the proposed project.

(5) The effectiveness the proposed organization may reasonably be expected to have in reducing inappropriate hospital utilization, containing health care costs, using medical and other health manpower, emphasizing early detection and treatment of illnesses, and achieving a better distribution and quality of care.

(6) The capability of the applicant

to organize and manage the project successfully.

(7) Evidence of the applicant's intended contribution to the project.

(8) Evidence of intent from providers expressing a willingness to be employed by or contract with the proposed health maintenance organization for the provision of basic health services.

(9) Evidence, in form of letters, from individuals, groups, or organizations indicating that they support the development and operation of the proposed health maintenance organization.

(10) The results of marketing efforts and the prospects for eventual economic viability as an operational health maintenance organization without continued Federal support.

(11) The inclusion of medically underserved populations in groups to be enrolled.

(12) Location relative to the number of organizations providing health services to a defined population on a prepaid capitation basis, which are already operating in the area.

(13) The percentage of anticipated total enrollment to be drawn from nonmetropolitan areas to be served.

(14) In the case of an existing organization operating on a prepaid capitation basis, the applicant's potential for expeditious transition into a qualified health maintenance organization.

(15) In the case of expansion projects, the potential rate of increase of expansion, or the potential increase in the area to be served by the expanded health maintenance organization.

(b) In considering applications under this subpart the Secretary will give priority to applications which contain assurances satisfactory to the Secretary that when the organizations become operational, not less than 30 percent of their members will be members of a medically underserved population.

§ 110.407   Loan guarantee provisions.

(a) *Disbursement of loan proceeds.* The principal amount of any loan guaranteed by the Secretary under this subpart shall be disbursed to the applicant in accordance with an agreement to be entered into between the parties to the loan and approved by the Secretary.

(b) *Length and maturity of loans.* The principal amount of each loan guarantee, together with interest thereon, shall be repayable over a period of 20 years, beginning on the date of endorsement of the loan guarantee by the Secretary. The Secretary may however, approve a shorter repayment period where he determines that a repayment period of less than 20 years is more appropriate to an applicant's total financial plan.

(c) *Repayment.* The principal amount of each loan guarantee, together with interest thereon, shall be repayable in accordance with a repayment schedule which is to be agreed upon by the parties to the loan and approved by the Secretary prior to or at the time of his endorsement of the loan. Unless otherwise specifically authorized by the Secretary, each loan guaranteed by the Secretary shall be repayable in substantially level combined installments of principal and interest, to be paid at intervals not less frequently than annually, sufficient to amortize the loan through the final year of the life of the loan. Principal repayment during the first 36 months of operation may be deferred, with payment of interest only by the applicant during such period.

Subpart E—Loans and Loan Guarantees for Initial Operating Costs

§ 110.501	Applicability.

The regulations of this subpart, in addition to the regulations of Subpart B, of this part are applicable to loans and loan guarantees awarded pursuant to section 1305 of the Act.

§ 110.502	Definitions.

(a) "Operating cost" means any cost which under generally accepted accounting principles or under accounting practices prescribed or permitted by State regulatory authority is not a capital cost and which is incurred on or after the first day of the applicable period of operation or expansion as defined in paragraph (b) of this secton: *Provided,* That payments made by a health maintenance organization during such applicable period to reduce balance sheet liabilities existing at the beginning of such period are operating costs to the extent that they are expressly approved by the Secretary at the time the loan or loan guarantee is made. In addition, when deposits of funds to restricted reserve accounts are required by State authority, deposits made during such applicable period are operating costs.

(b) "First 60 months of operation or expansion" means the 60 month period beginning on the first day of the month during which the health maintenance organization first provides services to members, or in the case of significant expansion, first provides services in accordance with its expansion plan.

§ 110.503	Eligibility.

(a) *Eligible applicants.* (1) Any public qualified health maintenance organization is eligible to apply for a loan under this subpart.

(2) Any nonprofit private qualified health maintenance organization is eligible to apply for a loan or a loan guarantee under this subpart.

(3) Any private (other than a nonprofit private) qualified health maintenance organization which will serve a medically underserved populations is eligible to apply for a loan guarantee under this subpart.

(b) *Eligible projects*—(1) *Loans.* In the case of public or nonprofit private qualified health maintenance organizations, loans may be made pursuant to section 1305 of the Act and the regulations of Subpart B of this part and this subpart to eligible applicants to assist them in meeting the amount by which their operating costs during a period not to exceed the first 60 months of their operation exceed their revenues in such period, or in meeting the amount by which their operating costs, which the Secretary determines are attributable to significant expansion in their membership or area served, as defined in § 110.-202(c), and which are incurred during a period not to exceed the first 60 months of their operation after such expansion, exceed their revenues in that period which the Secretary determines are attributable to such expansion.

(2) *Loan guarantees.* Loan guarantees may be made pursuant to section 1305 of the Act, and the regulations of Subpart B of this part and this subpart to guarantee to non-Federal lenders payment of the principal of and the interest on loans made to any nonprofit private qualified health maintenance organization or any private (other than a nonprofit private) qualified health maintenance organization for the amounts referred to in paragraph (b)(1) of this section: *Provided,* That any such private (other than nonprofit private) qualified health maintenance organization will serve a medically underserved population.

§ 110.504	Project elements.

An approvable application must provide:

(a) Statements which describe in detail:

(1) The applicant's adequate accomplishment of feasibility survey, planning, and development activities; and

(2) The health maintenance organization's management capability.

(b) Detailed information on the health maintenance organization's marketing plan and enrollment forecasts and experience.

(c) A detailed narrative statement describing:

(1) All existing and planned provider arrangements including copies of all executed contracts; and

(2) All facilities to be used in the delivery of health services.

(d) Financial information in such detail as the Secretary may prescribe.

(e) Evidence that any certificate of need required under State law for the operation of the health maintenance organization has been obtained by the applicant.

§ 110.505   Reserve requirement.

The applicant receiving a loan or loan guarantee under section 1305 of the Act shall establish a restricted reserve account beginning at the point when the revenues and expenditures of the health maintenance organization reach the break-even point, or by the end of the 60 month period following the making of the loan or the guarantee under section 1305 of the Act, whichever is sooner, unless a longer period is approved by the Secretary. This reserve shall be so constituted as to accumulate no later than ten (10) years following the endorsement of the loan or loan guarantee, an aggregate amount equal to one year's principal of and interest on the loan, as determined under the terms of the loan made or guaranteed.

§ 110.506   Evaluation and award.

Within the limits of funds available for such purposes, the Secretary may award loans or loan guarantees to those applicants whose projects will, in his judgment, best promote the purposes of section 1305 of the Act and the regulations of this part, taking into account:

(a) The ability of the health maintenance organization to achieve financial viability;

(b) The ability of the health maintenance organization to make repayments of the principal and interest when due and to have additional funds to defray the remaining operating deficits;

(c) The comments, if any, of the appropriate health systems agency or State health planning and development agency;

(d) The relative distribution of qualified applicants with respect to the following factors:

(1) The inclusion of medically under-

served populations in the groups to be enrolled;

(2) Location relative to the number of organizations providing health services to a defined population on a prepaid capitation basis, which are already operating in the proposed area; and

(3) The percentage of anticipated total enrollment drawn from nonmetropolitan areas served or to be served by the applicant.

§ 110.507   Funding duration and limitation.

(a) In any fiscal year the amount disbursed to a health maintenance organization under section 1305 of the Act and this subpart (either directly by the Secretary or by an escrow agent under the terms of an escrow agreement or by a lender under a loan guaranteed under section 1305 of the Act and this subpart) may not exceed $1,000,000.

(b) A loan or loan guarantee under section 1305 of the Act shall be limited to two-thirds of the Secretary's projection of the amount by which operating costs during a period not to exceed the first 60 months of operation exceed revenues for such period, except as approved by written waiver by the Secretary for such higher percentage of the total operating deficit.

(c) The approval of any loan or loan guarantee shall not obligate the United States in any way to make any additional loan or loan guarantee with respect to the approved application or portion thereof, except as may be otherwise set forth in the agreement between the United States and the approved applicant.

(d) In considering applications for loan guarantees under section 1305 of the Act and this subpart, the Secretary will give special consideration to applications for health maintenance organizations which will serve medically underserved populations.

§ 110.508   Loan provisions.

(a) *Disbursement of loan proceeds.* The principal amount of any loan made or guaranteed by the Secretary under this subpart shall be disbursed to the applicant in accordance with an agreement to be entered into between the parties to the loan and approved by the Secretary.

(b) *Length and maturity of loans.* The principal amount of each loan or loan guarantee, together with interest thereon, shall be repayable over a period of 20 years, beginning on the date of endorsement of the loan, or loan guarantee by the Secretary. The Secretary may, however, approve a shorter repayment period where he determines that a repayment period of less than 20 years is more appropriate to an applicant's total financial plan.

(c) *Repayment.* The principal amount of each loan or loan guarantee, together with interest thereon, shall be repayable in accordance with a repayment schedule which is to be agreed upon by the parties to the loan or loan guarantee and approved by the Secretary prior to or at the time of his endorsement of the loan. Unless otherwise specifically authorized by the Secretary, each loan made or guaranteed by the Secretary shall be repayable in substantially level combined installments of principal and interest to be paid at intervals not less frequently than annually, sufficient to amortize the loan through the final year of the life of the loan. Principal repayment during the first 60 months of operation may be deferred, with payment of interest only the applicant during such period.

Subpart F—Qualification of Health Maintenance Organizations

§ 110.601 Applicability.

The regulations of this subpart apply to any entity seeking a determination by the Secretary under section 1310(d) of the Act that it is a qualified health maintenance organization. (See § 110.109 concerning the requirements for a health maintenance organization with members who are entitled to insurance benefits under Title XVIII (Medicare) of the Social Security Act or to medical assistance under a State plan approved under Title XIX (Medicaid) of such Act. See § 110.110 concerning the requirements for a health maintenance organization with members who are enrolled under the Federal Employees' Health Benefits Program.)

§ 110.602 Definitions.

In addition to the terms defined in § 110.101, as used in this subpart:

(a) "Operational qualified health maintenance organization" means a health maintenance organization which the Secretary has determined provides basic and supplemental health services to all of its members in accordance with Subpart A of this part and is organized and operated in accordance with Subpart A of this part.

(b) "Traditionally qualified health maintenance organization" means an entity which operates a prepaid health care delivery system and which the Sec-

retary has determined meets the requirements of § 110.603(b). (A transitionally qualified health maintenance organization is deemed a "qualified health maintenance organization" for the purpose of compliance by an employer which has a contract with such health maintenance organization with the requirements of section 1310(a) of the Act so long as the health maintenance organization complies with its time-phased plan approved by the Secretary under § 110.603(b)(2) (iii).)

(c) "Pre-operational qualified health maintenance organization" means an entity which the Secretary has determined will, when it becomes operational as a prepaid health care delivery system, be an operational qualified health maintenance organization.

§ 110.603 Requirements for qualification.

Upon the basis of an application submitted in accordance with this subpart and such additional information and investigation (including site visits) as the Secretary may require:

(a) The Secretary will determine that an entity is an operational qualified health maintenance organization, if he finds that the entity meets the requirements of Subpart A of this part and if the entity provides written assurances that it:

(1) Provides and will provide basic and supplemental health services to its members;

(2) Provides and will provide such services in the manner prescribed by section 1301(b) of the Act and Subpart A of this part;

(3) Is organized and operated, and will continue to be organized and operated, in the manner prescribed by section 1301 (c) of the Act and Subpart A of this part;

(4) Under arrangements which will safeguard the confidentiality of patient information and records, will provide access to the Secretary and the Comptroller General or any of their duly authorized representatives for the purpose of audit, examination or evaluation to any books, documents, papers, and records of the entity relating to its operations as a health maintenance organization, and to any facilities operated by the entity; and

(5) Will continue to comply with any other assurances which the entity has given to the Secretary under §§ 110.203 (e); 110.303(b); and 110.403(b).

(b) The Secretary may determine that an entity is a transitionally qualified health maintenance organization if the entity currently is organized and currently is providing prepaid health services as described in this subparagraph, and provides assurances satisfactory to the Secretary that it will:

(1) With respect to all new group and individual (non-group) contracts which it enters into after the date of the Secretary's determination that the entity is a transitionally qualified health maintenance organization, provide basic and supplemental health services to members enrolled under such contracts and will provide such services in the manner prescribed by Subpart A of this part and will with respect to such members, be organized and operated in accordance with § 110.108.

(2) With respect to its group and non-group contracts which are in effect on the date of such determination, and which are renewed or renegotiated during the period approved by the Secretary under paragraph (b)(2)(iii) of this section in accordance with the plan so approved;

(i) Provide at least those services specified in the following sections of this part except that these services may be limited as to time and cost: § 110.102(a)(1) (physician services); § 110.102(a)(2) (outpatient services and inpatient hospital services); § 110.102(a)(3) (medically necessary emergency health services); and § 110.102(a)(6) (diagnostic laboratory and diagnostic and therapeutic radiologic services);

(ii) Be organized and operated in accordance with § 110.108 (except that it need not assume full financial risk for the provision of basic health services as required by § 110.108(b), and need not abide by the limitations on insurance of § 110.108(b)(1) and (3)) and provide that payment for basic health services shall be in accordance with § 110.105 (except that it need not comply with the community rating system as required by § 110.105(a)(3), and need not comply with the limitations on copayments of § 110.105(a)(4), and the requirement of § 110.106(b) that supplemental health services payments which are fixed on a prepayment basis be fixed under a community rating system);

(iii) Implement a time-phased plan acceptable to the Secretary which specifies definite steps for meeting, on a contract-by-contract (or category of contracts) basis, within a period not to exceed 3 years from the date of the Secretary's determination of qualification, all the requirements of Subpart A of this part; and

(iv) Upon completion of the time-phased plan;

(A) Provide basic and supplemental health services to all of its members;

(B) Provide such services to all of its members in the manner prescribed by Subpart A of this part; and

(C) Be organized and operated in the manner prescribed by Subpart A of this part.

(3) A health maintenance organization which has more than one regional component, as defined by § 110.101(l)(4), will be considered qualified for those regional components which have signed assurances in accordance with paragraphs (b)(1) and (b)(2) of this section: Provided, That all of the regional components have signed such assurances within one year of the date on which the first of the regional components signs these assurances. In the event that not all regional components have signed these assurances within this one year period or if any of them have failed to comply with the time limitation of paragraph (b)(2)(iii) of this section, the qualification of the entire entity will be terminated.

(4) The assurances specified in paragraphs (b)(1) and (b)(2) of this section need not be executed on behalf of the entity until it has been notified that the application is otherwise approvable. At such time, the applicant must specify the date on which such assurances will be made effective and must execute the assurances accordingly. The Secretary's approval of the application will be effective on the date so specified.

(c) The Secretary may determine that an entity is a preoperational qualified health maintenance organization if it provides assurances satisfactory to the Secretary that it will become operational within 30 days following the Secretary's determination of qualification, and will, when it becomes operational, meet the requirements of Subpart A of this part. Upon notification by the entity to the Secretary that the entity has become operational, the Secretary will, within 30 days of such notification, make a determination whether the entity is an operational qualified health maintenance organization; in the absence of such a determination the organization is not an operational qualified health maintenance organization even though it becomes operational.

§ 110.604   Application requirements.

(a) An entity seeking a determination that it is a qualified health maintenance organization pursuant to this subpart shall apply to the Secretary at such time and in such form and manner as the Secretary may prescribe.[1] The application must be executed by an individual authorized to act for the applicant and to assume on behalf of the applicant the obligations imposed by the statute and the regulations of this part. The application shall provide a complete description of how the entity meets or will meet the requirements of Subpart A of this part and applicable sections of the Act as set forth in a separate application form[2] provided by the Secretary.

---

[1] Applicants should be aware that provisions of the Freedom of Information Act, 5 U.S.C. 552, may require disclosure of certain official Government records. Regulations of the Department of Health, Education, and Welfare, 45 CFR 5.71, provide exceptions to disclosure. Applicants submitting material which they feel is covered by these exceptions should label such material "Privileged" and include a concise explanation of the applicability of 45 CFR 5.71. In the event that the Secretary determines that such material is not appropriately labeled "Privileged" under 45 CFR 5.71, he will inform the applicant of such determination and, if the applicant does not concur, allow the applicant to withdraw his application. Otherwise, the Secretary will not voluntarily disclose such material and will notify the applicant of any court process or subpoena to compel such disclosure.

[2] Application forms and instructions may be obtained by writing the Office of Health Maintenance Organizations Qualification and Compliance, Assistant Secretary for Health, Department of Health, Education, and Welfare, 5600 Fishers Lane, Rockville, Maryland 20857 or the Regional Health Administrator in the appropriate Regional Office of the Department of Health, Education, and Welfare at the addresses set forth at 45 CFR 5.31(b).

(b) In addition, each application shall describe interrelationships, if any, between the entity and any of the entity's contractors which provide a professional health service or administrative function or service to the entity. Such description should include identification of interrelationships such as common financial or beneficial ownership, or common directorship or trusteeship. However, descriptions or contracts for nonmedical services are required only if the interrelationship represents, in the aggregate, dollar amounts in excess of 5 percent of either party's income or expenses, whichever is smaller. If no such interrelationships exist, the application shall so state.

§ 110.605   Evaluation and determination of qualification.

(a) The Secretary will evaluate applications submitted under this subpart, and may obtain such additional information as he may require, employing site visits, public hearings or any other procedures determined appropriate by him and will determine whether the applicant meets the appropriate requirements of §§ 110.603 and 110.604, section 1301 of the Act, and Subpart A of this part.

(b) The Secretary will notify each entity applying for qualification under this subpart of his determination and the basis for such determination, and will publish in the FEDERAL REGISTER the names, addresses, and descriptions of the service areas of the newly qualified health maintenance organizations on a monthly basis, and a cumulative list of all qualified health maintenance organizations on an annual basis.

(c) Copies of lists published pursuant to paragraph (b) of this section may be obtained from, and additional information regarding qualified health maintenance organizations will be available for public inspection between the hours of 8:30 a.m. and 5 p.m., Monday through Friday at the Office of Health Maintenance Organizations Qualification and Compliance, Assistant Secretary for Health, Department of Health, Education, and Welfare, Parklawn Building, 5600 Fishers Lane, Rockville, Maryland 20857.

(d) Upon the denial of an application for qualification under this subpart, the Secretary will, in writing, so notify the entity making such application and shall provide such entity a reasonable opportunity for a reconsideration of such determination under paragraph (e) of this section or for a fair hearing under paragraph (f) of this section.

(e) A request for reconsideration shall be submitted in writing, within 60 days following the date of the notification of denial, addressed to the officer or employee of the Department of Health, Education, and Welfare who has denied the application, and shall set forth the grounds upon which such reconsideration is requested, specifying the material issues of fact and of law upon which the applicant relies. Reconsideration will be based upon the record compiled during the qualification review proceedings, materials submitted in support of the request for reconsideration, and other relevant materials available to the Secretary. Written notice of the reconsidered determination will be provided to the entity seeking reconsideration. Such notice shall set forth the basis for the determination and shall inform the entity of its rights to seek a fair hearing under paragraph (f) of this section.

(f) Any entity dissatisfied with an initial determination or a reconsidered determination of its application or qualification under this subpart may, within 60 days following the date of notification of any such determination, request a fair hearing. Such request shall be made in writing and shall specify the material issues of fact upon which it is based.

NOTE.—Pending promulgation of regulations governing fair hearings, applicants requesting a hearing will be provided a copy of applicable procedures.

[FR Doc.77–16002 Filed 6–7–77; 8:45 am]

RULES AND REGULATIONS

Subpart H—Employees' Health Benefits Plans

§ 110.801 Definitions.

In addition to the terms defined in § 110.101 and § 110.602 of this Part, as used in this subpart:

(a) "Employer" shall have the same meaning as that given such term in Section 3(d) of the Fair Labor Standards Act of 1938, as amended, (29 U.S.C. 203).

(b) "Bargaining representative" means a representative designated or selected for the purposes of collective bargaining under the National Labor Relations Act, as amended, (29 U.S.C. 151 *et seq.*) or under the Railway Labor Act, as amended, (45 U.S.C. 151 *et seq.*).

(c) "Employee" means any individual employed by an employer, whether on a full- or part-time basis.

(d) "Eligible employee" means an employee who meets the terms and conditions established by an employer or its designee to participate in a health benefits plan.

(e) "Designee" means any person or entity authorized to act on behalf of an employer or group of employers to offer the option of membership in a qualified health maintenance organization to the employer's eligible employees.

(f) "Service area" means the particular geographic area described by the health maintenance organization as its service area as part of its application for a determination that it is a qualified health maintenance organization (see § 110.604(b)(1)(xix) of this part), or such other area defined by the health maintenance organization and found by the Secretary to be the area within which basic and supplemental health services are available and accessible to members as required by section 1301(b)(4) of the Act and § 110.107 of this part.

(g) "Health benefits" means health benefits and services.

(h) "Health benefits plan" means any arangement for the provision of, or payment for, any of the basic and supplemental health benefits described in § 110.101(b) and (c) of this part offered to eligible employees, or to such employees and their eligible dependents, by or on behalf of an employer.

(i) "Qualified health maintenance organization" means an entity which has been found by the Secretary to meet the requirements of Title XIII of the Act and the applicable regulations of this part.

(j) "To offer a health benefits plan" means to make participation in a health benefits plan available to eligible employees, or to such employees and their eligible dependents, whether the financial contribution by the employer on behalf of such employees is made directly or indirectly (e.g., through payments on any basis into a health and welfare trust fund).

(k) "Group enrollment period" means the period of at least 10 working days each calendar year during which each eligible employee is given the opportunity to select among the alternatives included in a health benefits plan.

(l) "Collective bargaining agreement" means an agreement entered into between an employer and the bargaining representative of its employees, and includes such agreements entered into on behalf of groups of employers with the bargaining representative of their employees in accordance with the provisions of the National Labor Relations Act, as amended, (29 U.S.C. 151 *et seq.*) or the Railway Labor Act, as amended, (45 U.S.C. 151 *et seq.*).

(m) "Employer-employee contract" means a legally enforceable agreement (other than a collective bargaining agreement) between an employer and its employees for the provision of, or payment for, health benefits for its employees, or for such employees and their eligible dependents.

(n) "Health benefits contract" means a contract or other agreement between an employer, or its designee, and a carrier for the provision of, or payment for, health benefits to eligible employees or to such eligible employees and their eligible dependents.

(o) "Carrier" means a voluntary association, corporation, partnership, or other non-governmental organization which is engaged in providing, paying for, or reimbursing all or part of the cost of health benefits under group insurance policies or contracts, medical or hospital service agreements, membership or subscription contracts, or similar group arrangements, in consideration of premiums or other periodic charges payable to the carrier.

§ 110.802 Applicability.

(a) The regulations of this subpart apply in each calendar year to each employer which:

(1) Was required during any calendar quarter of the previous calendar year to

pay its employees the minimum wage specified by Section 6 of the Fair Labor Standards Act of 1938 (or would have been required to pay its employees such wage but for section 13(a) of such Act);

(2) During such calendar quarter employed an average number of not less than 25 employees;

(3) Offers, or on whose behalf there is offered, in the calendar year beginning after such calendar quarter a health benefits plan to its eligible employees; and

(4) Has received a written request for inclusion in the employer's health benefits plan from one or more qualified health maintenance organizations which operates in an area in which any eligible employee resides.

(b) For an offer to be effective under paragraph (a)(4) of this section, the request for inclusion in the health benefits plan shall be received by the employer at least 180 days before the expiration or renewal date of a health benefits contract or employer-employee contract and at least 90 days before the expiration date of a collective bargaining agreement, unless otherwise agreed to by the health maintenance organization and the employer or its designee. For employers with a collective bargaining agreement that is automatically renewable and without fixed term, or is for a fixed term but has provisions for periodically changing the wages, hours, or conditions of employment, such agreement shall be treated as renewable, for purposes of this subpart, on the anniversary date of the collective bargaining agreement if it has no fixed term, or at such other times not less than annually, as may be provided by such agreement for discussion of changes in its provision, whichever is earlier. Additionally, the request for inclusion in the health benefits plan shall:

(1) Be in writing and directed specifically to a managing employer official at the employer site being solicited or to the employer's designee;

(2) Provide evidence that the health maintenance organization has been determined to be qualified by the Secretary under subpart F of this part;

(3) Indicate whether the services of health professionals which are provided as basic health services are provided through health professionals who are members of (i) the staff of the organization or a medical group (or groups), or (ii) an individual practice association (or associations);

(4) Provide a current financial report;

(5) Describe the health maintenance organization's service area or the proposed service area, and give the dates basic and supplemental health services will be provided in such area or areas;

(6) Describe the location of facilities where, and give the dates and hours of operation when, health services are provided or will be provided at such facilities;

(7) Provide proposed contracts between the health maintenance organization and the employer, or its designee;

(8) Include sample copies of marketing brochures and membership literature;

(9) Identify the staff and ownership of the health maintenance organization and the physicians who will provide health services for the organization;

(10) State the payment for basic and supplemental health services to be required for various categories of memberships; and

(11) State the health maintenance organization's capacity to enroll new members and the likelihood of any future limitations on such enrollment.

§ 110.803 Offer of health maintenance organization alternative to employees.

(a) An employer subject to § 110.802 shall, at the time a health benefits plan is offered to its eligible employees or to such employees and their eligible dependents, include in such plan the option of membership in qualified health maintenance organizations in accordance with the provisions of this section.

(b) If more than one qualified health maintenance organization which provides services in an area in which eligible employees of such employer reside have requested inclusion in the health benefits plan as provided by § 110.802, and

(1) One or more of such organizations provides basic health services through professionals who are members of the staff of the organization or of a medical group (or groups); and

(2) One or more of such organizations provides such services through an individual practice association (or associations), then, of the qualified health maintenance organizations included in a health benefits plan of such employer pursuant to this section, at least one shall be an organization which provides basic health services as described in paragraph (b)(1) of this section and at least one shall be an organization which provides basic health services as described in paragraph (b)(2) of this section.

(c) An employer subject to this subpart shall offer the option of membership in additional qualified health maintenance organizations to its eligible employees, described in paragraphs (c)(1) and (2) of this paragraph, if such additional qualified health maintenance organizations demonstrate that their service areas include the place of residence of eligible employees:

(1) Who do not reside in the service area of qualified health maintenance organizations already included in the employer's health benefits plans; or

(2) To whom membership in qualified health maintenance organizations already included in the health benefits plan is not available because such organizations have closed their enrollment of additional eligible employees of such employer.

(d) An employer subject to this subpart is not required to include in the health benefits plan offered to eligible employees the option of membership in the specific qualified health maintenance organization which initiated the request for inclusion in the health benefits plan: *Provided,* That the employer or its designee selects, in a manner consistent with this section, one or more other qualified health maintenance organizations that may not have made a request within the time limit of § 110.802 (a)(4) but are willing to be included: *Provided further,* That such latter health maintenance organizations are of the same type (i.e., the type described in paragraph (b)(1) of this section or the type described in paragraph (b)(2) of this section) and serve, or will serve at a minimum, the same area (in which the employer's employees reside) individually or collectively as the health maintenance organization which submitted the timely request.

(e) An employer or its designee including the option of membership in a qualified health maintenance organization pursuant to this subpart as part of the health benefits plan offered to its eligible employees shall provide for a group enrollment period during which eligible employees may enroll in any qualified health maintenance organization or may transfer from a qualified health maintenance organization to any other alternative without application of waiting periods or exclusions or limitations based on health status as conditions of enrollment or transfer. Nothing in this subpart shall preclude the uniform application of coordination of benefit arrangements between the health maintenance organizations and the other carriers which are included in the health benefits plan at the official transfer time of the group enrollment period.

(f) During the group enrollment period in which the alternative of membership in a qualified health maintenance organization is offered to a group of employees for the first time, the health benefits plan alternative shall be presented to each eligible employee with the requirement that an affirmative written selection be made among the different alternatives included in the health benefits plan. In subsequent group enrollment periods, a selection among such alternatives shall be made available; however, such written selection is required only when the eligible employee elects to change from one alternative to another.

(g) In addition to the group enrollment period, the opportunity to select among different alternatives within a health benefits plan shall be made available to new employees, employees who have been transferred or otherwise changed their place of residence resulting in eligibility for membership in a qualified health maintenance organization for which they were not previously eligible by place of residence, or eligible employees covered by any alternative which ceases operation. At the time such employees are eligible to participate in the health benefits plan, such opportunity shall be made available without waiting periods or any exclusions or limitations based on health status as conditions of enrollment or transfer, and shall be presented to such employees with the requirement that they make an affirmative written selection among the different alternatives included in the health benefits plan.

(h) The employer shall provide each qualified health maintenance organization which is included in its health benefits plan with fair and reasonable access, not less than 30 days prior to and during group enrollment periods, to employees referred to in § 110.805, for purposes of presenting and explaining its program in accordance with § 110.108(c) of this part. This access shall include, at a minimum, the opportunity for distribution of educational literature, brochures, announcements of meetings, and other relevant printed materials meeting the requirements of § 110.108(c) to each such employee. The employer or its designee shall be given the opportunity to review, revise, and approve such materials before distribution. Revisions shall be limited to correcting factual errors, misleading or ambiguous statements, unless otherwise agreed to by the health maintenance organization and the employer or its designee, or as may be required by law. The employer or its designee shall complete promptly any such revisions in the offering material so as not to delay or otherwise interfere with the group enrollment period. In no event shall the access to eligible employees provided to s'ich qualified health maintenance organizations be more restrictive or less favorable than that provided other offerers of alternatives included in the health benefits plan, whether or not the representatives of the other alternatives elect to avail themselves of such access.

§ 110.804   Timing of the health maintenance organization alternative offer to employees.

The employer or its designee shall offer eligible employees the option of membership in a qualified health maintenance organization at the earliest date permitted under the terms of the existing contracts. Should such health maintenance organization's request for inclusion in a health benefits plan be received at a time when the existing collective bargaining agreement, employer-employee contracts, or contract for health benefits does not provide for including a qualified health maintenance organization in the health benefits plan, the inclusion of the health maintenance organization in the health benefits plan shall occur at the time that new contracts are offered or a new contract negotiated and shall be consistent with the following paragraphs:

(a) If an existing collective bargaining agreement is in force at the time the request for inclusion in the health benefits plan is made by the health maintenance organization to the employer or its designee, the request shall be raised in the collective bargaining process when a new contract is negotiated or if such agreement is automatically renewable, on its anniversary date or at such other times as may be provided by such agreement for discussion of changes in its provisions, or in accordance with a specific process to review health maintenance organization offers.

(b) In the absence of a collective bargaining agreement, if there is an existing employer-employee contract, health benefits contract or any other arrangement which provides for a health benefits plan, such option shall be included in any health benefits plan offered to eligible employees when the existing contract is renewed, or when a new health benefits contract or other arrangement is negotiated. If an employer-employee contract or health benefits contract has no fixed term or has a'term in excess of one year, such contract shall be treated as renewable on the earliest annual anniversary date of the contract. If the employer is self-insured, the budget year shall be treated as the term of the existing contract.

(c) For employers with multiple contracts or other arrangements included as part of the health benefits plan which may have different expiration or renewal dates, the offer shall be included for each contract or arrangement at the time such contract or arrangement is renewed or reissued or the benefits provided under such contract or arrangement are offered to employees.

§ 110.805   Employees to whom the health maintenance organization alternative must be offered.

Each employer subject to this subpart or its designee, shall offer the option of membership in a qualified health maintenance organization to each eligible employee, or to such employees and their eligible dependents, who reside within the service area of the qualified health maintenance organization being offered.

(a) For those employees of an employer represented by a bargaining representative, the offer of the health maintenance organization alternative is subject to the collective bargaining process.

(b) For those employees not represented by a bargaining representative, the offer of the health maintenance organization alternative shall be made directly to such employees in accordance with this subpart.

§ 110.806   Copayment levels and supplemental health services determination.

Each eligible employee's election of a copayment level and of supplemental health services to be contracted for is to be made as follows:

(a) For those employees of an employer represented by a bargaining representative, the selection of supplemental health services and copayment levels is subject to the collective bargaining process.

(b) For those employees not represented by a bargaining representative, the selection of copayment levels and supplemental health services to be offered to eligible employees shall be made through the decision-making process that exists with respect to the existing health benefits plan.

§ 110.807   Employer contributions for health maintenance organization alternative.

(a) The health maintenance organization alternative shall be included in the health benefits plan on terms no less favorable, in regard to an employer's monetary contribution or designee's cost for health benefits, than those on which the other alternatives in the health benefits plan are included: *Provided,* That the employer shall not be required to pay more for health benefits as a result of offering the option of membership in qualified health maintenance organizations than such employer would otherwise be required to pay for health benefits by a collective bargaining agreement or other employer-employee contract in effect at the time that the health maintenance organization is included in the health benefits plans.

(b) The amount of the employer's or designee's contribution shall be determined in a manner consistent with this section.

(1) Administrative expenses of the employer, or its designee, incurred in connection with offering any alternative in the health benefits plan shall not be considered in determining the amount of the employer's contribution to the health maintenance organization.

(2) The amount of the employer's contribution or designee's costs may exclude such portions of the contribution allocable to benefits (e.g., life insurance or insurance for supplemental health benefits) for which eligible employees or such employees and their eligible dependents will continue to be covered notwithstanding selection of membership in the health maintenance organization, and which benefits are not offered on a prepaid basis by the health maintenance organization to such employer's employees.

(c) Where the specific amount of the employer's contribution for health benefits is fixed by a collective bargaining agreement, by an employer-employee contract, or by law, the amount so determined shall constitute the employer's obligation for contribution toward the health maintenance organization dues or premiums on behalf of eligible employees or such employees and their eligible dependents.

(d) Where the employer's contribution for health benefits is determined by a collective bargaining agreement, but the amount so fixed includes contribution for benefits in addition to health benefits, the employer shall determine, or shall instruct its designee to determine, the portion of such employer's contribution applicable to health benefits in accordance with this section.

(e) In the absence of a collective bar-

gaining agreement or employer-employee contract specifying contribution for health benefits, the employer's contribution to the health maintenance organization on behalf of eligible employees or such employees and their eligible dependents, unless otherwise agreed to by the health maintenance organization and the employer or its designee, shall be based upon the total costs of such health benefits offered to the employees for the most recent period for which experience is available, reduced by such amounts identified in accordance with paragraph (b)(2) of this section. Such cost determination shall be consistent with paragraphs (a) and (f) of this section.

(f) For purposes of this section, an employer's contribution or its designee's cost for the alternatives within the health benefits plan other than the qualified health maintenance organization option shall be determined in the following manner, unless otherwise agreed to by the health maintenance organization and the employer or its designee:

(1) If the employer's contribution or its designee's cost for health benefits with respect to the non-health maintenance organization alternative is determined solely on the basis of a fixed prospective amount (not subject to retrospective adjustment), contributed by the employer or paid by the designee, then the prospective payment made by or on behalf of the employer to the non-health maintenance organization alternative for the provision of health benefits to eligible employees or to such employees and their eligible dependents under such alternatives shall be used as the basis for determining the employer's obligation for contribution toward the health maintenance organization dues or premiums.

(2) If the employer's contribution or its designee's cost for health benefits with respect to the non-health maintenance organization alternative is determined by a contract with a carrier on any form of retrospective experience rating basis, any billing contract arrangement, any plan of self insurance, any direct service plan provided by the employer or its designee, or any other form of health benefits plan wherein the actual cost to the employer or its designee is determined retrospectively, an estimated cost shall be used to determine the obligation for contribution toward the health maintenance organization's dues or premiums. Such esti-

mated cost shall be determined by the employer or its designee based on consideration of the following factors:

(i) The employer's or designee's cost experience for non-health maintenance organization alternative with respect to the most recent benefit period for which such experience is available at the time when the employer's prospective contribution or designee's obligation to the health maintenance organization is to be determined;

(ii) A reasonable allowance for inflation based on historical cost trends and anticipated future cost increases;

(iii) Where applicable and consistently applied, cost differences experienced in the provision of health benefits for separate regional or local areas of employment;

(iv) Anticipated changes in the composition and experience of the covered population actually being served by the non-health maintenance organization alternative attributable to the shift of enrollment to the health maintenance organization;

(v) Any changes in health benefits to be provided by non-health maintenance alternatives during the period for which the estimated contribution is to be determined; and

(vi) Any other anticipated material change in the experience rating basis under any health benefits contract for the benefit period.

(g) An employer or its designee shall retain for at least three years the data used to compute its level of contribution to the alternatives included in the health benefits plan. Such data may be reviewed by the Secretary either on his own initiative or in response to a request which sets forth reasonable grounds supporting such a request, to determine whether the level of contributions determined by the employer complies with this subpart.

§ 110.808   Relationship of section 1310 (a) of the Public Health Service Act to the National Labor Relations Act as amended and the Railway Labor Act, as amended.

The obligation of an employer subject to this subpart to include the option of membership in a qualified health maintenance organization in any health benefits plan offered to its eligible employees shall be carried out consistently with the obligations imposed on such employer under the National Labor Relations Act and the Railway Labor Act.

[FR Doc.75–28696 Filed 10–24–75; 8:45 am]

Index